Women and Medicine in the French Enlightenment

WOMEN AND MEDICINE IN THE FRENCH ENLIGHTENMENT

The Debate over *Maladies des Femmes*

LINDSAY WILSON

The Johns Hopkins University Press
Baltimore and London

© 1993 The Johns Hopkins University Press
All rights reserved
Printed in the United States of America on acid-free paper

The Johns Hopkins University Press
701 West 40th Street
Baltimore, Maryland 21211-2190
The Johns Hopkins Press Ltd., London

Library of Congress Cataloging-in-Publication Data

Wilson, Lindsay B. (Lindsay Blake)
Women and medicine in the French Enlightenment : the debate over
"maladies des femmes" / Linday Wilson.
p.   cm.
Includes bibliographical references and index.
ISBN 0-8018-4438-X (HC : alk. paper)
1. Medicine—France—History—18th century.   2. Women—Health and hygiene—
France—History—   3. Medical jurisprudence—France—History—
18th century.   4. Women's Health—France.   I. Title.
[DNLM: 1. History of Medicine, 18th century—France.   WZ 70 GF7 W7W]
R505.W55   1993
306.4'61'094409033—dc20
DNLM/DLC
for Library of Congress   92-15475

A catalog record for this book is available from the British Library

CONTENTS

ACKNOWLEDGMENTS

Scholarly life is often solitary, especially if one's research is based on archives. Nevertheless, gaining access to materials in distant places requires considerable institutional support, as does participating in forums where one's ideas can be tested and refined. The institutions whose support I wish to acknowledge here are Colby College, Stanford University and its Institute for Research on Women and Gender, and the National Endowment for the Humanities.

But the character of institutions is shaped largely by the people associated with them. Personal thanks go to Doug Archibald, Bob McArthur, Hal Raymond, Pete Moss, and Rob Weisbrot at Colby for encouraging me to pursue a highly ambitious research program over the course of many years. The final phases were expedited with the steady and cheerful assistance of Arielle Silver and Grace Von Tobel. At the Johns Hopkins University Press, Jacqueline Wehmueller immediately sensed the significance of this project and patiently guided me through each stage of the publication process.

I was able to make significant conceptual advances in my understanding of the social history of science and medicine with the help of Everett Mendelsohn, David Rothman, Steven Marcus, Stephanie Kiceluk, and Sander Gilman. Deborah Rhode, Sherri Matteo, Karen Offen, Susan Groag Bell, and Joan Cadden offered critical insights into women's studies. Special thanks go to Carolyn Lougee, who first introduced me to the world of Ancien Régime France, and to Sarah Hanley, whose generous and judicious criticism enabled me to bring this project to completion.

I am grateful to friends like Virginia Prystay, Allen Weiss, and Jack Archer in Paris and Terry Wilson and Esther Viscarello in the Bay Area who opened their homes and hearts to me. Randy Wilson and I embarked on a journey together eighteen years ago and I hope he will agree that it has been worthwhile, if a bit unpredictable. His support has been absolutely unwavering, as has his commitment to gender equity. This book is dedicated to two generations of Wilson women—to Carolyn, whose strength and love will always be an inspiration to me, and to Caroline, who is my hope for the future.

Women and Medicine in the French Enlightenment

Women's History and the Social History

of Medicine

It was Michel Foucault, in his books *Madness and Civilization, The Birth of the Clinic*, and *The History of Sexuality*, who first perceived the value of examining the history of medicine as a means of elucidating the evolution of politics and society in early modern France.[1] Not only did Foucault's approach provide a fascinating and provocative framework for interpreting history as a whole; it also laid the basis for a reappraisal of the history of medicine. Foucault provided a corrective to the traditional view of the history of medicine as consecutive chapters in the disinterested pursuit of truth, even as he aroused the indignation of traditional historians of medicine who accused him and his followers of indulging in polemic and neglecting the fact that medicine had an internal history that must be understood and respected.

Foucault identified the century of Enlightenment as a turning point in the history of medicine and civilization: the point at which the dialogue between reason and unreason was broken and irrationality came to be identified with immorality. Doctors, entrusted by an increasingly centralized state with the task of upholding the bourgeois moral order, were encouraged to distinguish the normal from the pathological in such a way as to reduce differences between social groups, repress vice, eliminate irregularities. Foucault questioned this use of medicine. He maintained that from the mid–eighteenth century onward, doctors, whatever their intentions, had come increasingly to judge rather than to observe, to punish rather than to heal, their patients.

Foucault's thesis—tantalizing, dramatic, and uncompromising as it was—was bound to provoke considerable interest and controversy. More significantly for the historian, it gave rise to a whole new school of historiography. In the 1970s, both critics and supporters agreed that Foucault's thesis required substantiation. Initially, the burden of proof fell not on the critics but on the supporters. Foucault had provided the theoretical framework; he bequeathed to other historians, most notably Jean-Pierre Peter, the task of engaging in the painstaking archival research necessary either to confirm or to disprove the theory.[2]

The results have been less than gratifying. For the most part, those historians who embraced the theory found themselves unable to interpret the archival data in any other light and were thus bound to confirm Foucault's hypothesis. Those who opposed the theory could do so on methodological grounds and thus had no need to return to the sources to suggest an alternative way of looking at eighteenth-century medicine. There seemed to be little possibility for dialogue between the two schools. Although this dispute among scholars of the history of medicine was never satisfactorily resolved, it has been largely ignored by later historians unfamiliar with the primary sources. Thus, in *The Body and the French Revolution*, Dorinda Outram elevates Foucault's thesis to the level of a historical truism, using it as a springboard for a dazzling, but problematical, interpretation of the larger political, social, and cultural currents of the Revolution.[3]

In the 1980s several works examined the cultural construction of illness and challenged the equation of science with morality and progress while avoiding the ideological excesses to which Foucault's followers have been prone. I am thinking specifically of Herzlich and Pierret's *Illness and Self in Society*, Gilman's *Difference and Pathology*, Coleman's *Death Is a Social Disease*, Latour's *Pasteurization of France*, and Proctor's *Racial Hygiene*.[4] These works, however, do not concentrate on the crucial early modern period. I propose reconsidering, in the light of such approaches, the connections among medicine, politics, and society in the eighteenth century. I regard the Enlightenment as a pivotal point in the history of medicine not because its legacy is clear, but rather because it is ambiguous. What characterizes Enlightenment thought is not its consistency but its diversity; during the Enlightenment, many formerly unexamined issues were opened for debate by an increasingly engaged public.

The enthusiasm for science which inspired the age of Enlightenment was nowhere more evident than in medicine. From Descartes and Locke to the Encyclopedists, champions of enlightenment linked health with happiness and believed that the progress of the new philosophy depended on the progress of medicine.[5] As Jean Meyer has observed, applied science was not considered an annex or by-product of pure science, but its true end.[6] First place among the applied sciences belonged to medicine because the liberation of the individual was thought to begin with the body. Diderot remarked that he read no books more willingly than books of medicine; that he found the conversation of no men more interesting than that of physicians. He translated Robert James's *Universal Dictionary of Medicine, Surgery, Chemistry, Botany, Anatomy, Pharmacy, Natural History, etc.* (1746) just before writing his *Pensées philosophiques* and beginning work on the *Encyclopédie*, in which medicine held the place of honor.[7]

But Diderot was not the only philosopher of the Enlightenment to take an interest in medicine; Montesquieu's reading included the Holy Scripture, Calvin, Seneca, Pliny, and the *Histoire de la médecine* of Dr. Freind, while Voltaire's library contained forty-eight works of medicine.[8] Indeed, medicine preoccupied nearly all the philosophes because so many of the questions they were asking dealt with the relationship between body and soul. They expected medicine to serve as a test and antidote to speculative philosophy and turned to it to settle debates about divine providence, the origin of the species, the hierarchy of nature, the immortality of the soul, and original sin. Their arguments for reform were predicated on the notion that law and morality should be brought into harmony with the underlying laws of nature.[9]

James's dictionary had envisioned medicine at a turning point. Following Harvey's discovery of the circulation of the blood in 1628, conflicting sects within medicine had presumably yielded to the consensus that "the general principles on which the treatment of disease is based are universally the same."[10] Doctors, like scientists, claimed privileged insight into truth, and the faculties and academies based their claims of the moral excellence of doctors and scientists on the epistemological certitude of their scientific method.[11] The eulogy of the physician Pierre-Antoine Marteau, crafted for the Academy of Sciences, Letters, and Arts of Amiens, is typically grandiloquent: "Medicine is a science so vast that it touches all the sciences and has no bounds other than nature herself. The knowledge it demands seems to be reserved only to spirits capable of embracing the universe."[12]

Physicians tended to be among the enlightened elite in both Paris and the provinces. They constituted approximately one-fourth of all the academicians in provincial academies throughout France and were second in strength only to justice and administration professionals. The prestige physicians enjoyed within the academies stemmed from their long, costly studies; their esprit de corps; their commitment to public service; and a reputation for close observation and analysis, established as much through their teaching as through their practices. Their influence was especially broad because they penetrated all social milieu.[13]

3

As the authority of the church declined over the course of the eighteenth century, the influence of the medical community increased. The state asked doctors to rule on very difficult medical issues with profound religious, social, and political implications. Their increased influence on the courts and the family was evidenced by the rise of medical jurisprudence and of new medical specialties focusing on the diseases of women and children.[14]

Yet even as medicine was equated with enlightenment and the medical community relished the prospect of enhanced power, an unprecedented crisis in medical authority loomed. It was precipitated by simultaneous attacks on the epistemological certitude of medicine and the corporative structure of the medical community. These attacks reflected broad changes in thought and social structure which characterized the final fifty years of the Ancien Régime, namely the dechristianization of culture, the disintegration of corporative society, and pervasive skepticism regarding the validity and utility of the ideology of absolutism.[15]

In centuries past, medical theory had been rooted in theology, while medical practice had been governed by the faculties, colleges, and corporations. The Faculty of Medicine of Paris had brooked no challenge to its infallibility and had not hesitated to assert its right to censorship over all medical works. A consensus on moral as well as theoretical issues was both assumed and expected of members of the medical community. But the eighteenth century saw a decline in the Faculty's power to command conformity. The ideals of arbitrary authority and enforced conformity, though a source of security for some, were antithetical to the new spirit of inquiry with which philosophy and science were infused by the Enlightenment. More progressive members of the medical community, while rejecting the Faculty's power to enforce conformity or to serve as the sole voice of authority in medical matters, nevertheless did not abandon their conservative colleagues' ideals of consensus and authority—indeed, consensus and authority were considered the necessary foundations of the new science.[16] They merely sought to ground adherence to these ideals on the principles of reason and observation rather than on faith or deference to tradition. But reason did not immediately provide a new standard upon which to base authority, and the issue of authority could not be confined to the theoretical domain.

After decades of bitter debate in the middle of the century, doctors and surgeons had arrived at an uneasy truce based on carefully defined separate spheres of competence. Throughout France, each group jealously guarded its prerogatives against the other and against their common enemy: the mass of charlatans, empirics, priests, and women who dabbled in medicine without the faculties' or corporations' authorization.[17]

The challenge that charlatans, empirics, and folk healers of all sorts posed to the professional medical community in the late eighteenth century was not new, but it seemed more threatening at a time when the larger corporative social structure seemed to be failing and was becoming the object of increased criticism by philosophes and administrators. The charlatans' and empirics' attacks on professional privilege reverberated through the popular press, eliciting considerably more public involvement than had earlier disputes between the Paris Faculty and provincial graduates or between the Faculty and Théophraste Renaudot.[18] Here, as in the theoretical domain, a new basis for authority had to be forged. The medical community was expected to legitimize its authority not by asserting traditional claims to privilege, but by demonstrating that its insights and methods were indeed superior to those of the charlatans and empirics. The superior knowledge of doctors and surgeons should presumably result in more successful cures.[19]

But the revolution that would transform medicine in the late nineteenth century was only a distant dream in the eighteenth. True, advances were being made in hygiene which would lead ultimately to a lowering of mortality rates. Yet doctors and surgeons, whatever their differences in training and world view from the charlatans and empirics, frequently remained unable to demonstrate the superiority of their techniques or the greater efficacy of their cures. Their lack of success was particularly striking in the area of the *maladies des femmes*.

Maladies des femmes are defined here as disorders thought to be derived from the sexuality of women. The complications attending menstruation, pregnancy, and menopause were the most common subjects addressed by the many medical writers on the subject of the *maladies des femmes* in the late eighteenth century. The issue of late births falls under this rubric, as do the influence of the imagination of women on the formation of the fetus, and convulsions or hysteria. The mechanics of reproduction and the causes and proper treatment of nervous disorders remained areas of mystery to the medical community and the lay public alike. It was in these areas that popular superstitions seemed to abound and that the cures of charlatans and empirics were most likely to be employed, sometimes with startling success, sometimes with equally dramatic failure.[20]

To Parisian doctors associated with elite teaching or research institutions, the *maladies des femmes* were a source of considerable perplexity. Many doctors held women responsible for the confusion over the *maladies des femmes* thereby undermining the medical community's understanding, placing it, at best, on a par with that of charlatans and empirics. This was an era when doctors did not always examine their patients directly but often made diagnoses by correspondence, relying on patients and family members to present the relevant facts of the condition accurately.[21]

5

Because women were thought to have poor judgment, a large segment of the medical community as well as the courts received their testimony with suspicion. They were suspected of misrepresenting their illnesses through either ignorance or deceit.

While doctors associated with the elite faculties, societies, and academies of medicine regarded women's misrepresentations as an obstacle primarily to the theoretical development of an enlightened science of medicine, their more obscure provincial colleagues regarded the apparent ignorance of women as a threat to their very subsistence. As the guardians and transmitters of the traditional beliefs and remedies that these doctors and surgeons were intent on supplanting, women were accused not only of constituting the charlatans' greatest clientele but of illicitly practicing medicine themselves.[22] As both clients and practitioners of charlatanry, women were thought to present a distinct obstacle to the progress of medicine and to the medical community.

Women and their illnesses thus figured prominently in the struggle for authority being waged between the professional medical community and the charlatans. Until now historians have not taken much note of this fact. Typically, American historians of French medicine have seen the battle over charlatanry as an early phase in the process of professionalization and have relied on a substantial body of work by such sociologists as Ernest Greenwood, William Goode, Geoffrey Millerson, and Eliot Freidson to provide the theoretical tools to make sense of the battle.[23] This orientation has led them to concentrate on tracing the evolution of medical institutions and their regulation by the state.

Certainly politics shaped the development of medical institutions, but I am convinced that the parameters of eighteenth-century politics need to be defined more broadly than has so far been done by historians of medicine like Matthew Ramsey and Toby Gelfand.[24] The story of the dynamic role that medical debates played in focusing public attention on fundamental conflicts confronting society and the state cannot adequately be told if one confines one's inquiry to the acts of legislative committees and regulatory bodies and relies primarily on sources in governmental and medical archives. The late eighteenth century witnessed a significant shift in the center of politics from the institutions of court and *parlement* to the journals, theaters, and streets. As Keith Baker and Sarah Maza have demonstrated, a politics of contestation was emerging in which public opinion would be hailed as the ultimate court of appeal, superseding the authority of the king.[25]

I have thus drawn material for this study of medical causes célèbres focusing on women from a large variety of sources. I have consulted technical medical treatises, medical topographies, official reports of the academies, laws, projects for medical reform, and judicial archives, as well as the correspondence between Parisian and provincial doctors of the Royal Society of Medicine and the letters, memoirs, and educational treatises of eighteenth-century women. The juxtaposition of published and manuscript sources affords an unusual glimpse into contradictions between the public and private faces of medicine. I have referred to numerous specialized studies on law, labor, journalism, science, and art in order to explore the complex interplay between theory and practice.

The professional medical community's view of medicine and society in France at the end of the eighteenth century determined the initial focus, but not the circumference, of this work. Scientific, and above all, medical, issues were a source of continuing fascination to all sectors of society during the Enlightenment. Discussion of medical causes célèbres figured prominently in the learned and provincial journals, as did advertisements for remedies and debates about their efficacy. Books on medical topics constituted 30 percent of all books reviewed in the *Journal des savants* and 25 percent of books reviewed in the *Mémoires de Trévoux*.[26] Because they were so alluring, appealing to the experience and conscience of each reader, medical case histories were published in both the learned and popular journals. They mingled science with literature, the real with the bizarre, instructing as they entertained.

Cases involving medical jurisprudence were of concern not just to members of the medical community but to jurists and the general public as well. Hence legal compilations are as important a source for understanding some medical debates as are the medical consultations. Advertisements for these compilations figured prominently in journals, and women writers on education urged women to study law in order to preserve themselves and their families from destruction. Until recently, historians of medicine have ignored these sources. Social and intellectual historians interested in the history of publishing or jurisprudence have recognized their value but have not focused on medical issues.

Reliance on such a variety of sources affords us unique access to the dialogue that was continually conducted between the medical community and the lay public on a number of medical issues with important social and political ramifications. The fact that much of the literature generated by medical debates in this period is highly polemical does not detract from its value to social historians of medicine; it merely emphasizes the significance of these issues to the rest of society. As Jeremy Popkin has argued, eighteenth-century journals were often more widely read than the famous texts of the philosophes. Moreover, because they offered an opportunity for readers to register their views, the journals are an indispensable guide to public taste and outlook, especially in the last quarter of the eighteenth century, which saw an efflorescence in the publication and circulation of journals throughout France.[27]

The chapters that follow examine a number of key debates involving various *maladies des femmes*. The debates span the half-century preceding the Revolution, beginning with the Convulsionaries of St. Médard in the 1730s, continuing with late births in the 1760s, and concluding with mesmerism in the 1780s. In each of these debates, the state called upon the medical community to offer a judgment on a medical issue having profound social and political repercussions.

The fact that both sides in each debate initially favored appealing to the medical community to offer a definitive ruling is evidence of the increasing authority accorded medical opinion. Such recognition coincided with the emergence of a new medical speciality, that of medical jurisprudence. As Jean Lafosse, author of a plan for a treatise on medical jurisprudence and of articles on medical jurisprudence published in the supplement to the *Encyclopédie*, made clear, the ambitions of late eighteenth-century practitioners of medical jurisprudence and their supporters were grand. Lafosse defined medicine as nothing less than knowledge of human nature and of the physical laws of nature. He conceived of medical jurisprudence as the science relating legislation to medicine, and he believed that medical advice should be solicited wherever it might be useful.[28]

Medical jurisprudence had two functions. First, medical jurists sought to advise legislators on how to make good laws that would serve as a kind of preventive medicine, preserving the social body from the illnesses of crime and social disorder. Next, they aimed at assuring the good application of laws in order to protect the innocent from judicial errors.

Specific tasks were assigned to each function. Preventive medicine was to take the form of medical experts issuing what Lafosse termed political or economic reports on a wide range of subjects. Reports were needed on the physical education of children in public institutions; on the examination of mercenary nurses; on inoculation; on the effect of working conditions on health; on the quality of food and water; on clothing and habitation; on environmental hazards emanating from swamps, slaughterhouses, tanneries, mines, and cemeteries; and on experimental remedies.[29]

Judicial reports, intended to keep courts from making potentially disastrous judicial errors, covered an equally broad but different range of subjects. Judicial reports were to be issued in cases involving deformed fetuses, abortions, cesarean section, abnormally short or prolonged pregnancies, signs of pregnancy, infanticide, impotence, rape, virginity. They were also solicited in inquiries into causes of death, the effects of torture, the validity of miracles, and medical malpractice.[30]

The development of medical jurisprudence was supported by reformers and defenders of the traditional order alike. While reformers saw medical jurisprudence as pivotal in their campaign to transform the structures of society and the state, defenders of the Ancien Régime hoped that medical jurisprudence might point the way toward modest reform without undermining the basic principles and institutions on which their power was based.

The debates on the Convulsionaries of St. Médard, late births, and mesmerism all involved *maladies des femmes* that fell within the domain of the emerging science of medical jurisprudence. In the case of the Convulsionaries of St. Médard, medical experts were asked to rule on the legitimacy of the supposedly miraculous cures experienced by Jansenist critics of the Catholic church. Whether the cures were indeed legitimate and not the work of deception or were simply the effects of natural healing, they could be interpreted as a vindication of the Jansenist cause.[31] Thus the controversy over the Convulsionaries involved more than an effort to sort out true miracles from false, saints from sinners. Medical reports had been solicited for this purpose for centuries without much ado, but at issue in this case was nothing less than the legitimacy of the traditional institutions of church and state and of the principles of hierarchy, privilege, and patriarchy upon which they were based. The affair became a cause célèbre, arousing unprecedented popular fervor, enlightened critique, and institutional anxiety. It would also pose a stumbling block for Enlightenment thinkers sympathetic to the Convulsionaries' appeals for reform but repelled by the irrationality of the convulsionary behavior that placed the Jansenist cause before the public eye.

Thirty years later, a debate over the physical possibility and hence legitimacy of late births would preoccupy the medical community and capture the popular imagination in a similar way, emerging as another medical cause célèbre. The debate was precipitated by an inheritance dispute between a widow, Renée, and her husband Charles's collateral heirs. Renée claimed the right of her child to inherit, while the collateral heirs challenged the legitimacy of a child born ten months and seventeen days after Charles's death.

The debate over late births represented another challenge to the legitimacy of traditional institutions. This time, it was the integrity of the patriarchal family which was directly threatened. Governmental authorities took great interest in the resolution of this affair, for political policy was based on what Sarah Hanley has termed the family-state compact.[32] Framers of the family-state compact argued that the stability of society and the monarchy depended on the perpetuation of family lines and the defense of patriarchal authority. The integrity of the family was threatened by concealed pregnancies, abortion, infanticide, and claims to prolonged pregnancies like Renée's. The church also sought to limit such aberrations from what it regarded as the natural and divine order. For it, the stakes were even greater, involving not just the moral welfare of the family, but the spiritual salvation of infants dying without benefit of baptism.

Debate over the legitimacy of Renée's child led inevitably to debate over the legitimacy of the patriarchal family and lines of inheritance. Because the details of the case were recounted in a number of scholarly and popular journals, its influence was great, eliciting other cases of late births and shaping the theory and practice of medical jurisprudence on the subject for the next fifty years.

The final cause célèbre to be discussed in depth here is that of mesmerism, which arose in the 1780s. As Robert Darnton has persuasively argued, mesmerism in many ways marked the end of the Enlightenment in France.[33] Mesmer's unorthodox cures, because they challenged traditional medical remedies, cosmologies, and models of the physician-patient relationship, fell under the rubric of experimental remedies to be investigated by experts in medical jurisprudence. Members of the medical community were thus summoned to issue a judgment on the legitimacy of Mesmer's cures.

As was the case with the debates over the Convulsionaries and the possibility of late births, however, the focal point of controversy regarding legitimacy would shift dramatically from that envisioned by the state. Judgment of the validity of Mesmer's cures necessarily presumed judgment of the legitimacy of the traditional medical methods and institutions that Mesmer rejected. Medical experts thus found themselves in the awkward position of attempting to arbitrate a dispute in which they figured prominently as accused parties. The institution whose authority they were specifically called upon to uphold was not the church, the state, or the family, but the medical community itself and the whole corporative structure of society. Ultimately, however, the defense of corporative society entailed defending church, state, and family, for all were based on the principles of hierarchy, privilege, and patriarchy.

The debate surrounding mesmerism may strike the uninitiated reader as diffuse, for it touched on a number of apparently unrelated issues, including the desirability of mothers breastfeeding their children and the need for reforms in the education and regulation of midwives and charlatans practicing in the countryside. In the eyes of the debaters, these ancillary issues were not irrelevant at all. The controversy over mesmerism, as is perhaps fitting for the debate that culminates the series of medical causes célèbres discussed here, dramatically fused medical issues with social and political concerns. Diagnosis of individual illnesses was transformed into diagnosis of larger social illness and prescriptions for remedy. To many critics, the social illness to be diagnosed and cured seemed systemic, affecting all parts of the social body.

Mesmer's critics, finding it difficult to discredit all the healings, especially given his patients' fervent testimony, focused on another aspect of Mesmer's unorthodox approach: the doctor-patient relationship. Noting that the majority of Mesmer's patients were women and that cures were often effected through touch, the medical experts reporting to the state argued that the erotic overtones of mesmerist cures presented a major threat to public morality and health. They raised the specter of adultery and illegitimacy corrupting society in epidemic proportions.

Fears of adultery and illegitimacy also rose to the surface in contemporaneous debates regarding maternal nursing and midwifery and were incorporated into the mesmerist controversy. The severest critics of mercenary nursing accused mothers who sent their children out to nurse of being inhuman, impious, and adulterous because they were defrauding their children of their true mothers. Even more troubling than the loosening of moral bonds was the possibility that mercenary nurses might transmit venereal disease to the infant and its natural family. Such worries were not unfounded, for the medical archives and journals of causes célèbres detail cases in which infected nurses and infants were examined by medical experts to ascertain who had been the source of the infection—the nurse or the infant (and, by extrapolation, its parents).[34] Doctors and surgeons, united with church and government officials in a far-reaching campaign to reform the practice of midwifery in the countryside at the end of the eighteenth century, were similarly motivated by concerns over public health and morality. They argued that increased education and regulation of midwives were necessary in order to assure both the physical survival of mothers and children and their spiritual and moral well-being.

By educating and regulating midwives more closely, officials hoped to bring them and the women they served into conformity with patriarchal standards of morality enunciated by church and state and upheld by the medical community.[35] Certificates issued upon completion of midwifery courses reminded recipients of their dual loyalty: they were expected to serve parishioners, but they were also bound by law to preserve the life of the child and mother against any "unfortunate accident."[36] The phrase no doubt had more than one meaning, for in the late eighteenth century the fear that midwives and charlatans were those most likely to traffic in contraceptives, abortion, and infanticide became an increasingly powerful weapon in the medical community's assault on anyone unlicensed to practice medicine, including Mesmer's followers.

On the eve of the Revolution, however, the question of who was responsible for the degeneracy and disorder that seemed to penetrate every institution of the Ancien Régime remained unresolved. Were Mesmer, his followers, and the women whom they presumably held under their sway truly responsible for the impending social chaos, or were the traditional beneficiaries of the principles of hierarchy, privilege, and patriarchy to blame? Mesmer's defenders effectively turned the arguments of the medical experts reporting to the state against them, to be resolved only in the inferno of revolution.

By closely examining the debates over the Convulsionaries, the possibility of late births, and mesmerism, we can gain insight into the forces that were transforming the family, the church, corporative society, and the state on the eve of the Revolution. We are also better able to comprehend the challenges facing the medical community, so intimately implicated in upholding these traditional institutions, but dedicated at the same time to the movement for enlightened reform. In arbitrating the causes célèbres associated with *maladies des femmes*, doctors and surgeons confronted and attempted somehow to resolve the contradictions inherent in Enlightenment thought and corporative society.

In each cause célèbre, medical experts sought to establish authenticity: in the case of the Convulsionaries and mesmerists, the authenticity of claims to miraculous or unorthodox healings; in Renée's case, the authenticity of the assertion that a pregnancy could last more than ten and a half months. At the outset of each debate, it was assumed by virtually every individual and institution involved that doctors and surgeons were most suited to judge the validity of these claims because they had superior insight into the fundamental, unchanging laws of nature. Medicine seemed to offer conservatives and enlightened reformers alike the promise of certitude and the basis upon which to build a consensus regarding the laws and values that should govern a healthy and just society.

As each debate progressed, however, the epistemological issue of how truth was to be pursued became increasingly problematical. Although everyone affirmed the existence of universal laws of nature, it was unclear how these laws could best be perceived and interpreted. Should the judgments of the great classical authorities like Hippocrates set the standard? Or should the views of the majority of medical experts considering an issue prevail? Or should observation and experience serve as the ultimate authority? If the last, whose observations could be trusted? Did one need to be male, affiliated with a medical corporation, and a member of the social elite in order to make reliable observations? Could the observations of a woman drawn from the lower orders of society and lacking impressive academic titles and connections carry any weight?

The epistemological crisis recurring in all three medical debates coincided with the philosophes' reexamination of a key doctrine in the Enlightenment credo: the notion that the regular and immutable laws of nature should inform all social and ethical reform. Did such laws truly exist or was any rule of conduct simply conventional? wondered Voltaire. Was beauty indeed linked to goodness and truth? Or was the universe nothing more than an assemblage of monstrous beings, subject to unceasing change? asked Diderot.[37]

Such unresolved questions made certitude and consensus impossible, and the medical judgments that were supposed to settle the controversies surrounding the Convulsionaries, the problem of late births, and Mesmer instead created further tumult. Unable to act in unison, various medical experts used different criteria to come to radically different conclusions. They heatedly sought to expose the weaknesses of opposing methods and views, dramatically demonstrating the vulnerability of any medical judgment. It became clear that if medical judgments were not founded on some kind of superior insight into the laws of nature, then the authority of physicians and surgeons had to be called into question. And it was.

Given increasing public skepticism over the opinions of medical experts, the debates became open forums in which any interested party might air his or her views. As the paper wars heated up, rhetorical flourish was perceived to play an ever more important role in the public's evaluations of whose argument would carry the day, and medical experts faced a crisis of identity in which they had to sort out their commitment to varying roles and the accompanying modes of analysis and discourse. Were they primarily men of science, philosophes, or men of society? If these personae came into conflict, which should take priority?

But the crisis facing medical experts was not nearly as great as that confronting enlightened advocates of the transfer of power from the court and *parlements* of the absolute monarchy to the court of public opinion. How valid was this court of public opinion if it could be so easily swayed by emotion and riveted by spectacles dominated by bold and licentious women associated with men whose social position, religious orientation, or moral integrity were suspect? Was the goal of attaining consensus on political and social reform doomed to be as elusive as that of attaining insight into the fundamental laws of nature?

Ultimately, in each debate, as physical criteria for establishing truth failed, debaters concentrated on weighing the social and political repercussions of a judgment. In the absence of definitive physical proof, concern about the moral impact of a decision became paramount. In the cases of the Convulsionaries and mesmerism, medical experts turned from evaluating the authenticity of cures to noting their erotic overtones and the fact that so many followers were women. It was argued that the public spectacle created by dramatic healings in the streets or salons threatened the social and moral order.

The social condition of the women involved in the cures became a target for controversy. Critics of the Convulsionary cures drew attention to the women's humble social condition, suggesting that these women were feigning miraculous cures for the sake of publicity and financial gain. Debate over the Convulsionaries was thus transformed into debate over how to control the unruly lower orders in society. In contrast, Mesmer's critics noted that the majority of his followers were women drawn from families of considerable means or position and sought in Mesmer's spectacles a cure for boredom rather than for physical suffering.

Allusions to the gender and social condition of Mesmer's followers provided critics with the opportunity for broadening the scope of the debate considerably. Responsibility for the degeneracy and abuse of privilege which were perceived to be sapping the vitality of the upper orders was attributed to women's unjust and pernicious influence over culture and values. This focus, in contrast with that of the 1730s debate regarding the Convulsionaries, was in keeping with the different mood of the 1780s. At the end of the eighteenth century, social critics were considerably more preoccupied with the problem of restraining the abuse of privilege than with emphasizing the virtues of subordination.

The 1760s debate over late births occurred midway between the debates over the Convulsionaries and mesmerism and also centered on issues of gender and social position. Skeptics of Renée's claim to a late birth remarked that lawsuits such as hers arose only in cases in which a wealthy husband died without a direct heir and transmission of property was thus destined to go to the collateral heirs. They argued that assertions of a prolonged pregnancy were never made by poor families who had nothing to gain in producing a posthumous heir. At this point in the century, however, the moral disarray of the upper orders of society, which Mesmer's critics would later describe so vividly, seemed more a threat than a reality.

Sorting out the real objects of attack behind the rhetorical warfare waged in the medical causes célèbres provides us with some interesting case studies of how, as Joan Scott argues, gender can be used as a category of historical analysis to explore the various ways in which sexual symbolism is employed in the interests of maintaining the social order or promoting change.[38] But symbol and metaphor, if they tell us a great deal about larger social and political tensions, reveal little about the reality of sickness or the ways in which cultural constructions of illness affected the quality of health care available to women in the eighteenth century. It is for this reason that this book considers the larger problem of convulsions in a separate chapter. The numerous case histories of female disorders detailed in the consultations of doctors and surgeons provide unusual insight into the options of health care available to women and into the philosophies and attitudes toward women upon which each option was based. Counterbalanced by women's own reflections on health care, they lead us to examine the complex interplay between the images and realities of disease and to explore the gap in understanding which separated medical practitioners from their female patients.

Analysis of these medical case histories and causes célèbres reveals the influence that traditional values, largely prejudicial to women, continued to exert in early modern society. It demonstrates that the ghost of the medieval synthesis of medicine, ethics, law, and theology, whose influence on Renaissance thought has been so admirably traced by Ian Maclean, was not entirely laid to rest by the end of the eighteenth century.[39] Despite the fact that classical authority in the physical sciences had been effectively undermined centuries earlier, the amalgamation of Galenic and Hippocratic medicine, Aristotelian ethics, and Roman law, which had served as the foundation for medieval and early modern conceptions of women, would determine the point of departure for eighteenth-century medical debates concerning the *maladies des femmes*. According to this view, women represented the passions within the human soul and the potential for disorder in society. They had to be subjected to the authority of men, whose reason was presumably strong enough to prevail over the passions, bringing harmony to the soul and order to society.

But if traditional values continued to influence the ways in which people thought about society and medical experts approached medical problems, they did not go unchallenged during the eighteenth century. As Maclean notes, "For a synthesis to be effective, it must embrace the whole encyclopaedia of knowledge, and must account for all known evidence, using a method adaptable to each individual discipline."[40] The debates over the Convulsionaries, the possibility of late births, and the mesmerist cures presented medical experts and the general public with evidence that could not be reduced to the single scheme that had informed the medieval synthesis. A new scheme would have to be elaborated, perhaps one more in keeping with the approach to knowledge of the eighteenth-century Encyclopedists. The editors of the *Encyclopédie*, arguing that their chief contribution to the progress of the human mind lay in their ability to organize and disseminate knowledge in new ways, prided themselves on their dramatic departure from the hierarchical and theological principles that had governed the structure of earlier encyclopedias.[41]

The Enlightenment in France needs to be seen as an era in which all assumptions were thrown open to an increasingly engaged public for discussion, disputation, debate. The role women could play in the court of public opinion should not be underestimated. The medical causes célèbres studied here reveal that women took an active role in shaping public sentiment on issues of concern to them, notably health and religion. Their involvement in the Convulsionary and mesmerist movements led them to offer new ideals of religiosity and the patient-doctor relationship which would challenge and ultimately transform traditional models.[42]

All Robert Darnton's arguments regarding the social dynamics of mesmerism notwithstanding, eighteenth-century medical debates cannot be reduced to a conflict between insiders and outsiders. Although critics of empirics and charlatans emphasized the need to bring them into subordination to the hierarchical structure of the Ancien Régime, the medical community cannot be seen as a cohesive unit acting authoritatively in defense of traditional institutions and in opposition to reform. Vocal defenders as well as critics of the Convulsionaries, Renée, and Mesmer could be found within the corps of medical experts and throughout the various social orders.

Nor can the debates, despite their rhetorical flourishes, be considered yet another skirmish in an unending battle between the sexes. Documents by women supporting the Convulsionaries, Renée, and Mesmer have entered into the historical record in far greater numbers than have documents by women challenging them. This does not necessarily mean, however, that the majority of women whose voices have not been recorded were at odds with their fathers, husbands, and sons. Some women may well have been as appalled by the spectacles created by the Convulsionaries and mesmerists and by the debate over late births as were some men. But the underlying rationale for similar responses could vary. For example, female advocates of maternal breastfeeding and the regulation of midwifery did not necessarily see these reforms as efforts to restrict women more narrowly to the domestic sphere or to ensure their subjugation to the patriarchal order, though some women probably did see these issues in this way.[43] Others, like Mme Roland, used breastfeeding as an opportunity to enhance their relationships with their children or attain power over them. Enlightened men, too, had a variety of reasons for defending or opposing maternal nursing.

Finally, just as the perception of some absolute truth eluded the medical experts in each cause célèbre, so too must our judgment of who were the true heroes, heroines, and villains in each debate be clouded by the complexity of the issues, motives, and characters involved. This is as it should be if we are to come to grips with a period that has been too facilely categorized as an age of triumph—for either enlightenment or repression.

CHAPTER ONE

The Debate over the Convulsionaries of St. Médard, 1727–1765

Convulsions at St. Médard

When the Jansenist deacon François de Pâris was buried in the cemetery of St. Médard near the rue Mouffetard in Paris in 1727, he left behind a loyal following convinced of his saintly virtues and healing powers. Large numbers of people from his parish came to worship at his grave. They suffered from a wide range of disorders that had failed to respond to the arsenal of remedies traditionally applied indiscriminately to all manner of ailments, including fevers, scabies, rabies, rheumatism, suspension of menstruation, paralysis, deafness, and blindness. They left the cemetery proclaiming the sainthood of Pâris on the basis of the seemingly miraculous healings many of them experienced.

As news of the healings spread, crowds of suppliants and spectators were drawn to the little parish cemetery. Impressed with the healing power of Pâris and convinced of the legitimacy of the Jansenist cause that he had embraced, they organized an apocalyptic religious cult far more radical in doctrine than conventional Jansenism. Although the movement primarily attracted people of modest means, it found followers among the local notables, too. Socially diverse, the movement brought together the rich and the poor, the enlightened elite and the illiterate, the young and the old, males and females.[1] Committed to the goal of restoring Christianity to its original purity, Pâris's followers attacked the principles of hierarchy, privilege, and patriarchy upon which the church of the Ancien Régime was based. They advocated a return to the communitarian, egalitarian spirit that had characterized the early church. Although they recognized the uniqueness of the priestly function and the validity of the sacraments, they sought increased participation for the laity and increased responsibility for the lower order of clergy within the church.

Although innocuous enough at its inception, the cult became increasingly controversial as it attracted disciples from all parts of Paris and beyond and as the healings were accompanied by frenzied convulsions and the enunciation—with tears, screams, and groans—of apocalyptic visions. The Convulsionaries knocked their heads against walls, clawed at their breasts, or tore at their limbs before demanding a certain *secours*, which consisted of blows, even severe beatings, but left recipients curiously unharmed and in some cases deeply relieved or even ecstatic.

As Catherine-Laurence Maire notes, the little cemetery of St. Médard was transformed into a theater, a fair, a monastery, a Hôtel-Dieu, and a tribune.[2] The city of Paris became not only a stage for, but a witness to, spectacular corporal manifestations as the Convulsionaries acted out diverse scenes from religious history and contemporary church conflicts. Favorite subjects for representation were Christ's parables, stories of martyrs and persecution, and the mysteries of the faith. Toward the end of the century, certain Convulsionaries enacted scenes of pregnancy and birth in their performances.[3] The smallest details concerning the miraculous healings and convulsions were recorded in little inexpensive books, brochures, flyers, songs, and poems, often printed by women printers and circulated by women colporteurs in Paris and throughout the provinces. Never before in history had an ecclesiastical-political quarrel attracted so much publicity. More than sixteen hundred publications concerning the affair had been released by midcentury.[4]

Fearful of the potential for public disorder in these gatherings and responsive to the church's apprehension of religious scandal, the royal government strove to dismantle the cult by issuing lettres de cachet, making arrests, sponsoring medical inquiries into the authenticity of the healings and convulsions, and, as a last resort, closing the cemetery in 1732. For its part, the church threatened the cult's followers with excommunication, ordered the public burning of the biography attributing sainthood to Pâris, and attacked the notion that a divine impetus lay behind the supposedly miraculous healings through convulsions.

Although in the beginning many mainstream Jansenists defended the cult and regarded its healings as vindications of the Jansenist cause, they turned against the cult as the behavior of its followers became ever more bizarre. The church was not slow to recognize how it could use dissension within the Jansenist ranks to its own advantage. It encouraged publication of the tracts of Jansenist critics of the Convulsionaries. Doctrinaire Catholics could hardly have issued more virulent critiques of the Convulsionaries than did the Jansenist critics. To the church, the threat of the Convulsionaries was that they might serve as a vindication of the Jansenist cause. The church perceived, however, that what appeared to be a threat could be transformed into a blessing. The Convulsionaries introduced dissension among Jansenists, dividing the movement and doing much to discredit the Jansenist cause in the minds of Jansenists and doctrinaire Catholics alike.

Conservative Jansenists wondered why God would have chosen as his prophets women and girls who seemed to be in a trance and incapable of the free use of reason when they articulated their visions. The specter not just of irrationality, but of immorality, haunted them. "And how," they demanded, "can it be that God is supposed to communicate to girls who have themselves shaken, pulled about by men, suspended upside down in the air, and placed in shocking postures, and that he works through them in a miraculous manner in order to have them announce to the church some very great wonders?"[5]

Certainly the Convulsionaries deviated dramatically from traditional models of religiosity for women, which sought annihilation of the self through scrupulous obedience, constraint, and silence. From the moment of their entry into the novitiate, young girls were forbidden to play with their hats or belts; to jump down stairs; to look behind them or through windows to see who might be passing by; to laugh without reason; to lean their heads to one side or stretch their necks when praying to God. In Tronson's *Spiritual Exercises*, which set the standard of conduct of convents throughout early modern France, chastity was considered the paramount virtue, a privileged means of demonstrating one's union with God and of edifying one's associates. Girls were expected to bring their conduct in line with St. Augustine's advice: "Wherever you go, be sure to do nothing that could attract or serve as bait for anyone's disordered appetite. . . . You are not prohibited from looking at men, but from lusting after them or wanting to be lusted after by them. . . . However it is not only by touching, but also by the desire for affection and by glances that a woman is lustful and is lusted after. And do not say that your thoughts and affections are chaste if you look at men lasciviously, for the immodest eye is the messenger of a heart soiled by lewdness."[6] In keeping with these sentiments, one might infer that women's chastity was threatened by any entry into the public sphere.

Just as important to the traditional model of female religiosity as chastity was humility. Here, too, in the eyes of their critics, the Convulsionaries were guilty of the worst sort of transgression. Catholics and conservative Jansenists viewed the investiture of women with clerical functions as a visible profanation of the mysteries of the faith, an act expressly forbidden by God.[7] They found the prospect that power within the church should be transferred from men to women, that priestesses rather than priests should serve as the intermediaries between God and man, to be perhaps the most unsettling aspect of the Convulsionary movement.

If hierarchy within the church should be dismantled, conservatives reasoned, would the threat to authority not extend to secular society as well? Appealing to love of country as well as love of God, conservative Jansenist leaders reminded their followers that it was their duty as loyal subjects to the king to condemn this movement.

The Convulsionaries' defenders sought to defuse the critics' attack by making the Convulsionaries appear as unthreatening as possible. They distinguished the moderate from the more radical Convulsionaries, arguing that fanatics who encouraged the *secours*, preached a curious sort of millenarianism, and advocated the elevation of women to the priesthood could not be taken to represent the movement as a whole. In their efforts to make the movement more acceptable to the general public, the defenders downplayed the involvement of women and girls, noting that the Convulsionary movement included people of both sexes and diverse ages and social conditions.[8]

Yet even as the Convulsionaries' defenders repudiated the public displays of the *secours* and the exaltation of women to priestly authority, they affirmed the assault of the sect on traditional notions of social hierarchy within the church. God, they declared, brings man low in order to raise him up. Rather than disparaging the sex, youth, or social standing of the Convulsionaries, their supporters asserted that God had selected these very people in order to demonstrate his displeasure with man's false grandeur and pretensions to wisdom. The time for upheaval within the church, they announced, was at hand: "those who would lead must now follow; those who would follow must now lead."[9]

Many Jansenists regarded the Convulsionaries' discourses and miraculous healings as a divine indication of the truth of their doctrines and a justification of their cause. Certainly the notion of finding physical proof of divine intent appealed to many an ordinary man or woman who had little taste for subtle theological debate. As one writer observed, "I do not need the authority of the Pope to know if a man from my neighborhood has been paralyzed or made blind or deaf and dumb and healed by appealing to M. Pâris."[10]

But if the right of the Pope to determine the validity of a miraculous cure was disputed, nearly everyone—defenders and critics of the Jansenists alike—agreed that the judgment of the medical community on the question was crucial. Indeed, as the conflict between religious groups regarding the Convulsionaries increased, the judgments of doctors and surgeons became all the more significant. To the lay public, the task confronting the physicians seemed easy enough: the miracles were either false or true; the convulsions were either real or fake.[11]

Not all doctors and surgeons, however, were eager to become involved in the controversy. Some had refrained from giving an opinion on the issue because it seemed to belong more properly to the domain of theology than to medicine or surgery. Their critics argued that it was the duty of doctors and surgeons to serve as the deputies of the church by acting as competent and disinterested judges. To refuse to take a stand, they asserted, was to commit a crime against God, the church, and France itself as a Christian state, and anyone who did so should be barred from communion.[12]

While the threat of exclusion from communion seems extreme, it was true that the bonds between the church and the medical community in early modern France had been close. Doctors of medicine received their degrees in a religious ceremony and were required to swear an oath to defend the precepts of religion. They had traditionally been consulted by the church on the verification of miraculous healings and the authenticity of relics. In cases involving charges of witchcraft, they had been asked to determine whether someone was truly possessed or suffered from such purely natural disorders as melancholy or epilepsy. When confronted with a seriously ill patient of whatever religious persuasion, they were expected to notify a priest so that final confession could be obtained and the last rites administered. Doctors failing to abide by this regulation were to be fined for their first infraction, suspended for practicing medicine for three months for their second infraction, and threatened with permanent suspension for their third infraction.[13]

There were also cases of medical jurisprudence in which the church took an interest. In trials of women accused of concealment of pregnancy and infanticide, doctors and surgeons were summoned to determine whether the infants had been born dead or alive. The church became involved in these cases because the infants had generally not been baptized and had been denied a Christian burial by their mothers. Trials in cases of impotence were also a concern of the church because a confirmation of impotence might entail the dissolution of marriage. Here again, doctors and surgeons were arbiters of questions of importance to both the church and the state.[14]

The Judgments of Medical Practitioners

Given the precedents established for the right of the medical community to rule on matters in which faith, politics, and medicine intersected, it is not surprising that the critics and defenders of the Convulsionaries would succeed in drawing doctors and surgeons into the controversy. The medical community was expected to play a pivotal role in determining the nature of the Convulsionaries' illnesses, evaluating the authenticity of the miraculous healings, and implicitly, in judging the validity of the Jansenist cause. How, then, did the medical community respond?

In 1732 the lieutenant-general of police René Hérault, summoned twenty-four doctors and surgeons to the Bastille to examine seven of his Convulsionary prisoners. Because the medical consultants were asked to focus on the nature of the convulsions rather than on the illnesses from which the Convulsionaries had sought relief, very little was made of their illnesses.

The doctors and surgeons defined convulsions as violent, involuntary contractions or spasms of the muscles and sought to determine if the Convulsionaries' contractions were indeed involuntary or could be provoked at will. They discovered that, under duress, each of the Convulsionaries could induce contractions and concluded that because the convulsions were not involuntary, they were neither genuine nor inspired by a supernatural source.[15]

On the basis of the medical consultants' report, Louis XV issued an ordinance dated January 27, 1732, denouncing the convulsions as a threat to civil as well as religious order and closing the cemetery of St. Médard. He hoped, by this ordinance, to put an abrupt and definitive end to the spectacle of convulsions and to the large gatherings they attracted.

The report was not, however, greeted with equanimity by the Convulsionaries' supporters, who challenged the impartiality of the doctors and surgeons on the grounds that several of them had ties to the police and the court. Many believed that the so-called confessions of the Convulsionaries had been forced and that few of them had actually received any sort of medical examination. Rumors that one of the Convulsionaries immediately upon release from the Bastille retracted his admission that the convulsions were voluntary and that one of the doctors involved in the examinations renounced the conclusions of the report on his death-bed only strengthened these suspicions.[16]

Issues of bias apart, critics challenged the methodology of the consultants. They considered the handful of Convulsionaries studied to be too few to justify the consultants' sweeping conclusions. They protested the effort of the medical community to naturalize the convulsions as well as the miraculous healings that came from them, arguing that the doctors and surgeons lacked the necessary religious sensibility to comprehend how the power of God might overcome obstacles of nature which had defied the most trusted medical remedies.[17]

It should be noted that although the twenty-four doctors and surgeons agreed in their assessment of the convulsions, the medical community was itself divided on the issue. From 1727 to 1735, numerous claims to miraculous cures were made by Convulsionaries, supported by the testimonies of acquaintances, and documented by doctors and surgeons.[18] As a result, in 1735 Archbishop Vintimille directed his inspector general, Nigon de Berty, to conduct an inquiry into the cases provoking the greatest controversy.

Nigon de Berty began his report by remarking on the human propensity to believe in the fantastic and urged particular circumspection in examining claims to healings of the poor and obscure, who had shown themselves to be particularly superstitious. Because the miracles had become a rallying point for the Jansenist cause, he said, special caution was needed in assessing the Convulsionaries' claims to miraculous healings.

Nigon de Berty thus established certain well-defined conditions that the Convulsionaries' healings would have to meet if they were to be accepted by the archbishop.[19] The illness had to be incurable or cured in a manner that defied the ordinary laws of nature. The healing had to be sudden, perfect, and without relapse. It had to be linked temporally to an act of religion with no admixture of physical remedies. More than one witness was necessary to substantiate the healing; witnesses had to be of good character; and their testimonies could not contradict each other. Finally, the person healed had to be cognizant of all the facts and details attending the healing.[20]

Nigon de Berty's strategy for undermining the validity of the miraculous healings of the Convulsionaries may be explored by examining his treatment of one case, that of Marie Mossaron. Mlle Mossaron was a young woman who suffered an attack of convulsions which degenerated into apoplexy and then into paralysis. After using remedies prescribed by a doctor, surgeon, and pharmacist for eighteen months with no success, Mossaron resolved to seek the intercession of Pâris and was healed.

Nigon de Berty focused first on the medical substantiation of Mossaron's claim to a miraculous healing. He was particularly critical of her doctor's judgment that her condition was incurable, coming as it did only twelve days after the onset of paralysis. In addition, although the doctor acknowledged the miraculous quality of Mossaron's cure, he admitted that he had not actually examined her until several weeks after the healing. The surgeon and pharmacist were similarly faulted for having failed to follow the disorder throughout its eighteen-month course and assuming that the healing had been both sudden and complete.

The contradictory statements of the other witnesses regarding Mossaron's healing prompted Nigon de Berty to wonder if she hadn't feigned the gravity of her illness in order to make the miracle more striking. "Everything," he exclaimed, "revolves on the uncertain sincerity of this girl. However, is a miracle founded on such a support, a proven miracle?"[21] Nigon de Berty did not believe so, and to refute Mossaron's claim he appealed to the judgments of wiser and more enlightened, but anonymous, medical consultants.

Finally, Nigon de Berty likened the illness suffered by Mossaron to that of Anne Le Franc, one of the first Convulsionaries to publicize her miraculous cure. In the case of Le Franc, seven doctors and surgeons brought in for a consultation had dismissed the illness as hysteria induced by a suspension of menstruation. Convulsions resulting from menstrual irregularities were, these consultants contended, frightening and sometimes dangerous, but hardly incurable. Often enough, in young women like Mossaron and Le Franc, such irregularities, as well as the convulsions that accompanied them, terminated quite abruptly—the result of a "revolution in nature." To just such an occurrence Nigon de Berty attributed Mossaron's seemingly miraculous cure.[22]

In the conclusion to his report, Nigon de Berty dismissed any notion of the divine character of the healings and convulsions and urged the archbishop to warn all good Catholics against a dangerous credulity regarding the Convulsionaries' claims to miracles. As a result of their credulity, he declared, they had exalted natural healings into miracles and acknowledged as acts of God frightening convulsions that could only be the "visible effects of a premeditated deception, of an overactive imagination, or of the malice of the Devil."[23] Blind belief had, he maintained, consecrated spectacles of convulsion which were puerile, cruel, shameful, and impious, threatening the moral as well as the religious order.

Under the pressure of Nigon de Berty's inquiry, Mossaron's surgeon and pharmacist retracted their validation of her miraculous healing. They admitted that they had not followed the case closely, relying to a great extent on Mossaron's description of the events leading up to her healing at St. Médard. They contended that the issue had finally to be reduced to the question of how much trust doctors and surgeons could place in their patients' testimony. How, they demanded, could they have tested Nigon de Berty's theory that Mossaron had feigned the severity of her condition toward the end in order to make her healing appear more dramatic? Any blame, they maintained, lay with her, and not with them.[24] Like the surgeon and pharmacist, Mossaron's physician refused to take responsibility for his apparent error. Because the testimonies of Mossaron, the pharmacist, and the surgeon upon which he had relied were flawed, the doctor reasoned, he could not help going astray. In light of Nigon de Berty's report, the doctor, too, withdrew his validation of Mossaron's healing.[25]

Mossaron responded by publishing a letter accusing her medical practitioners of bad faith in retracting their original statements. She went on to protest Nigon de Berty's reliance on anonymous medical experts having no direct knowledge of her case and his assumption that her condition had been identical to Anne Le Franc's. Attributing such careless marshaling of the medical evidence to Nigon de Berty's uncritical acceptance of gender stereotypes, Mossaron demanded, "Would he thus have regarded the opinions of the experts who appeared in the Anne Le Franc affair as a protocol of judgment for all the illnesses that can befall people of my sex?"[26] She reminded the public that this tactic had been used for centuries to undermine women's claims to miraculous healings and attributed its success to the fact that women were reluctant to discuss such intimate matters publicly.[27]

But Mossaron, like so many of the other Convulsionaries, refused to remain silent, and the paper wars continued. She denied suffering any menstrual irregularities during her illness and stood by her claim that her condition had been incurable and the healing complete, perfect, immediate—in short, miraculous. The original statements of her doctor, surgeon, and pharmacist should, she maintained, be granted more validity than retractions made under political pressure.[28]

As the polemical strategies employed in Nigon de Berty's report and in Mossaron's reply indicate, the evaluation of the medical community regarding the Convulsionaries was a crucial factor in conditioning public understanding of the convulsions and healings and in justifying the efforts taken by church and state to suppress the movement. The Convulsionaries' critics made the most of the fact that although the authority of the medical community was acknowledged by both sides, medical judgments were quite fragile. Under close scrutiny, they could easily be challenged and revised.

Theologians like Nigon de Berty were concerned primarily with proving what the convulsions were not—expressions of the divine will; therefore, they did not seek to determine what was responsible for the convulsions, although they offered a number of explanations ranging from the devil to the deceit or overactive imagination of the Convulsionary to some sort of physiological disorder suffered by the Convulsionary. The last option was offered somewhat tentatively, as if to mitigate some of the harshness of the critics' denunciation of honest, if misguided, Convulsionaries. Nigon de Berty hinted that some of the Convulsionaries were truly afflicted and in need of medical assistance. The majority, however, were to be censured as charlatans who had conspired either with the devil or simply with their fellows to deceive and defraud the public, undermining the moral order and subverting the authority of church and state in the process.[29]

The Naturalization and Moralization of Convulsions

While theologians were preoccupied with determining what divine or demonic impulses did or did not lie behind the convulsions, doctors and surgeons looked for natural causes. They regarded the convulsions as disorders to be healed rather than as phenomena to be feared, admired, or excoriated. The centuries-old tradition in which people speaking in tongues had challenged the validity of Catholic doctrine was thus ostensibly set aside. Medical practitioners would devise another framework for understanding the phenomenon of convulsions.

Naturalization did not, however, entail the suspension of individual responsibility for having entertained the convulsions. Although a physiological basis to the convulsions was acknowledged, it was thought to have its roots in an eroticism that many doctors believed could be—indeed, had to be—controlled by the will of the individual. Alternative physiological explanations for the Convulsionaries' behavior which might be advanced by twentieth-century physicians or students of the history of medicine figured not at all in the analyses of early eighteenth-century physicians. No diagnoses of anorexia, ergotism, or shock were made by either the Convulsionaries' defenders or their critics, and the case histories provide insufficient grounds upon which to make a retrospective diagnosis. Early eighteenth-century physicians concluded that those who failed to master the impulse toward convulsion were to be pitied for their lack of fortitude, while those who simply refused to master it were to be denounced for their depravity. In this period, naturalization of the convulsions thus involved moralization as well.

The Jansenist physician Philippe Hecquet was the most prolific and authoritative medical writer to attempt to naturalize the convulsions. His interest in the Convulsionaries was no doubt related to his lifelong fascination with the relationship between religion and medicine. By 1736 Hecquet would publish five books on the subject; four more remained in manuscript when he died in 1737 at the age of seventy-six.[30] Hecquet was also the author of a large and diverse corpus of works including three volumes on medicine, surgery, and pharmacy for the poor; an influential treatise on smallpox which condemned inoculation as a crime against God, nature, and the state; a book on the obligation of mothers to nurse their infants; and a translation of Hippocrates' aphorisms.[31]

Too infirm to attend the Convulsionaries' assemblies, Hecquet based his judgments on the testimony of faithful friends and enlightened physicians. Such diagnoses from afar were by no means unusual in the eighteenth century. Hecquet's justification of his method is summed up in an anecdote of a dialogue he had with a friend on the opposing side. The friend said, "It is said, Monsieur, that you are studying the Convulsionaries." Hecquet replied, "Studying, Monsieur? Do you think that I, after having practiced medicine for more than fifty years, would still need to learn about disorders as common as convulsions? No, Monsieur, I am not studying them; but I have studied them for a long time; and as for you, I advise you to go study them."[32]

Fearing that the phenomenon of convulsions would do much to discredit the Jansenist cause, Hecquet sought to dissociate mainstream Jansenism from the peculiar cult of the Convulsionaries. Hecquet is an important source because he was the only doctor to write extensive theoretical works on the Convulsionaries of St. Médard. The views he articulated on this phenomenon were not peculiar to him, but reflected the findings of a vast preexisting corpus of medical works on vapors.[33]

Like Nigon de Berty, Hecquet feared the destructive power of Convulsionism, though he preferred to employ his own medical terminology to dramatize the threat it posed. Thus one of his most important works on the Convulsionaries was titled *Le Naturalisme des convulsions dans les maladies de l'épidémie convulsionnaire*. While the contagion this epidemic threatened was the contagion of imagination rather than of physical organisms, the term *epidemic* was adroitly chosen to inspire public trepidation and distrust of the Convulsionaries as well as to place the resolution of the crisis firmly in the hands of doctors. Such rhetoric, employed for a similar purpose, would recur in the works of late eighteenth-century critics of mesmerism and of nineteenth-century crowd psychologists like Taine, Tarde, and Le Bon.[34]

Like the medical consultants cited by Nigon de Berty, Hecquet regarded convulsions as symptoms of the vapors or hysterical affections, which were thought to be sexually based disorders peculiar to *personnes du sexe*, an appellation routinely applied to women.[35] Because hysteria was regarded as a concomitant of female sexuality, no woman was thought to be immune to it, though some were more successful in resisting it than others.[36] Men who were subject to convulsions were considered effeminate, peculiarly sensitive individuals inclined to melancholy and the intense introspection brought on by an excess of studies. Their malady was diagnosed as hypochondria, the male parallel to hysteria in women. The important difference between the two lay in the frequency with which the two sexes were afflicted, itself a function of the differing degrees of constitutional fortitude manifested by the two sexes. Thus Hecquet observed, "But there are only accidents with respect to men, while the dispositions are innate or natural and universal among women."[37]

Hecquet located the physiological basis of hysteria in the reaction of the overly sensitive nervous system of women to upsets in the circulatory system. He identified two kinds of hysteria, one the result of a disorder in the red blood cells, the other of a disorder in the white. Vapors derived from derangements of the red blood cells were thought to be linked to the suspension of menstruation in young women or the onset of menopause in older women and to be accompanied by a painful and feverish upheaval of the whole constitution. Vapors derived from derangements of the white blood cells gave rise to convulsions that, although exhausting, were not accompanied by fevers and were not thought to attenuate health.[38] These vapors were thought to be stimulated by the passions, for good or for evil. A misguided religious zeal could provoke vapors, as could lust.[39]

While acknowledging that the vapors experienced by some of the Convulsionaries could have been the result either of menstrual irregularities or of harmless passions, Hecquet believed that the vapors experienced by most Convulsionaries had an erotic base.[40] Terming these vapors "shameful" and "criminal,"[41] Hecquet noted that they were often experienced by young girls, young widows, and old spinsters. He regarded these vapors as a manifestation of the women's sexual frustration and considered them shameful only because the women's fantasies had not been acted out within socially accepted channels. Marriage, in the mind of Hecquet and his contemporaries, was the obvious cure. For those for whom this solution was either impossible or unpalatable, recourse could still be had to the whole arsenal of traditional methods, including bleedings, baths, hemlock, opium, and tobacco.[42] Such remedies might be unpredictable but were not without effect.

For the majority of Convulsionaries, however, Hecquet's judgment was more severe. Hecquet suspected that the aroused imaginations, vanity, and greed of many of the Convulsionaries were more responsible for their convulsions than any imbalance in their blood cells. These girls came from hard-working, obscure families of modest means. Upon entering the Convulsionary cult they were quickly ennobled by virtue of their healing powers into priestesses who were neither expected nor obliged to continue in their former occupations.[43] Hecquet had no sympathy for such sudden, unwonted changes in social status, particularly when they signified a shift from a formerly productive to an idle role in society. Deducing mediocre virtue of the girls from their mediocre fortunes, he suspected most of them of a self-seeking duplicity that put them in a long tradition of hysterical connivers, including the Ursulines of Loudun. "It is not necessary to be very knowledgable in the affairs of the world," he observed, "to know how many astonishing scenes have been presented to the public throughout all time by hysterical or vaporous girls or women, whose enthusiastic operations have appeared so extraordinary that some have been attributed to God, others to the Devil. But even so, these creatures, often of mediocre virtue, have perpetuated a fraud, making a considerable profit for themselves and others whom they have lured by their tricks even as they have satisfied their vanity in the world."[44]

Hecquet's proposed treatment for these Convulsionaries was to remove them from theological controversy and spectacle and place them firmly under the supervision of physicians like himself. The women were to be isolated, intimidated, flagellated, and dunked in cold water. Such treatment, Hecquet hoped, would bring an abrupt end to the vapors and might even revive the women's modesty.[45]

Even as Hecquet emphasized the medical nature of convulsions and identified a physiological link between female hysteria and female sexuality, it is important to note that he shared the attitude of the theologians that hysteria typically reflected a disequilibrium in the moral rather than the physical constitution. This moral diagnosis and cure, rather than banishing theological perspectives from medicine, affirmed their centrality. The medical assertion that women possessed an innate and universal disposition toward hysteria was not so far removed from the moral assumption embedded in the Christian tradition that the nature of woman is to sin and deceive men. Hecquet did not hesitate to make either assertion, appealing to medical authority to substantiate the former and to scriptural authority to substantiate the latter. "The supremacy of malice which is in woman," he wrote, "when she lets herself go along with the natural penchant of her sex toward seduction is proven, for Scripture says that there is no malice comparable to that of a woman who wants to be evil."[46]

Hecquet's citation of Scripture gives dramatic testimony to his conviction that religion was central to the theory and practice of medicine, enduing it with nobility and dignity. To Hecquet, the study of medicine was the occasion for appreciating the glory of God, while the practice of medicine provided a lesson in humility for man. Nature was often inscrutable and doctors found themselves in a quandary as to how to read it. Rather than chafing at these limits, Hecquet extolled them. Through faith, he maintained, doctors learned to penetrate some of the mysteries of nature and to admire what they could not comprehend.[47]

Hecquet's notion of the centrality of religion to medicine informed his conviction that it was the duty of the doctor to serve as a moral exemplar, healing the moral as well as physical complaints of his patients. He typically began his visits to patients by asking them to join him in praying to God. Some were even urged to retreat to a convent in search of moral and spiritual reform. In difficult or terminal cases, Hecquet always advised his patients to put their spiritual affairs in order and sent for a clergyman.[48] Outlining the appropriate training for the young student of medicine, he wrote, "Finally, we have included the science of morality among those which ought to form a good doctor. For a good clergyman can be an excellent priest without a great knowledge of literature, but a Doctor will be a dangerous scholar if he does not have more religion and morality than science."[49]

Morality was especially important in regulating relations between the physician and his female patient, and Hecquet urged his fellow physicians to hold themselves in the restraint, knowledge, and modesty of the profession, "bearing in mind the contagion of the sexes."[50] Despite his conviction that it was women's nature to sin and deceive, Hecquet did not advocate restricting their role in attending births. It was fear that women would become accustomed to being touched by strangers that prompted Hecquet to argue vehemently against the employment of male accoucheurs.[51] In Hecquet's mind, such close association between male medical practitioners and female patients evidently posed a greater threat to morality than did the possibility that midwives would fail to uphold the patriarchal principles of the family-state compact. But he was writing before 1750, when the medical community, the clergy, and the courts, appalled at empiric practices that they claimed led to a large number of feticides, renewed their campaign to educate midwives and subordinate them to the higher authorities.[52]

Conclusion

Analysis of the medical consultations concerning the Convulsionaries reveals the authority the medical community commanded in the 1730s, but also the fragility of medical judgments and the lack of consensus among medical practitioners. Because evidence regarding *maladies des femmes* was based primarily on the testimony of women and therefore was considered suspect, medical judgments could be easily overturned.

Hecquet's solution to the quest for certitude lay in religious faith. Although he favored naturalizing the convulsions, his approach to medicine was grounded in a Christian perspective that identified Scripture as the ultimate source of truth regarding human nature. Such faith would continue to inform the writings of some mid-eighteenth-century physicians, most notably Astruc, who took up the issue of late births in the 1760s.

But to many, grounding medical judgments on the truths of religion would seem anachronistic by midcentury. In 1778, devotion to religion and propensity for polemic of the sort displayed by Hecquet decades earlier made official spokesmen for the medical faculties uneasy. Thus, in his biography of the most famous members of the Faculty of Medicine of Paris, Hazon praised Hecquet's charity but criticized his traditional approach to medicine and his tendency to let himself be carried away by fire, genius, and enthusiasm when attention to method would have served him better.[53] In accordance with this judgment, Hazon excised all references to convulsions or theological medicine in his otherwise extensive bibliography of Hecquet's works.

Even in the 1730s, Hecquet's emphasis on the moral qualities required of the physician and his refusal to separate matters of faith from medicine presented obstacles to the medical community's efforts to resolve the controversies surrounding the Convulsionaries. Like Hecquet, doctors and surgeons issuing consultations on the Convulsionaries frequently allowed their sympathy or distaste for the Jansenist cause to determine their judgment of the nature of the convulsions and attendant healings. Rather than focusing on the character of the healings to which the convulsions seemed to give rise, they addressed the threat to public morality which they believed the convulsions posed. Rather than examining a broad cross section of Convulsionaries, they focused on those individuals, mostly women, whom they believed vulnerable to attack.

By emphasizing the threat of moral degeneracy and sexual chaos which the Convulsionaries posed, the church and state, with some help from the medical community, managed to discredit the Convulsionaries and to undermine the unity and strength of the Jansenist movement. Not all Jansenist supporters wished to effect the same changes in the church and state hierarchies nor expected change to be executed at the same pace. Many were, however, united among themselves and with their critics in opposition to the perceived threat to the moral order posed by any changes in the sexual hierarchy. They endorsed a traditional view of religiosity for women which emphasized obedience, humility, and chastity, aiming at union with God through utter self-abnegation.

The subtle diversionary tactics employed by the church and state proved successful. As the fundamental issues regarding authority within church and state raised by the Convulsionary movement were obscured, the movement was defused of its potential political explosiveness. Yet the authorities' response to the Convulsionaries did little to solve the social, economic, and psychological problems facing young, unmarried women in early eighteenth-century Paris. As incendiary as the rhetoric regarding women's involvement in the Convulsionary movement became, statistics assembled by Catherine-Laurence Maire and Eliane Gabert-Boche confirm the fact that young, unmarried women comprised the majority of people receiving miraculous cures. Healings were reported by 81 women, 23 men, and 12 children for a total of 116 people. Only 25 of the women were married; 39 were single; 14 were widows.[54] Of 200 people experiencing convulsions in 1731–32, 70 percent were women, especially young, single women, the daughters of artisans and craftsmen.[55] Of 250 Convulsionaries arrested between 1732 and 1760, 60 percent were women, many of them booksellers.[56]

Gabert-Boche finds the fact that so many unmarried women were drawn to the Convulsionary movement unsurprising, given the large number of unmarried women in Paris at the time. Many girls delayed marriage or remained single because their families were unable to arrange a dowry or feared a mésalliance. Thus, in his *Tableau de Paris*, L. S. Mercier counted four unmarried women for every one married.[57] Maire interprets women's involvement in the Convulsionary movement as the reflection of profound social dislocation. She believes these women were feeling the contradictions of a society that pushed them into celibacy without providing them with a symbolic function within the religious domain or an assured social identity.[58]

Some historians have argued that women were drawn to the Convulsionary movement because it offered them power and authority and an opportunity to be heard free of the censorship of a father, husband, or confessor. Jean-Claude Pie cites one Convulsionary in particular, Anne Charlier, whom all Paris, even the king, hurried to see and hear. Pie casts Charlier in a heroic light, arguing that she prefigured women of today who refuse to be defined and legislated over by others, whether doctors or the state.[59]

Yet if a few women were able to establish a social identity for themselves through convulsions, many more would suffer from the image of women articulated so forcefully by the Convulsionaries' critics. This image would haunt Enlightenment writers and their conservative critics throughout the eighteenth century and continue to serve as a source of speculation for physicians like Charcot and Richet in the nineteenth century.[60] Diderot in particular was affected by the memory of the Convulsionaries, for he lived near the church of St. Médard from 1744 until 1746 and had his second baby baptized there. Finding the memory of St. Médard both disturbing and unsavory, he was drawn repeatedly to the subject of the Convulsionaries in his *Pensées philosophiques*.[61]

The Convulsionaries came to assume a paradigmatic quality for Diderot and other philosophes as the link between nervous disorders in women and religious fanaticism. The philosophes' image of the Convulsionaries thus perpetuated the association of women with frailty and irrationality, if not debauchery. Diderot regarded the Convulsionaries with considerably more compassion than did Hecquet, and he refrained from making women an object of moral censure, deploring instead the social conditions that created vice.[62] Still, Diderot considered women, regardless of differences in social condition, to be susceptible by nature to nervous disorders and superstition.

By midcentury, women's crucial role in stimulating philosophic discussion in the salons would give critics grounds for questioning the philosophes' commitment to the pursuit of truth and lead to conflict even among enlightened reformers about how much cultural influence women should have.[63] These concerns would figure prominently in the 1760s debate over late births and the 1780s controversy over mesmerism.

It is important to note that more than the memory of the Convulsionaries would remain alive decades after the cemetery of St. Médard was closed. Although the Convulsionary movement was pushed underground by the repressive measures taken by the state in the 1730s, it was not destroyed. In the provinces, young women would continue to claim miraculous healings effected through faith in the Jansenist cause, but late eighteenth-century physicians and surgeons were considerably more reluctant than their predecessors to have their authority and reputation brought to bear in ecclesiastical disputes that they believed lay outside the purview of medicine.[64] In Paris, the movement became more clandestine and eccentric. Stories of the excesses of the *secours* and miraculous healings continued to circulate in the 1750s and 1760s, piquing the curiosity of authors, poets, artists, and publishers. Doctors like Barbeu du Bourg and Morand and philosophes like La Condamine and d'Alembert attended secret meetings to see the *secours* for themselves.[65]

The responses of these visitors varied. La Condamine was especially struck by the suffering the female Convulsionaries inflicted upon themselves even as they denied feeling any pain. They were living proof, he declared, of the steadfastness and courage that fanaticism could inspire.[66] Other philosophes were drawn to the idea of convulsions as theater. D'Alembert argued that if the convulsions were made public, they would lose their appeal and fall into obscurity. Like the lieutenant-general of police, Bertin, he advocated accentuating the theatrical character of the Convulsionaries by putting them in the fair between the tightrope walkers and jugglers and charging spectators money to watch.[67] Voltaire employed the theater metaphor to a different purpose, observing that these farces had had serious consequences in less enlightened times and commenting wryly that being nailed to a cross in order to convince the world of the absurdity of a certain papal bull was a rather too costly form of persuasion.[68]

Yet because the Convulsionaries' assemblies continued into the 1760s, it was difficult to declare the triumph of enlightenment. As long as the specter of contagious convulsions remained, it would constitute a stumbling block to the philosophes' ideal of an enlightened public, the authority of whose opinions would ultimately supersede that of king or pope.

The Convulsionaries posed an interesting dilemma for the philosophes: even as the latter were skeptical of the Convulsionaries' miraculous cures and deplored their fanaticism, they realized that their stance could be construed as a defense of royal power and the Catholic hierarchy.[69] Still, not everyone was so finely or consistently attuned to the complexities of the issue, and in the 1760s both critics of the Enlightenment like Fréron and advocates like Voltaire would dismiss their opponents—Jansenists, Jesuits, or philosophes—authoritatively and indiscriminately by referring to them as Convulsionaries. The word had become the consummate symbol of fanaticism.[70]

33

CHAPTER TWO

The Debate over Late Births, 1764–1806

The Context

In 1764 the legitimacy of a child born ten months and seventeen days after the death of the husband of its mother was challenged by the collateral heirs of the husband before the Parlement of Rennes. Were the child declared illegitimate, the bulk of the estate of the husband would pass to the collateral heirs rather than to the wife as trustee for the child. The case was identified simply by the first names of the couple, Charles and Renée.

The attorney for the collateral heirs was M. de Villeblanche, who served as *procureur général* in the famous La Chalotais case. Representing Renée was M. Gerbier de Vaulogé, a member of the same family of lawyers as J. B. Gerbier, a Parisian lawyer known for concluding his cases with eloquent pleas to the judges to listen to the voice of nature, see the tears of the defendant, and then judge. These tactics proved unsuccessful in the La Pouplinière case, a contemporaneous case in which the inheritance of a child born after the death of its father was at stake, though legitimacy was not the pivotal issue.[1]

Both attorneys had made a name for themselves among their peers, the philosophes, and the reading public through their involvement in earlier causes célèbres. During the Enlightenment cases drawing public attention to social injustice, judicial inefficiency, and abuse of authority spearheaded the movement for reform.[2] Nicolas Toussaint Moyne (better known as Des Essarts) and François Richer, among others, capitalized on public interest in controversial cases by editing journals of causes célèbres which were eagerly read, especially by women. The cases were presented with considerable rhetorical flair and made what had traditionally been considered intimate family matters public. Merging the genres of history, tragedy, and the novel, the tales elicited strong emotions, including pity, indignation, and horror; held readers in suspense; and never failed to provide a moral.[3] Some were even transformed into plays and brought to the stage. They could create such a commotion that, as in the case of the *Prisonnier Anglois*, the theater had to be closed.[4]

But let us return to the case of 1764. The marriage of Charles and Renée fit the prototype of those December-May unions which, as a reading of Chaucer or Boccaccio demonstrates, were rich perennial sources of comic literature and neighborhood gossip. At the putative time of conception, Charles was seventy-six years old; Renée, thirty-four. The marriage had been infertile throughout its four-year duration. During the last few months of his life, Charles was afflicted with a serious illness that further decreased the possibility of fertility. One month before he died, Charles had to be attended by nurses day and night and the odor of gangrene rendered his room uninhabitable to Renée.

Neither Charles nor Renée had given any indication before Charles's death that Renée might have become pregnant. Charles made no provisions for the birth of a child in his will, but instead left his estate to his collateral heirs. Renée herself waited an inordinate three and a half months after Charles's death before declaring pregnancy. Appearances notwithstanding, Renée boldly asserted that the child was Charles's; the collateral heirs dared her to prove it in the public forum of the courts.

Both sides solicited consultations from distinguished doctors of the Faculty of Medicine and from surgeons of the Royal Academy of Surgery, who were asked to evaluate the possibility of *naissances tardives* (late births) in general and of this late birth in particular. Both those who argued for and those who argued against late births agreed that the average or normal length of pregnancy was nine months. The question they were asked to resolve was whether a pregnancy could last substantially longer than nine months and, if so, how much longer and under what circumstances. As the debate progressed and the arguments of each side were subjected to increasingly intensive scrutiny, the frailty of all the standard criteria would become evident. Ultimately, concern over the social and political ramifications of a judgment would take priority over strictly medical considerations.

Abridgments of the consultations of the Parisian medical experts appeared in medical journals like the *Journal de médecine, chirurgie et pharmacie* and the *Gazette salutaire* and reverberated in journals with such disparate philosophical orientations and audiences as the *Journal des sçavans*, the *Mémoires de Trévoux*, the *Journal encyclopédique*, *L'Avantcoureur*, Grimm's *Correspondance littéraire*, Bachaumont's *Mémoires secrets*, and Fréron's *L'Année littéraire*. References to the latest consultation could be found interspersed amid news of the protracted maneuverings of the Calas and Sirven affairs,[5] the publication and condemnation of Rousseau's *Emile* and Voltaire's *Dictionnaire philosophique*, and the controversy over inoculation.

Although the case originated in Brittany, it quickly gained an audience in Paris and throughout the provinces. Surgeons, midwives, and laypersons eagerly joined in the debate, submitting to the journals letters in which they defended or challenged various consultations on the basis of their own observations of unusual pregnancies, whether of human beings or of chickens.[6] Jurists offered their opinions, too, emphasizing the social significance of a definitive ruling on the issue of late births and expressing anxiety over the medical community's lack of consensus. The Encyclopedists saw in the debate the beginning of a salutary effort to establish a new science of medical jurisprudence.

Women constituted an important audience for this debate, which focused on issues affecting their goods, their honor, their very lives. Judicial and family archives are filled with references to the protracted and expensive disputes over marriage contracts and succession, which, like property itself, seemed to be passed down from generation to generation.[7] In their letters and memoirs, women reflected upon the latest cases,[8] discussed their dread of being portrayed as comic protagonists if they should themselves be involved in a case,[9] and recounted incidents in which they had deceived parents by following the example set by a cause célèbre.[10]

A number of women writers on education, including Mme de Genlis, Mlle d'Espinassy, and Mme de Miremont,[11] hoped to improve on the seventeenth-century educational manuals of Fénelon and Mme de Maintenon by emphasizing the importance of instructing women in matters of law lest they plunge themselves or their families into ruin. Mme de Puisieux went further still, arguing that all the liberal professions, including law and medicine, should be opened to women, while Mme de Coicy urged admission of women to the judiciary because it had proved so lucrative to men.[12]

For the medical experts, however, the focus of the 1764 case was epistemological before it was social or political. This case challenged the medical community to refine its criteria for perceiving truth and to develop a truly enlightened science of medicine. Whatever their differences, the defenders and opponents of late births, like the supporters and critics of the Convulsionaries, were united in their quest for certainty and consensus in medicine. In this debate, however, the honor of the medical community

36

was more clearly at stake than had been the case thirty years earlier. Physicians and surgeons of the 1760s were intent on restoring dignity to medicine by purging it of the multitude of extravagant and incredible observations they believed had dishonored it.[13]

Superstitions regarding sexuality and procreation abounded. Among the lay public, stories circulated of a woman who was impregnated by the memory of her dead husband and of other women who gave birth to fish, frogs, or rabbits.[14] Rumor had it that fetal deformities could be caused by upheavals in the mother's emotional state, that difficulties encountered in lactation might be the result of spells cast by gypsies, that the source of hysteria lay in movements of the womb; that menstrual fluid was poisonous.[15]

Descriptions of monsters appeared regularly in provincial journals, and caused women to puzzle over how a fetus could be born without a neck or with two heads and two torsos.[16] Confronted with these and other unsolved mysteries of gestation, pregnant women proved easy prey to charlatans like the one who visited Alby in 1782 waving an artificial fetus with twice the usual number of arms and legs and pushing an elixir aimed at preventing the birth of such a monster.[17]

While ignorance regarding the mechanics of reproduction fueled the superstitions of common folk and enhanced the business of charlatans, it spurred the nobility to fabricate increasingly elaborate myths about their origins. In response to the steady erosion of their position over the course of the eighteenth century, nobles sought a physical basis for their claims to power, privilege, and patronage. They argued that they were the descendants of great men and that the virtue of their ancestors gave them the mark of nobility. This virtue was supposedly contained in the seminal fluid. Thus De la Roque declared in his *Traité de la noblesse*, "There is in the seed I know not what force and I know not what principle which transmits and continues the inclinations of fathers in their descendants."[18]

Rumors of widespread promiscuity and illegitimacy among the nobility of the sort purveyed by Métra in his *Correspondance secrète* and Bachaumont in the *Mémoires secrets*[19] would, of course, undermine this myth. Bastardy, once regarded as a sign of noble's potency, had come increasingly to be seen as a sin and a sign of disorder.[20] The nobility thus had an interest in seeing if the medical community could use Renée's case to set clear standards for determining legitimacy. The definition of such standards could call into question the validity of the Grande Chambre's ruling of 1693 that the father of a child conceived during marriage is the husband of the mother.

Although enlightened members of the medical community might regard the superstitions of the public and the myths generated by the nobility skeptically, they too found themselves perplexed by the mystery surrounding the mechanics of reproduction. Their uncertainty is reflected in the titles of theses presented to the Faculty of Medicine of Paris from 1752 to 1764. One thesis posed the question whether or not procreation was a secret of nature. Another asked if menstruation was the result of an excess of blood in the circulatory system. A third wondered if the imagination of a pregnant woman could have a detrimental effect on the development of the fetus. A fourth addressed the issue of variations in the length of pregnancy which confronted the medical community in Renée's case.[21]

The questions surrounding sexuality and reproduction posed inherently greater challenges to the medical community than had the Convulsionary healings. In the case of the Convulsionaries, medical experts had been able to dismiss claims to miraculous cures simply by attributing the cures to natural causes. They had not been required to define precisely what the natural causes were or how they operated. The 1760s inquiries into sexuality and reproduction attempted to go much further—to distinguish clearly the natural from the unnatural and explain *why* something could or could not occur. The challenge came from outside the medical community as well as from within, with philosophes like Voltaire demanding, "Novice philosphers, you seek in vain to discover how an infant is formed and you want me to know how it is deformed?"[22]

Throughout the early modern period, even the most progressive medical experts found themselves frustrated when it came to understanding the mechanics of reproduction. Nor could experimentation be counted on to solve the riddle. As Paul Hoffmann has observed, William Harvey, who had used experimentation with great success in his research on the circulation of the blood, found his observations on generation misleading and was forced to retreat to a metaphysic of occult forces similar to Aristotle's.[23] It was not until 1826 that advances in instrumentation would enable Carl von Baer to observe the mammalian egg; in 1875, Wilhelm Hertwig would be the first to observe the fecundation of the ovum by the sperm.[24]

In the analysis that follows, I will explore how physicians, surgeons, midwives, and laypersons attempted to determine the limits of nature in one quite circumscribed matter—the length of pregnancy. Their debate over late births touches on many of the themes associated with the debate over the Convulsionaries, including the fragility of medical judgments, the continuing influence of Christian morality on medical views of women, and the importance of rhetoric, but carries them much further. Once again, we will see how the medical community and the public attempted to sort out the various physiological, philosophical, moral, and legal criteria for resolving a perplexing medical issue with provocative social implications. The context in which discussion took place, however, had changed significantly since the 1730s, as had the primary social concerns of the debaters. The focal point of the debate over late births was not the legitimacy of the church but the legitimacy of the patriarchal family. By the 1760s, the declining authority of the church was being felt throughout the institutions of corporative society. In this period, traditional theological arguments would prove much less effective in responding to challenges to the principles of hierarchy, privilege, and patriarchy than they had in the 1730s, and debaters would find themselves immersed in an unprecedentedly intense and far-reaching consideration of alternative principles upon which to govern society and the state. Nor could the state step in authoritatively to control the crisis or contain the controversy, as it had by closing the cemetery of St. Médard in 1732.

Let us turn now to an examination of the specific individuals and issues involved in the initial phases of the debate.

The Key Personae

Opinion on the possibility of late births was divided among those who opposed it, those who supported it, and those who attempted to mediate between the two groups. This last position would become ever more difficult to sustain as opponents and proponents grew increasingly impatient to arrive at a definitive resolution. In seeking such a resolution, both sides would find themselves taking ever more extreme positions than the medical evidence at hand seemed to warrant, and the prospects of arriving at a compromise would become increasingly remote.

The opponents of the possibility of late births found their spokesmen in three distinguished members of the Parisian medical community: Michel Bouvart, Antoine Louis, and Jean Astruc. Bouvart (1707–87) had been received by the Faculty of Medicine of Paris in 1738 and became an associate member of the Royal Academy of Sciences in 1743. He held a chair in medicine at the Collège Royal, but once his skills as a polemicist gained him a reputation outside the medical community, he abandoned teaching to tend to an ever expanding and lucrative medical practice among the Parisian elite.[25]

At the beginning of his memoir, Louis (1723–92) presents his credentials as a professor of surgery, royal censor, and consulting surgeon to the royal army. He was already a prolific author, having written on such diverse topics as the surgical treatment of wounds, the relationship between soul and body, hereditary diseases, venereal disease, and the certitude of signs of death. He published a refutation of the subordination of surgeons to doctors in 1748 and was named secretary of the Royal Academy of Surgery in 1764. A contributor of more than a hundred articles to all seventeen letterpress volumes of the *Encyclopédie*, he became increasingly interested in medical jurisprudence, obtaining a degree in law in 1769 and searching for medical grounds on which to vindicate the Calas and Sirven families, whose causes Voltaire championed so indefatigably.[26]

Astruc (1684–1766) was equally well known. He had served as consulting doctor to the king in 1730, taught at the Faculty of Medicine of Paris, and occupied the Geoffroy chair at the Collège Royal from 1731 to 1766. An erudite scholar and master logician, Astruc frequented the salon of Mme de Tencin and became known, along with Fontenelle, Marivaux, Mairan, Mirabaud, De Boze, and Duclos, as one of her seven sages. He had gained a reputation in the 1720s for combatting the plague, attained fame for his work on venereal disease, wrote texts on obstetrics and inoculation, and took the opposite side from Louis on the question of the subordination of surgeons. The son of a Protestant minister who converted to Catholicism after the revocation of the Edict of Nantes, Astruc had an interest in religion which would continue throughout his life, leading him to write two dissertations on the immortality of the soul and an inquiry into the textual authenticity of Genesis.[27]

The most prominent proponents of the possibility of late births were Antoine Petit (1718–94) and Jean Le Bas (?1717–97). Having attained the title of *docteur-régent* of the Faculty of Medicine of Paris in 1746, Petit taught courses there in anatomy and surgery for at least a year. Buffon chose him to be royal professor of anatomy at the Jardin du Roi, where he attained a reputation for eloquence. Public esteem for Petit's teaching and medical practice would prove to be important factors in his election to the Royal Academy of Sciences in 1760. Petit was unusual in that he had studied at both the College of Surgery and the Faculty of Medicine and was accomplished in both fields. Like Bouvart, he was not a prolific writer or a particularly productive scientist. His most important works, in addition to his writings on late births, included a report in favor of inoculation which he presented to the Faculty of Medicine in 1764 and a project for the reform of medical practice which was composed during the Revolution.[28] Petit was joined in the debate by Le Bas, a surgeon and royal censor.

Twenty-three doctors and surgeons co-signed Petit's consultation; eleven co-signed Le Bas's. Included in the list were professors of medicine, members of the royal academies, physicians to the king and royal household, and surgeons holding important posts within the hospitals. The consultations of the opponents were similarly co-signed by a number of prominent doctors and surgeons, also representing the full range of medical and scientific institutions within the city of Paris.[29] Despite their differences in perspective, the supporters and opponents of late births did not differ significantly in professional background or accomplishment. The debate within the medical community did not split along hierarchical lines; that is, doctors and surgeons who enjoyed relatively less power or prestige did not take sides with the public in an onslaught on the prerogatives of the medical establishment.

Rather than social position, perhaps the most important difference between the proponents and opponents was in epistemological approach. Whereas opponents of the possibility of late births focused on the importance of referring to the authority of Hippocrates and of affirming the existence of universal laws of nature, the proponents devoted their attention to exploring the physical, rather than the philosophical, possibilities of late births. They meticulously reviewed the long history of reports of late births, analyzing each case and trying to fit it into a comprehensive and convincing theory of reproduction.

Proponents and opponents also differed significantly on the meaning of enlightenment as it pertained to medicine. Both sides were committed to the goal of enlightenment, but whereas the supporters identified enlightenment with the broad dissemination of medical knowledge, the opponents were intent on developing an enlightened science of medicine free from popular error and superstition and comprehensible only to a highly educated scientific elite. While the supporters hoped to improve health care by supplying the people with simple medical precepts that would enable them to take care of themselves, the opponents believed it was dangerous to entrust such knowledge to nonprofessionals.[30]

This difference in approach was reflected not merely in the debate over late births, but in the debate over inoculation which occurred simultaneously. Astruc, Bouvart, and Petit figured prominently in both debates. Astruc and Bouvart viewed inoculation as a deadly lottery and opposed it on the grounds that insufficient experimentation had been done to justify the risk of exposing children unnecessarily to smallpox.[31] Petit, in contrast, regarded the risks of inoculation as negligible in the face of the death, deformity, mutilation, and blindness to which everyone who had not been inoculated was exposed. He believed that the decision to inoculate resided properly with the family rather than the state and sought to make the complex subject of inoculation clear enough so that the *mothers* of every family could understand and follow the discussion.[32]

As polarized as proponents and opponents of the possibility of late births were in their epistemological approaches, a few people attempted to mediate between the two sides. The most important were Marie Plisson and Jacques Barbeu du Bourg. The daughter of a Chartres lawyer, Plisson (1727–88) developed a taste for literature at a young age and, entirely self-taught, published various pieces of prose and poetry in local journals, including a series entitled "Provincial Promenades," which appeared in the *Mercure* of 1755–56. These promenades dealt with the theme of bringing enlightenment to the countryside and considered both the positive and negative images associated with medicine. One hundred copies of her *Ecologue* were printed and distributed in Paris and Versailles, where they were reportedly well received. Plisson's odes on the births of the Duc de Bourgogne and the Duc d'Aquitaine were mentioned in the *Journal des dames's* catalogue of notable works by women writers in 1764.[33]

Plisson embraced midwifery as a vocation while continuing to cultivate an interest in letters, the natural sciences, and philanthropy throughout her life. After a series of devastating floods in the Chartres regions, she published *Projet d'une société pour soulager les pauvres de la campagne* in 1758. It was the desire "of rendering service to my sex; . . . I have always loved and pitied this unhappy sex to which I belong,"[34] she wrote, that prompted Plisson to publish her reflections on the late births controversy.

Plisson acknowledged that many would consider it unseemly for a woman to involve herself in a public debate like this, much less challenge the opinions of medical experts. Women had ventured to reflect publicly upon the subject of late births before this debate, but only with great caution. Writing a treatise on the duration of pregnancy in 1753 for Mme la Marquise de M——, Pierre Pajon de Moncets, under the pseudonym of Mme Corron, alluded to the severe censure risked by revealing one's thoughts on this secret of nature. Discussion of the topic put women inside the sanctuary of sciences and the fine arts which had almost been forbidden them. The very act of writing could be regarded as a means of protesting men's unjust usurpation of the sciences and of demonstrating women's capacities for contributing to the accumulation of useful knowledge.[35]

As if to mitigate the threat that such writing posed or perhaps to expose the absurdity of the prejudice against women writing, Plisson played on the image of the excessive sensibility of women. Everyone, she noted, had uncontrollable quirks. Some people abhorred the sight of a cat, others the shadow of a mouse. She confessed to feeling an uncontrollable aversion to bad reasoning. "I have had," she wrote, "from infancy such a great horror of it that I was in danger of falling into an epileptic fit from it."[36] Writing, she explained, was a remedy for her, a way of mastering the small convulsive movements she felt in her right hand when she read an illogical work. She thus effectively and humorously reversed the image of convulsions associated with the Convulsionary spectacles of the 1730s. Rather than manifesting irrationality, convulsive movements could reflect reason's rejection of irrationality.

Plisson's contribution to the debate differed from that of the doctors and surgeons in the value it placed on common sense, as opposed to erudition, and in the sensitivity it expressed to the concerns of women. Still, Plisson was no doctrinaire defender of any woman's claim to a late birth. She believed that each case had to be evaluated critically on its own merits.

Like Plisson, Barbeu du Bourg (1709–79) was drawn simultaneously to letters, science, and philanthropy. He studied ancient languages, theology, and law before embarking on a career in medicine. A regent of the Faculty of Medicine, Barbeu du Bourg taught courses in pharmacy, surgery, and botany and edited the *Gazette d'Epidaure*, a journal aimed at simplifying and clarifying the theory and practice of medicine. His journal was filled with letters, announcements, remedies, medical curiosities, racy stories, and philosophical speculation. Barbeu du Bourg was also a vocal supporter of inoculation; a translator and editor of Benjamin Franklin's scientific work; and the author of a work on botany which eschewed Latin classifications and proved especially popular with women. Like Plisson, Barbeu du Bourg was impressed by how uncertain medical understanding of the mechanics of reproduction was and by how polarized the two factions debating late births had become.[37]

Criteria for Reaching a Judgment

As had been the case with Marie Mossaron in the 1730s investigation of the Convulsionary cures, medical knowledge of Renée's condition was indirect, resting primarily on Renée's own testimony. When Renée made a declaration of pregnancy before the courts, she refused to allow a doctor, surgeon, or midwife to confirm her condition and refrained from seeking medical assistance until the birth of the child several months later.

Given the lack of countervailing testimony in this case, opponents argued against the possibility of any late birth, especially those that had been recognized by the courts. In his analysis of legal precedents, Bouvart focused on an act of Parlement of September 6, 1653, which declared legitimate the child born to Renée de Villeneuve eleven months after the death of her husband. This act was based, according to the jurist Dufresne,[38] on a consideration of the good moral character of the widow and on the opinions of ancient doctors and philosophers regarding the physical possibility of late births. At this early stage in the debate, Bouvart chose not to discuss the issue of the widow's moral character, though he confided that he thought Renée's conduct could be discredited and advised the collateral heirs to do so. Instead, he turned his attention to the medical opinions that had informed the act of 1653. He was convinced that these opinions would not be accepted by any self-respecting doctor in 1764. Proof that the opinions of the ancients on which the earlier court decisions had been based were invalid would, he hoped, establish that the case of 1764 had no valid legal precedent.

In 1653 the court had accepted Renée de Villeneuve's claim that she experienced labor pains nine months from the date of conception but gave birth only a full two months later. The court, in establishing the legitimacy of the child, attributed the delay of the birth to three factors: the weakness thought inherent in the female sex of the child, the distress experienced by the mother at the death of her husband, and the advanced age of the husband at the time of conception.

Bouvart dismissed as fantastic such factors, arguing that in a more enlightened age such superstitions deserved no credence. There was no evidence that a female child caused a prolonged pregnancy or that the fetuses of older fathers developed more slowly or were less robust than the offspring of younger men. Nor was there any proof that the emotional state or physical condition of the mother could prolong a pregnancy beyond its natural term. That these factors, as well as continued menstruation during pregnancy or consumption in the mother or fetus, could influence fetal development Bouvart did not deny, but he believed the effect was invariably to advance rather than to prolong the pregnancy. The result would be miscarriage or premature, not delayed, birth.[39] He could not conceive of a birth as late as eleven months from which both mother and child would emerge in perfect health.

The primary authority cited in the medical opinions of 1653 was Aristotle; later authorities including the Riolans, Fontanus, Dulaurent, and Skenkius had apparently based their opinions on their reading of Aristotle. In his refutation of these opinions, Bouvart urged that medical knowledge be derived from careful observations rather than inherited, without critical reflection, from preceding generations. Although Aristotle might still be consulted on poetry, Bouvart observed, he had been thoroughly discredited in matters of physic. No self-respecting court should accept his authority in the 1760s.[40]

Bouvart's attack on the authority of the ancients was not, however, unequivocal. Knowledge of classical texts was, after all, what distinguished doctors educated in the faculties of medicine from their empiric rivals. Even as Bouvart appealed to enlightened readers' impatience with the superstition and errors of the past, he reflected the ambivalence of the age toward the authority of the ancients. Bouvart criticized Aristotle for mingling in matters beyond his ken in much the same way that he attacked contemporary charlatans for presuming to practice medicine. At issue was the question of medical expertise, not the obsolescence of the ancients' judgments.

In contrast to Bouvart's rejection of the medical opinions of Aristotle was his near adulation of the work of Hippocrates, who was generally held in high esteem by eighteenth-century physicians. Praising the "Father of Medicine" for his strikingly modern predilection for observing rather than prescribing laws of nature, Bouvart contended that the judgments of Hippocrates were unassailable. Appealing to the self-esteem of his colleagues, he declared that surely the 280-day limit to the duration of pregnancy which Hippocrates had calculated had to be acknowledged by the wisest doctors as the most just and the most sure.[41] But even opponents of late births admitted that there were problems with adhering to the authority of Hippocrates. First, Hippocrates' pronouncements on the possible duration of pregnancy were inconsistent. Although he had set 280 days as the norm, he had remarked upon pregnancies lasting ten or eleven months. Were these months lunar or solar? Were all the various and conflicting Hippocratic treatises genuine or had some been erroneously attributed to Hippocrates by Aristotle, Galen, or Avicenna and the errors perpetuated for centuries by Arab and European doctors?[42]

A second problem with following the authority of Hippocrates was that so many of his views regarding reproduction seemed primitive, indeed superstitious, resembling the perenially popular but largely discredited compendia of secrets which had been published since medieval times under the title *Albert Le Grand*.[43] In order to ascertain whether a woman was pregnant, Hippocrates had suggested giving her a drink of mead before she went to sleep. Ensuing stomach pains were a sign of pregnancy. To determine whether a woman was sterile, Hippocrates had advised fumigating all parts of her body; if the fumes permeated her whole body up to her mouth and nose, it was proof, he explained, that she was not sterile. Responding to parents' curiosity about the health of their unborn child, Hippocrates had warned that if a woman carrying twins had a sagging breast, one of the fetuses would be aborted. A sagging right breast indicated the fetus in danger was male, whereas a sagging left breast betokened an endangered female fetus.[44] The significance of this correspondence between the sides of the body was that Hippocrates believed that males occupied the right, more desirable, side of the womb, whereas females occupied the left side.[45] Because male offspring were generally favored over female, numerous measures had been devised for ascertaining the sex of the child before birth. Hippocrates' technique was to monitor the complexion of the pregnant woman. Women enjoying ruddy, healthy complexions during pregnancy were probably the mothers of boys, while women who appeared wan and sickly were more likely to give birth to girls.[46]

Such allegations, in the minds of the supporters of late births, lacked sufficient supporting evidence, especially since they contradicted a tradition of opinion received among women from the time of Hippocrates.[47] Thus Petit suggested that reason and experience, the two principles for which Hippocrates stood, should be given the title "Prince of Medicine," rather than Hippocrates himself. The mediators in the debate, Plisson and Barbeu du Bourg, agreed and proposed pursuing case histories as a more fruitful avenue for resolving the question.

Rather than examining contemporary case histories, however, the opponents chose another criterion for rejecting late births: the existence of certain uniform and immutable laws of nature. Striving to establish a science free from superstition, Bouvart, Louis, and Astruc postulated a nature whose laws were constant and invariable, a nature free from fabulous and monstrous aberrations, a nature devoid of connection with the supernatural. Whereas Bouvart based his belief in these laws of nature on Hippocrates, Louis, in keeping with his close ties with the *Encyclopédie* and deep interest in the law, emphasized their verifiability. The laws governing procreation were, he asserted, just as uniform as those governing any other process of nature and applied equally to humans and animals. Although the duration of pregnancy varied among species, it did not vary within them. The term of pregnancy was invariably set at nine months for humans and cows, eleven months for horses and asses, eight months for deer, five months for sheep, sixty days for dogs, thirty days for rabbits, and twenty-one days for chickens.

Citing anthropological data from Greenland, Lapland, Senegal, and Guinea, Louis agreed that variations in climate and custom could affect the nubility and fertility of women in different parts of the globe, but not the term of gestation.[48] Nor did he give any credit to the view popularized in the almanacs and journals that the violent passions and disordered imagination arising from a mother's dissipated life-style could have a detrimental effect on the development of the fetus. Emphasizing the mechanical nature of the reproductive process, Louis maintained that the mother had very little conscious (or unconscious) control over the course of her pregnancy: "It is manifest that the violence of the passions to which women abandon themselves, the diverse adventures that befall them, the disorder in their manner of living, can cause a change in the course and distribution of nutrition to the infant only with great difficulty. It forms, grows, and develops like the chicken. The mother provides it with warm heat and gives it asylum. The immutable laws of the animal economy do the rest."[49]

In describing the mechanics of reproduction Louis's prose assumed the tone of an ode to nature and a prayer to God. He paused frequently in his memoir to admire the harmony, order, and purposiveness apparent in nature and to worship the Creator responsible for such a work. He emphasized his belief that only those who understood very little about the workings of nature would acknowledge anomalies like late births. Such deviations impugned the very notion of the immutability of the laws of nature which Louis sought to demonstrate. They formed part of a picture of nature in which instability and chaos went unchecked, defying science's efforts at understanding and control and challenging religion's image of an omnipotent and omniscient Creator. Take a more expansive view, Louis urged, and "the more things are examined in their entirety, the better the physical impossibility of late births is understood. One does not put forth boundaries to nature. One respects its author when one recognizes the true limits which he has himself given in all his sovereign wisdom."[50] In Louis's mind, all that was fortuitous or anomalous might be possible, but it was not natural, and it thus lay outside the scope of medical doctrine or practice.

Louis put so much emphasis on the existence of universal, immutable laws of nature for two reasons. First, such laws were the foundation upon which his concept of an enlightened science of medicine was based. If one acknowledged aberrations in nature, he protested, "it would be necessary to say clearly that there are actions without principles and effects without cause—something repugnant to all reason."[51] Indeed, it was just this problem—of assigning causes to apparently remote effects and arriving at a systematic understanding of nature—that perplexed physicians most in the eighteenth century.[52] Second, Louis believed that the laws of society could be justified only insofar as they reflected the laws of nature. He dreaded to imagine what chaos would be unleashed in science and society if the belief in absolute laws of nature were overturned.

Proponents of late births like Petit shared Louis's concern with maintaining coherence in science and law and order in society but were more humble in their approach to understanding nature. Rather than insisting that the facts be reshaped to fit the theory, Petit believed that the theory could be enlarged to conform to the facts. "If nature herself has determined nothing precise on this subject," he remarked, "by what right do Physicians intrude? It is not for them to give laws to nature; their office is limited to observing and grasping that which she has established."[53]

Unlike Louis, Petit did not think that anomalies existed outside the natural order, though he admitted that they might seem to lie beyond the scope of human understanding. He believed that the scientific conception of what was natural had to be expanded to encompass the extraordinary as well as the commonplace in nature. He regarded late births as an aberration from the normal, but not necessarily from the natural, order of things.

In response to Louis's fear of acknowledging actions without principles and effects without causes, Petit maintained that the effects of phenomena could not be denied, even if their causes were unknown. Such an approach was in keeping with the skeptical empiricism of both Voltaire and Diderot, who believed that it could lead to precious therapeutic knowledge.[54] Petit likened the uncertainty over the causes of late births to the uncertainty surrounding the equally mysterious and equally disputed causes of magnetism and electricity: "You do not know of any illness capable of producing the indicated effect. . . . When one does not know the reason for something, is it necessary to reject it? Do you know the cause of Magnetism or Electricity? Do you know why intermittent fevers return to the same men? Does that prevent you from recognizing the existence of these fevers?"[55]

Petit's ally in the debate, Le Bas, was even more determined to dispute Louis's image of nature, even if it meant challenging the notion of perfect symmetry according to which the order and hierarchy of nature were reflected in society. Le Bas did not believe that an enlightened science could comprehend, much less dispel, the disorder inherent in nature and preferred to characterize nature as capricious and marvelous, ready to astonish even the most tireless and truthful investigators, as well as the vulgar public. "Generation," Le Bas declared, "is one of the most mysterious productions of nature. Can one decide constantly, certainly, and infallibly on such a mysterious operation?"[56] Le Bas thought not and was joined in his skepticism by the editors of the *Journal encyclopédique* and the *Mémoires de Trévoux.*[57]

This was not simply a battle over abstractions. Le Bas was prepared to offer evidence to throw the notion of universal laws of nature into doubt. He pointed out that because humans were the most voluptuous of all creatures, capable of conceiving in all seasons, the analogy between human and animal reproductive patterns was flawed. Nor could harmony in nature be affirmed when some women about to give birth found themselves deprived of milk, while others began lactating after the fifth month of an imagined pregnancy.

Plisson, the mediator, agreed with Petit and Le Bas that the invariability of the laws could not be supported by common sense and observation. Analogies between animals and humans aside, Plisson believed that Louis's claim to order even within the animal realm could not be sustained. The pregnancies of cats, she noted, had been observed to last six weeks by the eminent Buffon, but as many as eight weeks by the charismatic popularizer of science, Valmont de Bomare. She herself had a cat that she had tended carefully and whose pregnancy has lasted seven weeks and four days.

The opponents of late births had focused on the authority of Hippocrates and the doctrine of universal, immutable laws of nature in hopes that these two criteria could serve as the basis for consensus within the medical community. Indeed, Astruc regarded consensus as a guarantee of validity, quoting Cicero to the effect that the consensus of all is the voice of nature.[58] But the refutations of the supporters of late births revealed that the medical community was nearly as divided on the authority of Hippocrates or the existence of universal laws of nature as it was on variation in the duration of pregnancy.

In light of the opponents' failure to resolve the debate by such external criteria, each participant offered a slightly different limit to the duration of pregnancy. While Louis held the line at nine months, Astruc believed it should be ten, and Bouvart was willing to go as far as ten months and ten days. Petit argued that variations in the duration of pregnancy were the norm, noting that some women regularly gave birth early (at seven months) or late (at eleven months). Still, he saw no logical reason why pregnancies might not last a bit longer. Plisson extended Petit's limits on both sides, believing that births could occur anywhere from six to thirteen months after conception. Let us look briefly at the theories of reproduction offered by supporters and opponents in order to understand how they could come to such different conclusions.

Bouvart used the image of a pear tree to describe the mechanics of reproduction. He compared the relation between the womb and the placenta to the relation between the branch of the tree and the stem of the pear. The stem was separated from the branch, he explained, when the pear had come to its full development. Having received all the nutrients it could from the tree, the pear was unable to assimilate anymore. When the sap of the tree, continuing to flow toward the pear, found its passage blocked, it employed its force to separate the stem from the branch. In like manner, the force of the blood flowing from the mother to the fetus was directed toward separating the placenta from the womb once the fetus had absorbed all possible nutrients.

Plisson liked Bouvart's theory but believed it supported rather than precluded the possibility of late births. Continuing his pear tree analogy, she observed that some fruit remained on the tree longer than others before ripening. Such could be the case with fetuses, too. Plisson believed that two factors—the nutritive juices and the heat generated by the womb—governed the development of the fetus. For a normal birth, the two factors had to work in conjunction: with too many juices, the fetus would become putrid; with too much heat, it would become dessicated. Either way, it would perish. Variations between these extremes might accelerate or retard the fetus's development.

Le Bas rejected the pear tree analogy entirely, arguing that the constitutions of the parents determined not just the constitution of the newborn, but the duration of pregnancy as well. He contended that the seed of a young man was more likely to be fresh and robust, hence more disposed to grow promptly than was that of an old, enervated, infirm athlete.[59]

Barbeu du Bourg shared Le Bas's environmentalist bias but focused on how the development of the fetus was affected by fluctuations in the health, diet, emotional state, and activity level of the mother rather than the father. "Elegant ladies, who were the frivolous toys of a thousand diverse passions," were, he maintained, more likely to suffer complications of pregnancy than were unrefined women who "like the most unreflective animals," followed the instincts of nature automatically and experienced no difficulty bearing children.[60]

Technical points regarding reproduction were as elusive as was the larger picture. Thus Petit and Louis could not even agree on the determining factors of birth. While Petit regarded the irritation of the womb as the triggering factor, Louis attributed the hour of birth to a mechanical necessity attendant upon the perfect development of the organs of the fetus.[61] Because Petit's theory was based on the interrelation of the factors determining the hour of birth, it allowed for variations in the term of pregnancy which would have no ill effect on the health of either mother or child. Such variations, according to Louis's theory, had necessarily to result in serious injury to both mother and child.

Because all of the theories offered were highly speculative, each side in the debate was quick to criticize the other, demonstrating all too clearly the limits of medical knowledge. Petit objected to Bouvart's theory because it left too many unanswered questions. How, he asked, could it account for women who experienced miscarriages or for women who continued to carry fetuses that had died and petrified within the womb? How did it explain the length and effect of labor pains on the birth process? Le Bas was even harsher in his critique, asserting that anyone who had any knowledge of blood pressure would scoff at Bouvart's notion that it was strong enough to force the separation of the placenta from the womb.

Bouvart was equally severe in his assessment of his critics. He believed that Petit's theory was unacceptable because it incorrectly identified the variability of the term of pregnancy with the degree of sensitivity and extension of the womb. Le Bas's theory was, he pronounced, unworthy of review, and he dismissed it summarily as a flight of fancy. Indeed, given the lack of adequate instrumentation, all these theories contained some fanciful elements. Le Bas argued, however, that if his critics wanted to discredit his theory effectively, they would have to do so on the basis of countervailing evidence, not a priori reasoning.

Le Bas's position on this point was shared by all the supporters of the possibility of late births. Even an opponent like Astruc agreed with the proponents on the need for verification. He proposed a well-controlled experiment to solve the question. One need only confine forty young, married women to a house where they would be allowed to have intercourse with their husbands at specified intervals. Under such circumstances, the length of pregnancy could be accurately determined and, after five years, two hundred case histories could be assembled by which to establish a rule on the subject of duration of pregnancy.[62]

Astruc's proposed experiment met with varying responses. While Petit and Le Bas rejected it on the grounds that late births were so rare that the experiment would be too limited to yield significant results, the mediator Barbeu du Bourg supported the experiment but believed it would take a century to produce definitive results. But was Astruc's experiment practical or necessary? Petit and Le Bas pointed out that numerous case histories of late births recounted by women and documented by doctors, surgeons, midwives, and jurists already existed and were available for examination. Why were the opponents so reluctant to look at the evidence?

The answer to this question lies in the opponents' definition of an enlightened science of medicine. In their minds, the problem with relying on case histories of late births was that all of them depended on testimony provided by women. As Astruc exclaimed in reviewing the large number of case histories to be examined, "I confess that I would be frightened by the number of observations and I would scarcely regard them all as false if Physicians had made them, or at least had seen at their birth these supposed late infants of ten, eleven, twelve, thirteen months. But the Physicians have neither seen nor examined anything. Everything they report comes from women."[63] Restricting enlightenment by gender, Astruc continued, "It is said with reason that it is necessary to be very enlightened in order to make good observations. I am disposed to believe that Physicians are always enlightened, but I believe that women never are. Women are less enlightened on the length of their pregnancy than on any other subject. It is known that they often err through ignorance and even more because it is in their interest to do so."[64] Although Astruc appealed to reason rather than Scripture to support his premise that it was women's nature to deceive, his denunciation of women bore a striking resemblance to Hecquet's thirty years earlier.

Bouvart made the point even more emphatically. Reviewing a list of twenty-six authorities whom the supporters of late births had cited, he concluded that "all these stories are void of sense, and founded on no good reasons or observations (but only on the reports of *femmelettes*) which certain educated people have vigorously revised in order to give them an air of credibility."[65] Bouvart's choice of the term *femmelette* is significant, for it articulates the contempt with which the judgments of women were commonly viewed. Littré translates *femmelette* as a "weak, silly, ignorant woman" and quotes some seventeenth- and eighteenth-century uses of the term. The tendency to group all women regardless of differences in education and social position with the lowest, least educated groups of society was not peculiar to doctors, as a quote from Bossuet, Louis XIV's most ardent apologist for patriarchal authority and absolute monarchy, illustrates: "Their obvious error was nearly exposed by its own absurdity: this is why they assailed ignorant folk, artisans, *femmelettes*, and peasants." The notion that women were by nature gullible and superstitious is seen in a quote taken from Duclos's *Mémoires*: "Seeking to doubt the divinity, he [the duc d'Orléans] pursued soothsayers and fortune tellers and showed all the credulous curiosity of a *femmelette*."[66]

A century earlier, women were more likely than men to be suspected of sorcery. Sorceresses were considered monsters of a sort—women who defied the laws of nature.[67] Although women were no longer being burned at the stake for witchcraft in the mid–eighteenth century, the roots of suspicion were still alive. Sorcery was identified with charlatanry and prosecuted not as a crime of heresy but of fraud and deception. Fraud and deception were the very charges the opponents of late births would level against women who claimed to have experienced a prolonged pregnancy. Although the vocabulary had changed to fit this more enlightened age, the sentiment seemed to have remained the same, and the issue of late births itself strengthened the link between women and disorder.

Acknowledging the weight of this cultural tradition, the supporters of late births were quick to challenge such associations. What right, Petit demanded, did doctors have to presume that their judgments were always enlightened and women's never were? Unlike Astruc, Petit believed that on no other subject could the testimony of women be more reliable than on the duration of their pregnancies. To what could women be more attuned, he wondered, than to the changes occurring within their own bodies? To doubt the testimony of women on this subject was, for Petit, to doubt it on all subjects. Could men, he asked, provide more reliable observations about the course of pregnancies experienced by women than the women themselves?

More was at stake for the medical community here than the character or judgment of women or, as in the controversy over the Convulsionaries thirty years earlier, the legitimacy of the Jansenist cause. The opponents' rejection of women's observations was part of their larger rejection of the judgment of anyone who was not a graduate of a faculty of medicine or college of surgery. For the opponents, an enlightened science of medicine was inseparable from professional authority and demanded rejecting random observations by empirics, women, and graduates of foreign medical schools, where, it was rumored, diplomas could be had for a price. They believed that such observations had led in centuries past to an anarchy in which fact and fable were promiscuously intertwined in the works of even the most advanced medical practitioners. The goal of the opponents was to remove enlightened medicine from the taint of popular medical ideas.

Petit opposed the opponents on this point, countering their objections to relying on the testimony of women with the remark, "Besides, must one be extremely learned in Physic in order to judge that a woman, who quite distinctly feels her child move and who, consequently, is around four months pregnant, will have carried it for more than twelve if she gives birth eight months beyond this time?"[68] As Petit's remark implied, the subject matter of science, especially medicine, need not be abstract, but could be closely connected with domestic life. The science based on observation and experimentation, which he and the other supporters advocated, was inherently more democratic than was the science based on the authority of the ancients and a priori natural laws, which was favored by the opponents. It could not be monopolized by an aristocracy distinguished from the public by birth and knowledge of the classical texts.

With increased emphasis on observation, scientific speculation during the early modern period had been opening up to people of even modest origins, and it would do so in the debate over late births, too.[69] Such democratization of knowledge had political ramifications: if the average man or woman was capable of making valid judgments about the processes of nature, why couldn't he or she be equally capable of making valid judgments about the way in which he or she should be governed?

These contrasting views of science, medicine, and politics were not to be resolved during the debate over late births, but the proponents' pleas were sufficient to propel both sides toward a close look at the existing case histories. Although supporters and opponents surveyed a large number of medical case histories and judicial rulings on late births spanning centuries, the differences in their approaches can be seen by examining six cases on which they disagreed. Typically, the supporters cited cases and the opponents critiqued each case point by point.

The first case was reported to Le Bas in 1764 by Dr. Panenc, a practitioner of medicine in Aix-en-Provence. Over the course of their marriage, Panenc's wife had given birth to seven children—three boys and four girls, with the length of the pregnancies varying according to the sex of the child. She had carried the boys for nine months; the girls, for ten months and beyond. Because Panenc had followed these pregnancies carefully, Le Bas believed that any objection about the accuracy of the observations supporting this claim would have little weight. Nor would the question of motive be germane, for the legitimacy of the children was not contested.

Emphasizing the difficulty of determining the precise hour of conception and the ambiguity of the signs of pregnancy, however, both Bouvart and Louis questioned whether Panenc could be certain of the exact duration of his wife's pregnancies. His calculations were, after all, only approximate. Panenc had said that when his wife was pregnant with girls, the pregnancies had exceeded ten months, but he had not specified by how much. That was the critical question. Others had been known to err on this subject; why not he? In cases like this, where the symptoms were ambiguous and more than one diagnosis was possible, Bouvart urged doctors to prefer the diagnosis most in keeping with the normal order of things and to deviate only when they had demonstrable evidence of an aberration of nature.

The second case, recorded by the Royal Academy of Sciences of Rouen in 1753, concerned a woman of Jouarre who claimed to have remained pregnant three years before giving birth to a healthy, living son. The pregnancy was thought to have begun early in 1748. By February of 1749, the women's abdomen and breasts were quite enlarged. The woman did not, however, give birth until January of 1751. The case was verified by a notary and two surgeons.

Louis and Bouvart challenged the diagnosis of a three-year pregnancy, despite the fact that it had been confirmed by Winslow, one of the most celebrated practitioners of the day. They noted that swelling of the abdomen and breasts was not a definitive sign of pregnancy, but could be a symptom of some other disorder, most likely hydropsy (a disease characterized by an abnormal accumulation of fluid in the cells, tissues, and cavities of the body, which resulted in swelling). In support of their alternative diagnosis, Louis and Bouvart observed that the woman of Jouarre had stopped menstruating only in the last nine months of pregnancy, that no one but she had felt the quickening of the fetus in the eighteenth month, and that the size of the child was normal.

Louis's and Bouvart's alternative diagnosis was not at all unreasonable. Many of the medical causes célèbres of the late eighteenth century revolved around cases of unmarried women who had been thought pregnant but had in fact suffered from hydropsy and later recovered. Because the symptoms of hydropsy closely resembled those of pregnancy, some of these women were charged under the Edict of Henri II, composed in 1556 and reaffirmed in 1708, and tried for concealment of pregnancy and infanticide. The reverse error was also known to occur: women in the countryside who thought they were pregnant were misdiagnosed by provincial practitioners as hydropsic and administered violent remedies, which sometimes led them to abort.[70]

The third case involved a woman whose claim to late birth had been recognized by the Faculty of Leipzig in 1679: "My husband," she said,

died suddenly after supper a year ago last festival of St. Michel. I did not think I was pregnant, despite the conjectures many of my friends drew from the loss of flesh around my face and other ordinary symptoms of pregnancy. I realized it was true, however, fourteen days before the carnival. Being persuaded, according to my calculations, that I would give birth around the festival of St. Jean, I prepared everything that was necessary for the operation. I called the Midwife several times, but her help was useless to me. My belly swelled so prodigiously that I was unable to walk and I was forced to stay in bed for eleven whole weeks, during which I had a continuous discharge. At the end of this time I gave birth, by an act of Providence and with considerable difficulty, to a girl as large as a child of six months. This occurred a year and thirteen days after the death of my husband.[71]

This woman's testimony reveals how much the experiences of pregnancy and childbirth belonged to the private world of women. The advice and assistance of male doctors and surgeons were generally either not available or not solicited, and this woman was surely not unique in turning to Providence in her time of need. When a case like this came before the faculties or the courts, it often had to be decided solely on the basis of the testimony of women—the woman who had given birth, her female friends, and whatever midwife might have attended her.

Bouvart dismissed the ruling of the Faculty of Leipzig in this case because it contradicted an earlier decision they had made against a late birth of ten months and nine days. Surely the judgments of the doctors had been swayed by the power of the woman involved in the second case, Bouvart surmised. Why else would they reverse their earlier position against the possibility of late births?

While the testimony of the woman of Leipzig was impressionistic—her sense of time was determined by the passing of carnivals rather than by the passing of hours or days—the testimony provided by midwives could be more precise. The fourth case considered was submitted to Le Bas and a number of journals, including the *Journal de médecine, chirurgie, et pharmacie* and the *Gazette salutaire*, by the midwife Félicité Reffatin of Nevers. The daughter of a lawyer, Mme Reffatin had been sent to Paris to be educated with the girls of St. Thomas and later studied midwifery at the Hôtel-Dieu. She returned to Nevers to practice and instruct others in midwifery and was honored with the title of *pensionnaire* of the town of Nevers.[72]

Attentive to detail, Reffatin assiduously recorded the facts of her practice and frequently sent her reflections on particularly interesting cases to Le Bas and Levret. She prefaced her testimony with the following statement: "Permit me, sir, to add an observation I made last year; it is drawn from the twenty-third page of my register, marked and initialed by the Judge. I assure you that I have drawn it up, as I do all those observations I make each day, with the greatest exactitude. I love to observe scrupulously the movements of Nature and her variations in the period of gestation."[73] She then went on to report the case of a woman, Mme Renault, who had menstruated only three times during the course of her marriage. Each of these periods had been followed immediately by a pregnancy. The last pregnancy was thought to have lasted eleven months, beginning with the cessation of menstruation on February 20, 1763, and ending with the birth of the child on January 17, 1764. Le Bas included Reffatin's letter in his consultation not just to demonstrate the possibility of late births, but to refute the opponents' assertions that the observations of women, including midwives, lacked clarity, precision, and instruction.

In this case, as in the case of Mme Panenc, Bouvart emphasized the ambiguity of signs of pregnancy and the importance of preferring an explanation in keeping with the natural order of things. He suggested that Mme Renault had become pregnant several weeks later than she thought. He argued that the fact she had felt the quickening of the fetus in July and not given birth until January was not conclusive in itself. It was possible to feel quickening at three months even though four and a half months was the normal time. Mocking Petit's attack on the professional mystique maintained by doctors, Bouvart, demanded, "Must one be a great Physician in order not to overlook such a trivial thing? Is there nothing more unreasonable than to seize on the miraculous, when there is a very natural and plausible explanation? Would one want, finally, to persuade us that things most in conformity with the physical order have less right to be believed than the infallibility of the learned *matrone* Mme Reffatin?"[74]

Bouvart's oxymoron, "learned *matrone*" was intentionally ironic, for whereas *sage-femme* referred to a midwife who had received formal instruction, *matrone* was generally applied to midwives whose knowledge was derived from experience and secrets passed down from generation to generation. Since Reffatin had been trained at the Hôtel-Dieu, she was, contrary to Bouvart's designation, a *sage-femme*, not a *matrone*. As the tone of his critique indicates, Bouvart had considerably less sympathy with Mme Reffatin's error than with Dr. Panenc's. Presumption evidently held a higher place in his hierarchy of sins than ignorance. By assuming such a prominent role in the debate, Reffatin was violating the principles of subordination by profession, gender, and social condition which Bouvart and others believed were crucial to the preservation of the social order and the advance of science.

Bouvart's plea for greater circumspection was directed to doctors' assessments of the psychological as well as the physical dimensions of a case. Arguing that what was needed was not necessarily greater medical acumen but greater insight into human nature, he urged doctors to broaden their philosophical doubt to fit the peculiar needs of medicine.

He advised them not merely to examine the philosophical bases of knowledge, but to inquire into the sources of this knowledge. When applied to human affairs, skepticism was perhaps better termed suspicion. Doctors were urged to abandon courtesy in the pursuit of truth and assume the role of detective. "If the virtuous man (*honnête homme*)," Bouvart wrote, "in social relations should banish from his heart suspicions concerning the conduct of another, the Physician, for his part, should never take a step unarmed with that philosophical doubt with which Descartes gloriously inspired posterity."[75] Bouvart would provide ample illustration of how such doubt could be applied in his analysis of the last two cases.

The fifth case—involving a young girl who accused a rich young man of impregnating her—was related by Thomas Bartholin and cited first by Petit. Because the girl was suspected of fabricating the story, she was kept under strict surveillance in a *maison de force* for the duration of her pregnancy. After sixteen months, she gave birth to a child that lived for two days.

Bouvart maintained that, although Petit had provided the basic story line, he had not disclosed all the relevant details. Noting that in the original account Bartholin had referred to the mother as a prostitute rather than a young girl, that she had been held in prison rather than a *maison de force*, and that she had given birth to what appeared to be a still undeveloped embryo rather than child, Bouvart wrote, "We agree that one need be nothing less than a 'Great Physician' in order to adhere to [Petit's] opinion. It is for him to agree, in return, that one need only be a very mediocre moralist to suspect a young girl in captivity of having feigned a pregnancy before her detention in order perhaps to marry the young Plutus by whom she was made pregnant, or at least to obtain a pecuniary indemnity for the outrage done her honor."[76] Bouvart suggested that the girl had managed to be impregnated by one of the guards during her stay in prison and had given birth prematurely to an embryo that had no hope of survival.

The final case cited by Petit was drawn from a thesis written under the direction of Dr. Heister of the Faculty of Halle and related that the widow of a bookseller of Wolfenbüttel gave birth thirteen months after the death of her husband. The collateral heirs did not proceed against her because she was known to have led a retired life, seeing no one but doctors and other women during the course of her pregnancy. She later married a young bookseller and gave birth to two more children, both products of thirteen-month pregnancies. The duration of these later pregnancies was confirmed by her husband as well as by her doctor, the First Physician to the Duke of Brunswick.

Bouvart, observing that many of the case histories of late births had been recorded by Germans—a people known for their simplicity—made no apologies for his skepticism in approaching the history of the book-seller's wife. He sketched an alternative scenario that would account for why the woman might wish to deceive the doctor and others. The facts of the case were that the woman was twenty-nine years younger than her husband. An apprentice shared the house with them and married the woman several months after the death of her husband.

Bouvart speculated that the attraction between the wife and the apprentice had existed before their marriage and that the woman became pregnant shortly after the death of her husband. She attributed the pregnancy to her first husband, however, in order to retain the bookstore for her new husband. Bouvart presumed that she then pretended to experience a second thirteen-month pregnancy in order to still any doubts that might have lingered about the legitimacy of the first. This explanation, he asserted, was certainly preferable to the one offered by Heister because:

> Here everything accords with reason while in the system of Wagner and Heister, everything shocks and revolts it. There is nothing in their system which does not go against the sentiment of the wisest writers and most enlightened observers. Would it thus be necessary for us, out of respect for a renowned Anatomist and his student, to submit blindly to belief in a wonder in preference to a perfectly natural explanation? What, the wife of Meisner will have carried three children consecutively for thirteen months following the death of her first husband? It would make as much sense to say that the sun moved backward three times or that the rivers have three times returned to their source. This supposes an upheaval in the order of nature which violently offends reason."[77]

Plisson, in keeping with her role as mediator, sided with the opponents on some points and with the supporters on others. She concurred with Bouvart on the epistemological difficulty of ascertaining an approximate date of conception in humans, though not in his imaginative reconstructions of the latter two case histories. She disagreed with Petit that little skill was required for a woman to recognize the quickening of the fetus. Virtually all the signs of pregnancy, including the quickening of the fetus, were uncertain and ambiguous. Plisson cited from personal experience the case of a pregnant woman who had been misdiagnosed as hydropsic but gave birth two days later to a healthy boy. While agreeing with Petit that the judgments of the Faculty of Leipzig and of Panenc were well founded, she shared Bouvart's belief that alternative hypotheses could very well apply in the cases of the woman of Jouarre, Mme Renault, the girl of Leipzig, and the Wolfenbüttel bookseller's widow.

Petit and Le Bas were, however, unimpressed by Bouvart's imaginative reconstructions. Le Bas thought that the explanations of the observers of late births were at least as credible as Bouvart's and continued to prefer their eyewitness accounts to Bouvart's speculations from afar. Petit, too, found Bouvart's scenarios less credible than the recorded case histories and commented in his review of the case of the Wolfenbüttel bookseller's wife, "Heister has given us the history of the widow of Freitagius; you are going to give us the novel."[78] This is an interesting charge, especially given the increasing proclivity of both sides to engage in rhetorical flourishes designed to win public sympathy to their cause. By indulging in speculations about the march of passion or the diverse motives of various actors characteristic of the popular *causes célèbres* literature of editors like Dessessarts or Richer, doctors heightened human interest in the medical consultations, no doubt contributing to their circulation among an ever broader reading public. But were they abandoning their scientific integrity?

Although the positions of supporters and opponents of late births changed when it came to evaluating the criterion of observation, with the supporters now on the defensive and the opponents assuming the role of skeptics, the two sides' differing interpretations of the case histories revealed that, on this criterion, too, consensus was impossible. Petit and Le Bas continued to assert that the evidence for late births was convincing. If the opponents' demand for absolute proof were to become standard for all medical theories, they contended, investigators would have to give up trying to prove anything perfectly in matters of physic.[79] Yet, as Bouvart had demonstrated, the evidence was not perfect, and even an observer as sympathetic as Plisson to the impact of the debate on the position of women was partially persuaded.

Thus the debate would shift ground one last time as opponents made their final case against the possibility of late births. They did so not on the basis of any of the scientific criteria outlined so far, but on the social repercussions they predicted a decision in favor of prolonged pregnancies might have. The medical community's ultimate appeal to social rather than scientific criteria in Renée's case would thus directly parallel the final stage of the 1730s debate over the Convulsionaries.

Fearing that recognition of the possibility of late births constituted a significant threat to the stability of the family and the moral fabric of society, the opponents conjured up images of France inundated with illegitimate children, the miserable products of the immorality of women. The system of inheritance would, they warned, be thrown away as these illegitimate children usurped the patrimony of legitimate heirs.

In his reluctance to admit the testimony of women into medical reflections, Astruc had stressed his belief that women were likely to err, either through ignorance or because erring was in their interest. It was not uncommon for a married woman to experience a suspension of menstruation immediately before the onset of pregnancy. The symptoms of the two were similar, so that the woman might easily include the two or three months of suspension in her calculation of a pregnancy. If the woman were living with her husband at the time of conception, the child was presumed by law to be legitimate, and nothing was made of this error in calculation. In other circumstances, however, women might find it advantageous to make an erroneous calculation. Women who gave birth to an infant eleven, twelve, or thirteen months after their husbands' death would have to declare that they experienced a late birth if the children were to be acknowledged as legitimate. Women who gave birth during prolonged absences of their husbands faced a similar problem.

As Hecquet had done thirty years earlier, Astruc linked consideration of a woman's social condition to his evaluation of her testimony. Noting that claims to late births rarely arose among poor families in which there was little gain in producing a posthumous heir, he concluded that it was difficult not to suspect women who had something to lose of erring knowingly in pursuit of their self-interest.[80] If Astruc's pronouncement that all women who claimed a late birth after a husband's death were generally accepted, woe to the woman who made such a claim, for she would be presumed to be acting dishonorably. She risked suffering irreparable harm to her reputation and could hope for little chance of winning her case. If, on the other hand, she failed to file such a claim, rumor would undoubtedly have it that the child was illegitimate. To be sure, the number of disputes to be arbitrated would be drastically reduced and a social good therein attained. But the claims to late births would be silenced by social pressures based on questionable moral inferences rather than on reliable medical evidence.

Louis had hoped to circumvent the scenario outlined above by taking the matter of late births out of the hands of jurists and placing it firmly in the domain of medicine. If universal laws of nature indeed invariably set the term of pregnancy at nine months, then there would be no grounds for litigating claims to prolonged pregnancies. Unlike Astruc and Bouvart, Louis argued that the circumstances surrounding the pregnancy, the conduct or reputation of the woman claiming a late birth, and the fate of the children had no bearing on the medical facts of the case.

Louis's discomfort with the legal process centered on the presumption of paternity regularly accorded the husband in all cases in which a child was born during the course of marriage. Here, he believed, the formalism of the law came into conflict with the laws of nature and common sense. While based on a concern with preserving the social order by assuring the stability of the family, the presumption of paternity had, Louis argued, served to undermine both. The law was so formal that it refused to acknowledge the illegitimacy of a child even when it was admitted by the mother.[81]

Bouvart concurred with Louis's belief that late births violated the fundamental laws of nature, but he was not as ready to rule out the possibility of flukes. He reasoned, however, that statistically, late births accounted for very few of the total number of births. An occasional injustice caused by an arbitrary limit on the duration of pregnancy, he figured, was a small cost to pay for the greater good of preserving coherence in medical jurisprudence and stability in society. To admit the legitimacy of even a few claims to late births would open the doors to abuse and throw into disarray the honor of families and the order of successions.[82] Should women and midwives successfully collaborate to deceive families and the state regarding the legitimacy of children, the whole patriarchal system could be brought down.

The proponents offered three different responses to the specter of social chaos invoked by the opponents should the possibility of late births be recognized. First, Petit sympathized with the opponents' concerns and agreed that wisdom demanded all possible precautions to prevent the abuses they foresaw. Still, he differed with the assumption of Astruc and Bouvart and of Hecquet before them that preventing such abuses was the proper duty of doctors. Such matters should, he believed, be referred to magistrates and judges. Even the worst fears of the opponents did not justify doctors' rejection of late births on moral grounds alone.

Petit did not, however, share the fears of social chaos the opponents invoked, and he turned for support of his view to a review of the judicial precedents for late births. Almost all courts had at one time or another ruled children born of late births legitimate, yet these decisions had not brought about the decline in morals that the opponents of late births predicted. Nor did Petit think they would in the future. He did not share the belief of Rousseau, Grimm, or Restif de La Bretonne that theirs was a particularly decadent, because effeminate, culture. "Women today," he observed, "are as chaste, honest, and virtuous as they have ever been. They will continue to be so, whether our opinion is accepted or rejected."[83]

Finally, if social considerations were going to be taken into account, Petit and Le Bas wondered why the opponents seemed so much more concerned about the fate of the collateral heirs than about that of the woman and child. Whereas Astruc had evoked a frightening picture of the threat to the patrimonial estate posed by a widow's false claim to a late birth, Petit noted that he had not seemed equally concerned about the injury inflicted on a widow whose legitimate claim was dismissed peremptorily. Perhaps it was because Astruc implicitly attributed deceit to the widow, but never to the collateral heirs. Yet surely collateral heirs, propelled by the desire to seize a rich estate, might in bad faith contest a child's right to a legitimate succession.

This argument, perhaps because it deemphasized the conflict regarding women's social position and cultural influence underlying the debate over late births, was favored by the editors of both the *Mémoires de Trévoux* and the *Journal des sçavans*. Their concern was firmly centered on the fate of the child: "But if the child is declared illegitimate," exclaimed a reviewer for the *Journal des sçavans*, "the disgrace of the mother falls on him; he is a subject lost to society. Who can answer for the rest of his education and of his life? What a misfortune if he is truly the son of his father. What an injustice!"[84]

In contrast to the journal editors, Le Bas went directly to the gender issues raised by the debate, arguing that the social order was threatened more by rejection than by acceptance of the possibility of late births. He believed that the presumption of paternity attributed to the husband of a married woman should be applied to husbands who died just before the birth of the child as well, and for the same reason—to preserve the stability of the family. Given the uncertainty of proofs on each side, Le Bas urged his colleagues to weigh the impact of a decision on the family carefully. Wasn't it better politics, he demanded, to adopt a system that assures peace and tranquillity rather than one that introduces trouble, disorder, and uneasiness into the family circle?[85] Here he was directly attacking the fundamental precepts of hierarchy, privilege, and patriarchy that supported the family-state compact. The specter of bitterness, despair, and desolation which Le Bas associated with the compact was no doubt bound to strike a chord in a society in which so many families found themselves involved in conflicts over authority and protracted legal battles over inheritances or gossiping about the litigation of others.

Plisson shared Le Bas's concern for the impact that a ruling on late births was bound to have on the family. Observing that "certainly it has a bearing on the good order of society that women, who are already rendered unfortunate by the burdens of their social condition, not become more so by a system that has no rational basis,"[86] she contended that the demands of order and justice were more likely to be fulfilled if the social inequality between men and women were decreased rather than accentuated.

Plisson's emphasis on the emotional life and stability of the family is noteworthy. Clearly, affective bonds mattered to her, but she also emphasized the importance of a rational basis for judgment. Her focus was on being sure that justice was rendered in each case rather than on holding to an absolute standard of justice which might injure a few in preserving the well-being of the many.[87] The need for flexibility could be demonstrated by a hypothetical case history. Suppose, she conjectured, that a husband went to Paris on business for three and a half months and that his wife conceived the evening before his departure and gave birth six and a half months after his return. If the husband were to share the common prejudice, reinforced by Louis's consultation, he would believe that a late birth of ten months could not be legitimate and would suspect his wife of adultery. "How much mistreatment, how many indignities would follow, how many sorrows, suspicions, tears shed in secret!" Plisson exclaimed. "A system that entails such unhappiness—should it not be clearly demonstrated before being adopted?"[88]

In the absence of demonstrable medical proof, Plisson advocated exploring the particularities of each case in which a reasonable claim to late birth was made. Factors to be considered included the condition of the child at birth; the temperament of the mother; any upsets experienced during pregnancy; the mother's reputation and conduct both before and after the death of her husband; and her willingness to swear to the truth of her testimony.

The other mediator, Barbeu du Bourg, was also worried about the uncertainty of medicine regarding the possibility of late births and reluctant to see the medical community make a definitive ruling on the subject. He did not agree with the opponents that it was the responsibility of the medical community to set an arbitrary limit on the length of pregnancy simply because public order demanded one. Nor did he concur with the proponents that fear of unjustly depriving a child of its estate or of sullying the reputation of its mother justified a serious inquiry into claims to pregnancies as long as two years.

Instead, in direct contrast to Louis, Barbeu du Bourg urged his medical colleagues to trust in the wisdom of the legislators to weigh the demands of order and justice and to formulate equitable laws. The role of the magistrates, he believed, was to enforce these laws with more or less rigor, depending on the peculiar circumstances of the case. The role of doctors, surgeons, and midwives, he maintained, was to furnish these officials with facts that were true and worthy of their confidence and to respect the laws established. This was not to say that civil laws should take precedence over the laws of nature, but that the laws of nature had first to be perceived before they could be imitated.

Neither of the opposing sides would endorse Barbeu du Bourg's recommendation that authority on the subject of prolonged pregnancies be transferred from the medical community to the jurists. Nor did the editors of learned journals like the *Journal des sçavans* and the *Mémoires de Trévoux* advocate handing the matter over to the jurists, despite the fact that the pivotal criterion in the debate had proved ultimately to be the social repercussions a judgment might have.

As we have seen by exploring the various criteria by which supporters and opponents sought unsuccessfully to arrive at a consensus on the validity of Renée's claim to a late birth, the medical community was thrown into disarray by this debate. Not only did supporters and opponents disagree vehemently, but significant differences of opinion divided both camps internally.

But if the debate over late births demonstrated all too dramatically the limits of medical knowledge and the debilitating consequences of the eighteenth-century medical community's inability to arrive at a consensus, perhaps we should not judge it too harshly. Twentieth-century medicine is still unable to provide certitude on this point. *Black's Medical Dictionary* informs the reader: "It is generally accepted that pregnancy lasts about 280 days from the first day of the last menstrual period. In exceptional cases there may be considerable variation, but it is generally agreed that the shortest duration of a normal pregnancy is 240 days and the longest duration 313 days. The cause of these variations is not understood."[89]

The question to be explored in the chapter that follows is whether, once the debate over late births had come to center on the social and political consequences of a judgment, jurists could do any better than physicians and surgeons at weighing the consequences of the competing visions of society and the state which a ruling on Renée's case necessarily entailed.

CHAPTER THREE

Medical Causes Célèbres and the Development of Medical Jurisprudence

The Legal Context of the Debate over Late Births

While the editors of the learned journals provided professionals and amateurs throughout France with an open forum for recounting case histories, presenting experiments, and debating the physical possibility of late births, the jurists deplored any further temporizing on the issue, even in pursuit of so worthy a goal as enlightenment. They were impatient with the inconsistency and apparent arbitrariness of the rulings on late births made by provincial courts since the seventeenth century and repelled by the "scandalous researches" the disputes had provoked.[1] Thus they united as a group to urge that a maximum length for a legitimate birth be set and applied uniformly throughout the realm.

The jurists had little interest in the complex medical issues raised by the debate and did not share the medical community's preoccupation with ascertaining laws of nature that could serve as the basis for civil laws. They probably would have agreed with Vicq d'Azyr, secretary to the Royal Society of Medicine, that different epistemological standards governed medicine and law. Physicians, Vicq d'Azyr believed, were allowed more latitude for doubt than were lawyers, who were required to defer to custom and obliged to base their judgments on many contradictory laws and decrees.[2] The jurists would, however, have challenged the assumption of Vicq d'Azyr and opponents of late births like Louis that the simplicity and clarity of the laws of nature precluded any contradiction in human interpretations of them.

Observing the inability of the medical community to arrive at a consensus on the issue of late births, the jurists felt no compunction about intervening and insisting that the issue of legitimacy be distinguished from the question of the physical possibility of late births. While acknowledging the arbitrariness inherent in setting a fixed limit, the jurists argued that the decisions the courts were reaching in individual cases were equally arbitrary and potentially more damaging to the social order.

To understand the legal context in which the debate over late births took place, we begin by reviewing Jean Baptiste Denisart's *Collection de décisions nouvelles de notions relatives à la jurisprudence actuelle.* This was a text highly recommended by *L'Année littéraire* and other journals because it contained decisions on questions directly affecting their readers' material interests and strategies for family formation. Denisart gave graphic proof of the inconsistency that characterized rulings on late births by drawing up a table of ten cases adjudicated between 1626 and 1764. In four cases, the claims to late births had been recognized; in six, they had been rejected. In two cases (April 2, 1626, and September 6, 1653), the length of the pregnancies had been the same, but the rulings contradicted each other: the first infant was declared illegitimate; the second, legitimate. The court that judged the second case admitted that it had been swayed by attestations to the irreproachable conduct of the widow and by her testimony that she had begun to feel labor pains in the ninth month of her pregnancy.[3]

Suspicious of such affirmations of the virtue of women and skeptical of the validity of women's testimony, many jurists were unhappy with the favorable rulings. While the medical opponents of late births spoke of women as obstacles to the progress of medicine, jurists accused them of obstructing justice. Echoing the sentiments of Bouvart, the jurist Le Ridant remarked that women encouraged speculation and subtle reasoning in order to obscure the otherwise certain lights of practice. By alluding to the caprices of nature, they could hide the shameful effects of their disorderly conduct.[4] Le Ridant's remarks corroborate Sarah Hanley's thesis that women were, of necessity, prime participants in early modern family formation and state building, but threatened to undermine both by creating counterfeit cultures challenging the legitimacy of male models of authority.[5] Were the grounds for establishing legitimacy to hinge on the testimony of women, order within the family and the state could be severely compromised.

Thus, although very few cases regarding late births were likely to be brought before the courts, rulings on the matter could have significant repercussions. Worried that medical men had abdicated their responsibility to preserve the social order by allowing the testimony of women to cloud their medical judgments, Le Ridant was adamant that the jurists not follow suit. Quoting an earlier authority on jurisprudence, Le Ridant concluded his consideration of the issue with the remark, "To give the freedom of introducing such absurdities into justice is, according to Brillon, to make sport of both nature and the law, inviting women to engage in libertine conduct and compromising the honor and security of legitimate births."[6]

The prejudice Le Ridant articulated against the validity of women's testimony had deep roots in French jurisprudence. On the basis of the Roman legal theory that women's weakness made them susceptible to ignorance and deceit,[7] their participation in the courts had traditionally been circumscribed. According to both customary and written law, women were not allowed to serve as witnesses to wills or notarial acts. They were categorized and excluded as a group—along with prospective heirs, relatives, minors under twenty years old, monks, orphans, heretics, criminals, spendthrifts, the mad, the blind, the deaf or dumb—whose judgment was thought to be faulty or inconstant.[8] Although women could testify in criminal cases, by custom the testimony of two women was considered necessary to counter the testimony of one man. No law gave less weight to women's testimony; the task of determining the proportional significance accorded the testimony of men and women was left to the discretion of the judge.[9]

The inequalities of the laws as applied to women were so pronounced that some jurists felt obliged to explain and justify them. Houard, for example, maintained that such inequalities honored and protected women, saying nothing of the fact that the inequalities were socially desirable and politically advantageous to men engaged in the process of family formation and state building. In the article, "*Sexe*," in his *Dictionnaire*, he acknowledged that the customs of Normandy were in general very prejudicial to women and girls. But the privileges accorded the male sex need not be regarded as humiliating to females. Instead, Houard claimed, they attested to the respect and consideration the female sex had inspired in the first Normans. The mediocrity of the marriage portion accorded women had for its principle their love of retreat, of work, of modesty. Such virtues, it could be argued, constituted a better dowry than property because they gave women an impenetrable rampart against indigence. In Houard's view, Norman customs regarding marriage were to be praised for being both morally sound and politically prudent.[10]

It was true that, as Houard had observed, the laws favored the continuity and increasing prosperity of family lines and could protect women who never found themselves in conflict with this goal or with other family members. But what if family harmony should break down in a system established on the principles of hierarchy, privilege, and patriarchy? All too often in the eighteenth century, families found themselves torn apart by conflicts leading to extended litigation. The real disadvantages of the laws for females became evident when spouses separated; when the births of daughters were concealed in order to keep inheritances undivided; and when parents refused to accede to the marriage choices of their children.[11]

Despite the fact that abuses of paternal power were numerous, well publicized, and the subject of much gossip in the mid–eighteenth century, justifications of women's legal incapacity were penned not just by male jurists, but by enlightened women as well. How can we understand why a woman would support a system that gave men such power over the social condition and economic resources of women—all in the interests of preserving the family line and enhancing the power of the state? Let us consider the views of Mme Necker, who believed that women's legal subordination was grounded in the physical and moral orders and that it was the natural expression of women's superior moral position. "And if it is true," she wrote,

> that the first being in the order of nature is the one who is tied to other beings by the greatest number of relations, one does not injure women by presenting them in this light. . . . Women are thus more particularly destined never to have an isolated existence, but rather to become the complement of others; and in this respect, social institutions have reinforced nature, since the laws give to women no other rank than that of their husbands, and they are always obliged, to make themselves known, to draw near the hearth from which they derive their light.[12]

Concerned with preserving chastity and modesty, Necker regarded the laws as a necessary source of stability against the ethic of gallantry, which encouraged libertine, irresponsible behavior and broken families.[13] She viewed the prohibition of divorce as essential to maintaining morality and went beyond several jurists and some philosophes of the day in arguing that women's subordination was not merely socially necessary but in accordance with the laws of nature.[14]

In her reflections on women and the law, Necker looked to the laws of nature as a way out of the disharmony, instability, and moral chaos that threatened to engulf all institutions of corporative society. Yet, as the debate over late births made all too clear, the doctrine of universal, uniform laws of nature was itself being challenged—not just by physicians, surgeons, and midwives, but by the philosophes, government administrators, and the general public. In the minds of the jurists, the only possible response was to break the hypothetical connection between the laws of society and the laws of nature, and to advocate an authoritarian structure for family and state which would hold the chaos of both natural and social forces at bay.[15]

Nevertheless, although the jurists demanded, and the doctors and surgeons on both sides of the dispute desired, a resolution of the question of late births, a precedent-setting decision was not to come from Renée's case. Renée died a year after the case came to court—long before a resolution was possible—and the court declined to issue a judgment, thus denying both sides a victory.[16] While no uniform standard by which claims of late births could be judged emerged from the debate, the sound and fury generated by the five-year-long controversy was not without significance. The consultations issued by both sides were widely admired and imitated. Arguments from these consultations were incorporated in the briefs of the defenders and prosecutors of subsequent cases.

In his article, "*Accouchement*," for example, the jurist Houard discussed a case pending before the Parlement of Rouen in 1777 in which a son had been born to the widow Marie Rose l'Absolu eleven months and one day after the death of her husband Robert Le Sueur, a dry-goods merchant of Caudebad. The collateral heirs had succeeded in obtaining decisions in the lower courts against the legitimacy of this child. The attorney for the defense, M. Le Clerc, printed a memoir citing case histories of late births reported by Heister, Bartholin, Truey, and Dulignac and previously published in the consultations of the supporters of late births and in medical journals. He also marshaled to Mme l'Absolu's defense the arguments employed by Petit and Le Bas in favor of the possibility of late births.[17]

References to the consultations emanating from Renée's case were incorporated in new editions and revisions of important works of jurisprudence after 1770. Ferrière, in his *Dictionnaire de droit et de pratique*, reviewed the conflicting opinions of philosophers and the courts on the question of late births. Although Ferrière expressed a personal preference for a ten-month limit, he ended his summary inconclusively, referring his readers to the writings of "two of the most famous doctors of the Faculty of Paris, MM. Bouvart and Petit," whose writings touched a bit too much on personalities, but were "nevertheless filled with excellent research and very wise reflections."[18]

Still, the jurists were troubled by the uncertainty that continued to surround the issue of late births and frustrated by the continued inconsistency of rulings on individual cases. In his article on late births in the 1790 edition of his collection, Denisart classified the authors of medical consultations on the possibility of late births into three groups: those who believed the term had to be set at 280 days; those who argued that extraordinary circumstances could delay birth beyond the 280-day limit, but never beyond 300 days; and those who maintained that a birth could be delayed up to fourteen months. Denisart believed this diversity of opinion hindered the administration of justice and revealed only too clearly the disadvantages of variations in the law from province to province or, in this case, from court to court. "Suppose," he wrote, "that three children are born after the deaths of their fathers: the first, on the 275th day after the death of the husband of its mother; the second, on the 288th day; the third, on the 306th day. The first will be declared legitimate by all three opinions; the second will be declared a bastard by the first opinion and legitimate by the other two; the third will be declared a bastard by the first two opinions and legitimate only by the last."[19]

Denisart cited the case of Charles and Renée as a perfect example of the perplexities that lack of consensus within the medical community had introduced into jurisprudence. According to the consultations of Bouvart and Louis, a pregnancy of 320 days was physically impossible and Renée's child was illegitimate, while according to the consultations of Petit and Le Bas, such a birth could legitimately occur. In disputes over the legitimacy of infants born late, Denisart was concerned that the rights of citizens had no protection against the whims of judges who could find support from some segment of the medical community for any opinion they might decide to embrace. Acknowledging that no limit was based on demonstrable proofs, Denisart, like Ferrière, nevertheless believed that social utility required some set limit and favored compromising between extremes by setting a limit at ten months.

The same problem of conflicting judicial rulings based on a lack of consensus within the medical community plagued adjudication of the inheritance rights of children born prematurely. Denisart noted that traditionally three phases of fetal development at birth had been recognized. In the first, the infant could not be born alive. In the second, the infant could be born alive but could not survive. In the third, the infant would probably survive. A term of 122 days or less was generally attributed to the first phase, 123 to 181 days to the second, and 182 days or more to the third, but the courts did not rigidly apply these limits in evaluating inheritance claims.[20]

The law held that the collateral heirs of the husband were his apparent heirs until a child was born alive. It was difficult, though, for doctors (to say nothing of trained attendants) to determine whether a child was born dead or died shortly after birth. In addition, in some areas, it was necessary not just that the child be born alive, but that it be reasonably likely to survive. Inconsistency reigned. While an act of 1535 acknowledged the inheritance rights of an infant reputed to have been born alive, an act of 1635 rejected a similar claim. As in the case of late births, Denisart advocated introducing uniformity into judicial decisions on the inheritance rights of children born prematurely. He proposed setting a term of 182 days, before which an infant would be presumed born dead and after which it would be presumed born alive, particular appearances or circumstances to the contrary notwithstanding.

The Napoleonic Code

As the Ancien Régime drew to a close, resolution of the issues of the possibility of late births and the legitimacy of infants born late was as elusive as it had been at midcentury. Despite the social importance of legitimacy, there were no fixed principles for establishing it. Courts continued to issue contradictory rulings as they weighed fidelity to ancient traditions, the desire to avoid cases that could provoke a scandal, arguments based on a woman's moral reputation, and testimonial proofs differently.[21] The jurists distinguished themselves from the doctors and surgeons by urging that a compromise be arranged and some limit set. Both sides of the medical community desired such a limit, but each was unwilling to compromise. Hence, the issue was taken out of the hands of the medical community after the Revolution with the formulation of the Napoleonic Code.

As Diane Alstad has observed, the Napoleonic Code still invoked the idea of natural law but redefined and limited its implications by making a strong distinction between the laws of nature and the laws of society. Thus was the weakness inherent in Enlightenment dreams of reform recognized. One revolutionary legislator, Berlier, expressed his confusion and frustration by exclaiming, "The sacred rights of nature! Ah! I respect them; but isn't it advisable to define them?"[22] Another legislator, Peres, continued along the same lines, "Without doubt, nature has her rights; they are sacred, inalienable, imprescriptible; but these rights have a limit, and that limit is placed at the point where begin the conventions of a well regulated society."[23]

The Napoleonic Code would bring revolutionary experiments in divorce and recognition of the rights of illegitimate children to an end, reinstating a patriarchal model of the family which emphasized the legal incapacity of women. This restoration of patriarchy would have enormous repercussions on succeeding generations of women in France. As Yvonne Knibiehler and Catherine Fouquet have observed, the provisions of the code which regulated the lot of women as wives and mothers in the first decade of the nineteenth century would not be suppressed or replaced, only modified parsimoniously, over the course of the next two centuries. Article 312 of the code, aimed at ending adultery, declared that "a child conceived during marriage has for its father the husband of the mother," while article 340 forbade judicial inquiries into the paternity of children. This article was intended to avoid conflicts over inheritance; in effect it deprived unwed mothers and illegitimate children of the judicial recourse they had enjoyed under the Ancien Régime. No longer could fathers who were not husbands be held financially responsible for their offspring, the customary principle that "he who makes the child must feed it" having been abandoned. Young female domestic servants and factory workers were thus destined to become even more vulnerable to sexual exploitation of the sort described in chapter 6.[24]

The articles (312, 314, 315) of the Napoleonic Code which addressed the legitimacy of infants born prematurely or late admitted the inheritance rights of those born 180 to 300 days after conception. These provisions represented a victory for the jurists as well as for the more moderate opponents of late births. In his 1806 edition, Denisart lauded this legislation because it promised effectively to preclude all disputes concerning the social condition of children. "It has," he exclaimed, "fixed and narrowed the circle within which nature can still work her marvelous caprices, but which she can no longer cross at the expense of society."[25] Indeed, it seemed as though the articles of the code might have been written by Denisart himself before the Revolution. In fact, the source of these limits was not Denisart but Roman law. The provisions of Roman law had been cited frequently but observed only erratically during the early modern period, for they had always to be balanced against the weight of custom. Such was not the case with the Napoleonic Code.

The new articles were greeted with pleasure by some of the supporters of late births, too, for the code recognized in principle the possibility of late births. Reviewing the consultations submitted concerning the legitimacy of Renée's child, the editors of the *Encyclopédie méthodique* (1821) concluded that the opponents of late births had been more concerned with the moral and social consequences of legal recognition of late births than with their physical possibility. To them, the recognition of late births by the Napoleonic Code represented a philosophical advance in the study of nature as well as an improvement in jurisprudence.[26]

Not everyone, however, was happy with the new articles. There was some dispute over the exact meaning of the article concerning late births. The precise wording was, "The legitimacy of a child born three hundred days after the dissolution of the marriage *pourra être contestée*."[27] At issue was whether the word, "pourra" was meant to be conditional. Denisart interpreted the article to mean that any claim to legitimacy of a child born more than ten months after alleged conception would be rejected if it were contested. Since the state had no interest in disrupting the internal harmony of families, though, the legitimacy of these children would be assumed unless challenged by collateral heirs. "The law," he agreed, "is by no means called upon to reform that which it knows nothing about; and if the social condition of the child is not challenged, it remains sheltered in a silence that no one can desire to break."[28]

Two prominent authorities on medical jurisprudence during the Napoleonic era disagreed with Denisart's interpretations. Maurice Méjan and François Fodéré praised the authors of the code for ending legal disputes over claims of birth up to ten months after conception and interpreted article 315 to mean that only claims of birth after more than ten months gestation could be brought before the courts. The authors of the code had not stated that infants born before 180 or after 300 days had to be declared illegitimate on these grounds alone. Méjan and Fodéré believed that birth beyond ten months was physically possible and that the particular circumstances concerning a late birth had to be examined before a child could be declared illegitimate. "One sees," Méjan maintained, "that in expressing himself in this manner the legislator wanted to allow the possibility of contesting the child's legitimacy, but he also wanted it [the presumption of legitimacy] to triumph over all attacks that were not well founded."[29]

During the Napoleonic era, the courts themselves seemed unsure about how to interpret article 315, as Méjan's description of the reversal by Grenoble's Court of Appeals of a lower court's decision reveals. The case concerned Catherine Berard's claim to a late birth of 316 days. The lower court had interpreted article 315 in the manner suggested by Méjan, that is, that children born more than ten months after conception had a provisionary legitimacy that could be undermined only if illegitimacy were convincingly established by reference to the peculiar circumstances surrounding the late birth. The lower court had been convinced by the arguments of Mme Berard's attorney that a birth as late as 316 days was recognized by many doctors as physically possible and that the mistreatment she had suffered at the hands of the collateral heirs could easily have prolonged her pregnancy. Since the collateral heirs had introduced no testimony indicating that Berard was guilty of indiscretions, the court recognized her child's legitimacy on April 14, 1808.

The collateral heirs appealed the decision the same day. The Grenoble Court of Appeals reasoned that a thirty-day legal extension beyond the normal nine months had already been granted by the Napoleonic Code and that, while article 315 did not specify that all claims to birth after more than ten months had to be rejected, it did establish a legal presumption of illegitimacy in these cases. The court held that only extraordinary circumstances could be considered adequate to override this presumption of illegitimacy. It did not consider the circumstances surrounding Berard's pregnancy extraordinary enough to merit recognition of her child's legitimacy. On April 12, 1809, the higher court reversed the lower court's decision and decreed that the inheritance be apportioned among the collateral heirs.[30]

As difficult, perplexing, and ultimately inconclusive as the debate over late births from 1765 to 1769 had been, there is no denying the influence it had on the development and recognition of the new science of medical jurisprudence. One can measure this influence indirectly by examining editions of the *Encyclopédie* from 1751 to 1781. The 1751 to 1765 editions contained no references to legal disputes involving premature or late births or to the more general subject of legal medicine. By 1781, a special section was devoted to just these issues. The slow rate of development of medical jurisprudence over the course of the seventeenth and eighteenth centuries was not due, however, to a lack of interest on the part of the state. An edict of January 1606 had declared it the duty of the first physician to appoint one or two surgeons in each of the cities and market towns of France to report to the courts in cases where medical expertise was demanded. In February 1692 another edict required that a doctor be appointed and given sole authority to make medical reports in each of the cities and market towns. Concerned about the impenetrability of medical discourse to the courts, the authors of the edict urged doctors and surgeons making judicial reports to express themselves in intelligible and natural language. They needed to take into account the audience they were addressing: judges for the most part had no knowledge of the scientific anatomical terms and, consequently, a report written in scientific language tended to obscure rather than clarify the issues.[31] By the next century, demands for greater clarity would emanate from the general public, for whom the matters to be decided by the courts took on an ever greater significance.

The editors of the *Encyclopédie* of 1781, however, attributed the incomprehensibility of medical matters not to surgeons' erudition but to their immersion in the practical or empirical aspects of medicine and lack of philosophical and rational perspective. As a result, seventeenth- and eighteenth-century rulings on medical matters were often based on doctrines formulated by jurists or received through custom rather than on medical judgments.

Because the edict of 1606 made medical reports to the courts the domain of surgeons, medical jurisprudence was initially considered a branch of surgery rather than of medicine. The early practitioners of medical jurisprudence tended to be as unscholarly as most surgeons and were accorded the same lack of dignity and respect. The editors of the *Encyclopédie* of 1781 deplored the gullibility of most surgeons in matters of medical jurisprudence. "It is ignorance," they wrote, "that cherishes marvels and finds miracles everywhere. Without retreating to earlier times whose barbarism is a monument of humiliation for humanity, we see even today an absurd credulity among men who have been educated to know better."[32]

While enlightened doctors and surgeons like Petit, Le Bas, Louis, and Bouvart had established new standards of proof and argumentation for medical jurisprudence and defined new areas in which this science could be applied, many provincial surgeons still differed little from the empirics in medical expertise and world view. These surgeons continued to ground their notions of medical jurisprudence on deeply rooted popular beliefs in which the natural and supernatural were inextricably linked.

Stories of incredible pregnancies were commonplace in folklore and the popular press. In February 1637, a canard was circulated in the streets of Paris announcing that the Parlement of Grenoble, on the advice of doctors and midwives of the Faculty of Medicine of Montpellier, had recognized the legitimacy of Dame Madeleine d'Automont's child. The lady claimed to have conceived the child solely by concentrating on the memory of her husband, who had been absent for four years. The king's prosecutor of the Parlement of Paris decided to investigate this strange act and discovered that it had never, in fact, been issued. On July 13, 1637, the Parlement of Grenoble published an act declaring the reported act "false, contrived, libelous, and injurious to its honor."[33]

The story concerning Mme d'Automont was an egregious example of an extraordinary pregnancy and was officially denounced. Scarcely more credible tales continued to circulate over a century later, however, with the approbation of various doctors and surgeons. The editors of the *Encyclopédie* cited the example of Roederer (1726–63), a doctor who, in a dissertation awarded a prize at Petersburg, reported the case of his sister, who had given birth to a fish. His story was matched by that of a French surgeon who, caught up in the belief in sorcery, certified that a bewitched woman gave birth to several frogs.

Despite the apparent absurdity of some of these stories, the editors of the *Encyclopédie* did not find them at all amusing. They realized that what was recognized as absurd by doctors and judges in Paris might very well be accepted with all seriousness by provincial surgeons and the judges they advised. And they attributed to the credulity of these surgeons a number of what they termed "judicial murders": "These examples," they wrote, "which are only ridiculous, furnished bloody scenes in those ages in which the sovereign courts were less enlightened; but the lower courts and the first judges in small towns are often unsophisticated in matters of reasoning. Should a bad or inconsistent report move them, they can plague the innocent or leave the guilty unpunished. It is always the presumptuous half-science that gives to the false or uncertain the appearance of being true or evident."[34] In the minds of the editors, the success of enlightened reform depended on the development of an enlightened science of medical jurisprudence.

Even in cases where provincial surgeons were more sophisticated than the villagers they tended, public pressure to endorse wild speculation could sometimes seem insurmountable. Take, for example, the case of M. Dolignon, a surgeon practicing in Cressi en Laonnois. In 1774, he sent a letter to M. Dufau, a doctor, instructor in the art of accouchements in Soissons, and correspondent of the Academy of Bordeaux. Dolignon described the commotion created in his small village when a young woman named Catherine Berna filed a declaration of pregnancy with the local court, identifying the father as Nicolas Simon, a young man who had rejected her advances. Simon denied having impregnated Mlle Berna and declared that she would pay the devil for her lies by giving birth to four frogs. Berna's neighbors were so convinced of the power of sorcery that they believed they heard the frogs croaking in Berna's womb.

When the hour for the birth arrived, all the notables of the town, the mayor, the syndic, and hordes of women and children rushed to Berna's bedside, for the mayor had ordered that the birth would take place before the astonished eyes of the whole village. To the stupefaction and horror of these witnesses, the midwife, her hands washed in holy water, withdrew a frog from the birthing table. Three others followed in quick succession, as everyone but Dolignon rushed from the room in fright. Dolignon requested permission to examine Berna and discovered that the opening to the womb had remained virginal.

Public opinion was so strong in favor of trying Nicolas Simon on charges of sorcery that the justices of the court of Marle, although inclined to agree with Dolignon that the case was ludicrous, were compelled to hear it. For this reason, Dolignon had written to Dufau. "I am," he declared, "the only one who dares fight against the imbecility of the multitude. Deign, sir, to come here; you will soon see the deception. As demonstrator of the art of accouchements, you will instruct and enlighten the midwife and one of my colleagues who naively believe in such pregnancies. You like doing good deeds. This would be a very good one, freeing men of their illusions concerning the supposed facts of magic and spells."[35]

But was the education of midwives the solution to the problems posed by cases like Berna's? Some medical practitioners thought that more was at the root of such spectacles than a midwife's naïveté, and accused midwives attending such sensational and obviously unnatural births of collusion in abortion. Deploring the success of such ruses, Professeur du Bois of Brittany observed, "If they make her [the pregnant woman or girl] abort, they announce boldly that they have procured the exit of a toad and the ignorant public receives the news with the greatest credulity."[36] Even more worrisome for Bois than the perpetuation of popular superstitions was the prospect that such superstitions could be exploited to undermine patriarchal and corporative authority.

The editors of the *Encyclopédie* chose not to take up such charges, perhaps because they seemed to emanate as much from professional rivalries as from a concern with justice. Nor was the Berna case or more famous causes célèbres of the eighteenth century explicitly mentioned.

Still, there was general agreement that medical judgments offered by provincial surgeons in the trials of Calas, Sirven, La Barre, Montbailly, Chassagnieux, and Baronet were questionable, even negligent, based more on rumor and innuendo than on clearly defined standards of medical jurisprudence. Because they were dependent on the good will of members of their community to ensure a decent income, provincial surgeons too easily bowed to public pressure and, in especially controversial cases, came to conclusions based primarily on circumstantial evidence.

The potential of such reports to precipitate miscarriages of justice prompted experts like Louis and Lafosse to pursue extensive inquiries that would extend the theoretical framework of medical jurisprudence.[37] In some cases, notably that of Calas and Sirven, vindication of the innocent hinged on challenges to the medical opinions on which conviction had been based. The Sirven case merits analysis at this point because it reveals how miscarriages of justice could typically occur and ultimately, if tortuously, be reversed. The affair captured Voltaire's attention because of the epistemological and social issues it raised. It fascinated the public probably for less lofty reasons: it allowed them to enter the intimate, generally forbidden space of a family rumored to have been torn apart by religious fanaticism, madness, and finally murder.

The Sirven Affair

The Sirven affair began on March 6, 1760, when Elisabeth Sirven, daughter of Pierre-Paul and Toinette Leger Sirven, disappeared from the Sirven home in Castres. Pierre-Paul, a Protestant, was a *féodiste* employed by numerous nobles in the region to defend their feudal rights and privileges. When Elisabeth disappeared, he was summoned to the bishopric by Monseigneur de Barral, whose protection Elisabeth reportedly sought in her efforts to acquire instruction in the Catholic faith and, eventually, confirmation.

With her father's consent, the bishop placed the twenty-two-year-old woman in a convent under the protection of the *Dames noires*. This convent received both day and boarding students, many of whom were Protestants confined by *lettres de cachet* in the crown's efforts to bring them to its idea of the true faith. Throughout France, Protestant girls were often confined to convents like that of the *Dames noires* until they consented to marry Catholic men.[38]

Elisabeth's mental state and motives for seeking the bishop's protection on that day in March 1760 remain obscure. The sisters noted signs of derangement, madness, and half-wittedness in Elisabeth, interspersed with periods of lucidity. Stories circulated that she disrobed in the room of a superior and claimed to be communing with angels, and that she had to be isolated and whipped by a servant when she became agitated.

After seven months during which the *Dames noires* apparently made no progress in their efforts to convert Elisabeth, they returned her to her parents. The Sirvens claimed that Elisabeth returned disfigured, exhausted, emaciated, and covered with bruises. Once home, she experienced "crises" in which she threw linen out of the windows, tore apart whatever came to hand, and was found undressed and covered with excrement. The windows were sealed and Elisabeth was placed in restraining garments. Despite her confinement, she talked often of plans to marry a great lord. Her parents concluded that she had gone completely mad from having been confined to the convent for so long.[39]

Elisabeth's crises resembled those of the Convulsionaries thirty years earlier, though they were not invested with the same radical religious meaning. The *Dames noires* attributed the crises to the source to which Nigon de Berty had attributed the crises of Marie Mossaron and Anne Le Franc—menstrual irregularities. Elisabeth, they explained, suffered a suppression of menstruation the day she first presented herself to the bishop. A surgeon, Jean Durand, who was called to see Elisabeth after her departure from the convent, bled her and recommended baths morning and evening.

Claiming she had been cured, Elisabeth returned to the gates of the convent, apparently more eager than ever to convert. But why? Was she religiously inspired or did she simply want a husband? Lacroix, the Sirvens' lawyer, would later argue that although Elisabeth spoke often of marrying a Catholic, she had no suitors. Nor did her eccentric behavior make her an advantageous match. "Perhaps," he reasoned, "she considered marriage easier if she converted."[40]

The rivalry between church and family over who should determine Elisabeth's fate pitted the ideal of religious freedom against that of obedience to paternal authority. In an ironic reversal of the usual theological defenses of patriarchy, the sisters and vicar argued that the Sirvens were mistreating their daughter and urged the intendant to free Elisabeth from paternal rule and allow her to return to the convent for religious instruction. Their request clearly deviated from the rules of the family-state compact by recognizing the need in some cases to limit paternal power. Prolonged debate over Pierre-Paul Sirven's right to decide his daughter's fate would bring the family-state compact under increased scrutiny.

After moving to Saint-Alby in July of 1761 to escape further pressure, the Sirvens found themselves confronted by a curé and vicar sent by the intendant to investigate charges that Elisabeth was being mistreated. Before the bishop of Castres could consider the matter, Pierre-Paul left town on business on January 3, 1762, and Elisabeth once again disappeared from the family home. The next day, her body was found floating in a well.

Initially, most of the villagers believed that Elisabeth had committed suicide in a fit of madness. Witnesses would testify that she was simple, eccentric, subject to delirium. Some speculated that Elisabeth was desperate to find a husband because she was pregnant; others said that she wanted to marry in order to have children; still others whispered that she was possessed by the devil. Only after the medical experts issued their report was the notion of homicide taken seriously and the Sirven family brought under suspicion.[41]

The medical experts summoned were the doctor Jean Galet Duplessis and the surgeon Pierre Husson. They were asked to determine if Elisabeth had fallen into the well while alive or had been thrown in after she was already dead. Had she died from the fall, or drowned, or been strangled first? Galet Duplessis and Husson concluded that Elisabeth had not hurled herself into the well but had been thrown in dead, probably after being suffocated. They based their conclusion on the theory that if Elisabeth had drowned, her stomach and intestines would have been filled with water, but no water was present.[42]

Soon after the autopsy, Elisabeth's body disappeared from the town hall and an inquiry attempted to determine who the body snatchers were. Suspicions centered on Pierre-Paul Sirven as rumors circulated that the Protestant religion required parents to put to death any children who might desire to convert to Catholicism. It was said that a Protestant assembly had formulated this doctrine because Protestants were unhappy with the king's refusal to allow Protestant parents authority to punish children who renounced their faith.

Galet Duplessis and Husson actively contributed to these rumors. Galet Duplessis testified that Pierre-Paul Sirven's attorney, Jalabert, tried through threats and bribes to persuade him to disclose the conclusions of his report and to change it if it were unfavorable to Sirven. Declaring that he feared for his life lest Protestants mete out the same punishment to him that they apparently had to a child of theirs, Galet Duplessis appealed to the general prosecutor in Toulouse for protection.[43] Jalabert, claiming that his only goal had been to learn the details of the medical report, denied pressuring the experts to change their conclusions.

How unbiased was the experts' report? Clearly, Galet Duplessis gave some credence to the rumors regarding "Protestant justice," rumors fueled by accounts of the Calas affair being adjudicated in Toulouse even before the discovery of Elisabeth's body. Husson would later testify that on the day he opened the cadaver, Fabre, the regent of schools, told him that Elisabeth's mother was very harsh toward her, that she kept Elisabeth locked in a room, and that she beat her whenever she found her associating with Catholics. Another villager, Dame Françoise Paris, told him that Elisabeth's mother had declared that if her daughter abjured her faith, she would execute her.

Although doctor and surgeon both signed the medical report, Galet Duplessis would later dispute Husson's inference that because there was no water in the abdomen, Elisabeth had been suffocated before being thrown into the well. He would inform the court that drowning victims are suffocated not by water but by the pressing and contraction of organs attempting to receive the air necessary for life and would claim that the only uncontested proof of drowning was the presence of foam in the bronchi and lungs. Yet Galet Duplessis never had the chest of the cadaver opened to disclose the status of the lungs. Having observed certain marks on the neck of the cadaver, Galet Duplessis continued to suspect that violence had been applied to the body before it was thrown into the well.[44]

Was Galet Duplessis's critique of Husson's reasoning the reflection of more enlightened medical opinion, or was it, as Husson maintained, a response to pressure from Jalabert? Given the disagreement between the medical experts, the judge might have ordered a second visit by other experts, but he chose not to do so and, in the minds of some, the Sirven affair became the Galet-Husson affair.[45]

At this point, *monitoires* were read in churches urging people with knowledge supporting charges against the Sirvens to speak up. An inquiry of forty-five witnesses of Saint-Alby revealed that most villagers now tended to believe that Elisabeth had been of sound mind, hence unlikely to have contemplated suicide. Only twelve said that she appeared imbecilic or simple minded. A writ was issued against the Sirvens ordering them to be imprisoned, but they fled to Switzerland before the order could be executed. The tribunal of Mazamet nevertheless continued its inquiry and on March 29, 1764, found Pierre-Paul Sirven and his wife guilty of parricide. They were condemned to be hung and strangled in a public place; their two remaining daughters were required to witness the executions of their parents and then to be banished forever from Mazamet. Their goods were confiscated, and the sentence was carried out in effigy.

Reflecting on the verdict in the *Dictionnaire philosophique*, Voltaire would focus on the absence of definitive proof of a crime. The judges condemning Calas, Sirven, and other innocents were obliged, he emphasized, to be certain of their guilt. Certitude was not possible in the presence of alternative physical or moral explanations. Judges needed to consider the age, rank, and conduct of the accused; the motive he might have had in committing a crime; and the interest of his enemies in condemning him. Such judgments, Voltaire contended, were not the prerogative of medical experts, and he concluded, "It is indeed cruel that the life and honor of the father of a family should depend on an ignorant surgeon and an idiotic judge."[46]

The Sirven case was appealed to physicians associated with the Faculty of Medicine of Montpellier; to surgeons of the Royal College of Surgery in Montpellier; and to Antoine Louis, who was then serving as secretary of the Royal Academy of Surgery in Paris. All agreed that the report of Galet Duplessis and Husson was invalid. They argued that the two had neither known nor employed the means necessary to determine whether Elisabeth had died by drowning. The only means of determining this would have been to examine the lungs and bronchial cavity for water. Considering the marks on the neck of the cadaver, they agreed that there had been a fatal contusion. But it was not clear that the marks could only have been the result of foul play. Indeed the experts believed that marks on the body excluded all possibility that Elisabeth had been strangled. It seemed more likely that she had hit her head or neck on a rock or pail or on the sides of the well and had died as a result of hammering in her skull, fracturing her vertebrae, and twisting her neck in the fall.[47]

The consultations of the medical experts from Montpellier and Paris were issued in 1769 and would play a critical role in reversing the courts' condemnation of the Sirvens. Rehabilitation and restitution followed within two years. In the meantime, a number of important changes were occurring in the state's treatment of Protestants. In November of 1769, the Parlement de Toulouse repealed the denunciation and confiscation of goods of Antoine Benech, a Protestant who had refused last rites; in July of 1770, it affirmed the legitimacy of children born of Protestant marriages, without yet ruling on the legitimacy of Protestant marriages themselves.[48]

In the Sirven affair, little was made of the rumors that Elisabeth was desperate to find a husband because she was pregnant. Had the local medical experts and public opinion not been so preoccupied with stories of "Protestant justice" authorizing parents to murder children who abjured their faith, however, a very different scenario might have developed, one in which Elisabeth would have been condemned not just for having committed suicide, but possibly infanticide as well.

The Problem of Infanticide

Infanticide was a particularly sensitive issue in the 1760s because of the increased interest taken in it by the state, church, and medical community. At this time, the provisions of the Edict of Henri II were more likely to be enforced and to elicit the concern of philosophes like Voltaire, physicians like Louis and Petit, and women like Mme de Genlis, who feared that enforcement would only increase the number of judicial murders.

A product of interrelated efforts at family formation and state building, the edict, which was to be read by the curés in all the parishes of France every three months, condemned to death women who had concealed a pregnancy and deprived children who died shortly after birth of the Christian sacraments of baptism and burial. Directed at combatting the infanticides that often attended illegitimate births, the edict was one in a series of statutes aimed at tightening parental power over minor children, supervising publicly the female realm of pregnancy and childbirth, and empowering husbands to regulate the conditions of marital separation.[49]

Originally composed in 1556, the edict was reaffirmed in 1708. In order to preclude any suspicions that might arise from fatal accidents attending birth, widows and unmarried girls were urged to declare their pregnancies to the local magistrate. This provision was particularly burdensome, for it required unmarried pregnant girls to make an official confession of their lack of chastity and to expose themselves to public ridicule and mistreatment by their parents. Montesquieu had argued that is was as unreasonable to demand such a declaration from a girl as it was to ask a man not to defend his life. He proposed that the girls' confessions need extend no further than to members of their immediate family. Some of the local *parlements*, most notably the Parlement of Dijon, shared Montesquieu's view and determined that it was sufficient for a woman to reveal her pregnancy to other women or to her confessor.[50]

Fears of invasion of a woman's privacy and of the damage that might be done her reputation by overly zealous enforcement of this edict remained prevalent and were justified. In 1776 the Parlement of Paris found it necessary to rebuke the *officiers de justice* of Courcelles for making an unsolicited visit to ascertain the virginity of a young girl, Poulain. Rumors of Poulain's lack of morality had been circulated by a spurned lover who sought to prevent her from marrying someone else.[51]

Outside France, the public humiliation to which unwed mothers were exposed could be even greater. In her memoirs, Mme de Genlis expressed horror at the outrageous customs regarding seduction and infanticide which she encountered in Bremgarten, Switzerland. All seduced girls were required to make a public declaration and retreat to a hospice until giving birth. Six weeks after the birth, the unwed mother was subjected to a public ritual in which she was crowned with straw and made to walk through the town amid a crowd who flung mud at her. Hoots and insults accompanied her to the gates of the town, where the executioner gave her three kicks in the rear and ejected her from the town. She could return the next day, but often as not would be reduced to begging or prostitution to make a living. De Genlis considered the custom odious and predicted that it would only increase the rate of infanticide.[52]

Enforcement of the Edict of Henri II seems to have varied by region. My survey of cases before the Tournelle of Rennes from 1763 to 1766 produced four cases of women accused of concealment of pregnancy, clandestine birth, and infanticide; in one case, a death sentence was appealed.[53] Yvonne Knibiehler and Catherine Fouquet note that between 1735 and 1801, 83 declarations of pregnancy were made before 7 notaries of Vitteaux in the Côte d'Or and environs. Many of these declarations were made in an effort to compel fathers to pay support. The Parlement of Bourgogne made only three death sentences for those convicted of infanticide during this time; only one was carried out. In Paris, whipping and banishment were more common penalties.[54] Claude Grimmer observes that between 1775 and 1786, 107 convictions for infanticide were appealed to the Parlement of Paris; they represented only 1.1 percent of cases on appeal, a modest figure in comparison with the 6,297 cases of theft appealed at the same time.[55] Grimmer notes that in Aurillac, the edict was renewed with greater rigor in 1773; as a result, opposition to the law became more vocal.

Public debate on the matter would continue until the end of the eighteenth century, when revolutionary cahiers advocated dispensing with the Edict of Henri II and suggested, along the lines of Voltaire, that establishing hospices for unwed mothers and homes for abandoned children were better ways of dealing with the problems of illegitimacy and infanticide.[56] As was the case with much revolutionary rhetoric, however, the cahiers failed to acknowledge the extent of the problem. By the 1760s, the rate of illegitimacy had become so high and the number of abandoned children so great that hospitals and foundling homes in Paris and the provinces were overwhelmed. Chances of a foundling surviving in these institutions hovered around one in three.[57] Sympathy for the plight of the poor and projects for institutional reform could not avert these tragedies.

When women were charged with concealment of pregnancy and infanticide, medical evaluations were required, and doctors and surgeons were entrusted with the difficult task of determining whether the infant's death were natural or not. What appeared to be murder could very well have been a stillbirth or miscarriage. Because the symptoms of pregnancy and hydropsy were so similar, it was sometimes difficult to determine whether the woman had been pregnant.

On other occasions, doctors were asked to resolve delicate disputes between masters and servants. A lawyer representing a young female servant accused of theft by her master responded that she had been seduced and asked the Royal Society of Medicine if it were possible for doctors to determine whether a girl had given birth. The doctor assigned the task of answering this question turned to his colleagues and asked, "What should I respond?"[58]

Given the primitive state of medical analysis, there was ample room for error and abuse. As evidence of the misfortune that could result from the preservation of laws like the Edict of Henri II, Voltaire cited a case in which a young girl was suspected of concealing her dead baby. She was imprisoned, interrogated, and examined by midwives, who declared that she had been pregnant. Faced with the threat of torture, the girl confessed killing her child and was condemned to death. Yet she had not given birth; indeed, she was still pregnant and had the good fortune of giving birth at the very moment when the sentence was being read.[59] In recounting this incident, Voltaire may be suspected of having resorted to poetic license to make a point, but equally troubling cases can be found in medical consultations of the time.

Petit and Louis, although they had taken opposite sides in the debate over late births, joined forces in criticizing provincial surgeons for precipitous judgments in infanticide cases. A famous case in which they intervened involved Thérèse Ismère Famin, daughter of the postmaster of Mantes. When two newborn infants were found dead outside Gassicourt the morning after the swelling from which Mlle Famin had suffered for several months subsided, local surgeons were summoned to ascertain if she were their mother. They argued affirmatively. The judges ruled on the basis of this report, despite the lack of testimony from witnesses to support the surgeons' theory, and found Famin guilty of infanticide in 1767.

In evaluating the surgeons' report, Petit and Louis maintained that all the signs upon which the surgeons had determined that the girl had been pregnant were equivocal and that it was more likely that she had suffered hydropsy, as she claimed. There was no definitive proof that Famin had been pregnant, that she had given birth, or that the two infants found dead were her offspring and had been murdered by her. On the basis of their consultation, the court of appeals overturned the ruling of the lower court.[60] The reports of Petit and Louis were summarized in a number of journals, including *L'Avantcoureur* and the *Journal des dames*.

Disagreements like this did not cease with the inauguration of a new regime after the Revolution. Another case occurred in Troyes in the year VIII. Provincial *officiers de santé* concluded that a twenty-four-year-old woman, Mlle Granger, was guilty of infanticide, and the tribunal of l'Yonne condemned her to death. The case was appealed to the tribunal of l'Aube, and two famous experts on medical jurisprudence, Baudelocque and Bourdois, were asked to give their opinions on the case. They argued against the conclusions of the *officiers de santé*, maintaining that the infant's death was more likely the result of a miscarriage than of deliberate intent of the woman to harm her child. Eight local doctors and surgeons of Troyes concurred with Baudelocque and Bourdois in their judgment.

Another expert on medical jurisprudence, Fodéré, rebuked the *officiers de santé* for their injudicious conduct in the case, arguing that had the child not been illegitimate and had the woman not given birth in secret, charges of infanticide would never have been placed against her on the basis of the physical evidence at hand.[61]

In the Famin and Granger cases, rumors seemed to have had a greater role in influencing the local medical experts' interpretation of physical evidence than did the testimony of the young women themselves. Experts in medical jurisprudence like Petit, Louis, Baudelocque, Bourdois, and Fodéré successfully challenged the assumption of the local experts that women would always deceive if they had an interest in doing so. Unable to find convincing physical proof of infanticide, these authorities concluded that it was an injustice to declare Famin and Granger guilty. It should be noted, however, that skepticism regarding the interpretation of physical evidence did not necessarily serve the interests of women. While such skepticism could be effectively used to counter charges of concealment of pregnancy and infanticide, it could also be used to undermine accusations that women might bring against men for crimes like rape. As one authority observed, "As rape is perhaps of all crimes the most difficult to commit, it is also the one for which we must demand the most evident proofs."[62]

The editors of the *Encyclopédie* lauded the level of erudition attained by the consultations of Petit, Bouvart, and Louis and urged their dissemination throughout France in order that they might serve as a model for others.[63] The attention the *Encyclopédie* focused on medical jurisprudence led to reforms in the manner in which medical reports were constructed for the courts, and represented part of a larger movement toward the reform of medical education.[64] In his plan for the university, Diderot advocated specialties on the illnesses of women and children and envisioned a course in medical jurisprudence as the culmination of the curriculum in medicine. This course would include a discussion of the importance of medicine, its progress and history; the character and duties of the true physician; the incertitude of the signs of death; and late births.[65]

Still, progress toward reform was haphazard during the eighteenth century and was frequently the work of particular individuals rather than of the state or the faculties. Thus Petit, having amassed a considerable fortune as a result of an extensive medical practice, personally endowed chairs in anatomy and surgery at the Faculty of Medicine of Paris and gave 100,000 livres to his birthplace, Orléans, to establish a bureau staffed by four doctors, two surgeons, and two lawyers to give free consultations in medicine and jurisprudence to the indigent of the town and surrounding countryside.[66] It was not until after the Revolution that chairs of medical jurisprudence would be established in all three schools of health—Paris,

Montpellier, and Strasbourg. The law of 19 *ventôse an* XI on the organization of medicine would formalize the position of medical jurisprudence in the medical curriculum, leading to an efflorescence of texts on the subject in the first three decades of the nineteenth century.[67]

In the meantime, efforts at advancing medical jurisprudence were hampered by the slow pace of institutional reform and by difficulties in disseminating the ideas and techniques of Parisian experts to physicians and surgeons in the provinces. In addition, experts in medical jurisprudence like Sue and Lafosse came up against the same kind of vexing epistemological problems that had confronted the physicians and surgeons involved in the debate over late births. How could medical jurisprudence attain the degree of certitude necessary to avoid judicial murders and reassure the judge and the public against fear of error? In their pursuit of truth to be used in the service of justice, these physicians were troubled by the problem of scientific doubt. They came to wonder whether the ideal of mathematical certitude envisioned by Descartes lay within the scope of medicine.[68]

Descartes's interest in advancing medical knowledge was connected to his conviction that the mind was so closely connected to the body that improvements in the physical condition of humanity were bound to lead to mental advances as well. As the preceding analysis demonstrates, later Enlightenment figures, including Voltaire, Mme de Genlis, and the Encyclopedists, were equally eager to see medicine advance, but for different reasons. Were medical theory and practice improved, the miscarriages of justice which attended the Edict of Henri II and took such heavy psychological and social tolls on women, regardless of their marital status or social condition, might be prevented. In retrospect, this approach, however compassionate and well intended, did not go far enough, because it did not challenge the fundamental presuppositions of the family-state compact which had given rise to the edict. Although the revolutionaries would challenge patriarchal authority in the person of the monarch and make some changes in the laws of inheritance, legal commitment to paternal power within the family would be renewed after the Revolution and would inform family policy in France through the twentieth century.

CHAPTER FOUR

Science, Medicine, and the Salons:
A Struggle for Cultural Authority

Conflicting Visions of Science

The debates attending medical causes célèbres provided a forum for airing disagreements not just about the length of pregnancies, scientific method, or the relationship between medicine and jurisprudence but also about the ideals that should inform medicine and the role medical practitioners should play in society. Controversy over these matters drew the medical community into a larger eighteenth-century debate over the relationship between science and the Enlightenment. Should men of science embrace the ideals of the philosophes and commit themselves to enlightened reform? Were they pursuing power, recognition, and an authority that was ultimately derived from public esteem? Or was the true scientist someone who, committed to the ideal of the rigorous and necessarily solitary pursuit of truth, removed himself from the world? For this individual, authority was grounded not in public opinion but the voice of nature.[1]

Insofar as the medical debate over late births culminated in arguments over the social and political consequences of a judgment, it exposed the inadequacies of a model of science based on following the voice of nature. But if the voice of nature proved contradictory or even inaudible on the issue of late births, the alternative path, of following public opinion, seemed to many to be fraught with hazards. Such a solution represented a fundamental violation of the principles of hierarchy, privilege, and patriarchy upon which the institutions of the Ancien Régime were based.

Opponents of the democratization of science and politics likened the philosophes to charlatans—charlatans defined in the manner of Gouriet as those who were immortalized in the streets of Paris and idolized by women for their encyclopedic knowledge. Gouriet called charlatans France's first comedians because they never failed to turn heads and excite great enthusiasm.[2] To professional physicians and surgeons, of course, the term *charlatan* had especially troubling connotations. Charlatans were empiric, false physicians who set up stages in public squares, drawing people in by magical tricks and clowning in order to hawk their drugs more effectively before moving on to the next town.[3]

What would happen if the equation between philosophe and charlatan were to stick and if scientists and medical practitioners were to adopt the ideals of the philosophe?[4] If the success of philosophes, scientists, doctors, and surgeons depended on the esteem of women, cultural authority, too, would belong to women, who in the minds of many were least qualified to exercise it. To conservatives and even some of the most committed reformers, the Convulsionary cures of the 1730s had amply demonstrated women's irrationality, eroticism, and predilection for spectacle; Renée's claim to a late birth filled them with fear that matters of great social import would depend for resolution on the uncertain testimony and judgment of women. To see more precisely how the memory of the Convulsionaries and the controversy over Renée's claim stirred a much greater debate over who should exercise cultural authority, it is necessary to look beyond the literature of the medical causes célèbres to the writings of the philosophes, founders and members of the learned academies and faculties, and women.

The *Encyclopédie* article on the sciences written by the Chevalier de Jaucourt provides a point of entry into this debate. Jaucourt is an especially pertinent figure, for he straddled the worlds of medicine and the Enlightenment. With Tronchin, he had been a student of Boerhaave's in Leyden before becoming a prolific contributor to the *Encyclopédie*, writing numerous articles on medical topics.[5] In his article, Jaucourt acknowledged that the sciences were the work of the greatest geniuses, but that one needed to be a man of letters in order to profit from them *agréablement*. Scientific principles would be tedious if belles-lettres did not lend them their charms; conversely, letters would be condemned to an eternal infancy if they were not informed by the sciences. The *Encyclopédie*'s goal was to see the philosophical spirit of the sciences reign in men of letters and, through them, in the body of the nation.[6]

The Encyclopedists characterized themselves as a society of men of letters who formed the Republic of Letters, a novel concept in the eighteenth century. As Herbert Dieckmann has observed, this republic lay not outside, but within, existing society. It was the nucleus of the nation and of a vaster community that encompassed enlightened minds everywhere. Rejecting subservience to the church, the court, or a powerful patron, this republic addressed itself to a new forum that, in turn, it strove to develop and form: public opinion.[7]

But how could the sovereignty of public opinion be achieved? The Encyclopedists strove to communicate philosophic ideas and scientific discoveries clearly and simply so that erudition and theory could become matters of practical concern. Their purpose was to enable a public with no specialized training to speak competently on serious scientific, political, or economic issues. To achieve this purpose, they assured readers of their ability to understand and, by employing familiar genres like the letter, dialogue, or discourse, placed writer and audience on an equal level. They also expanded the media of discourse to include newspapers, pamphlets, and dictionaries, for as Voltaire had observed, one does not make a revolution with folios.[8]

It was hoped that emphasis on the literary would enable the Enlightenment to become a broad, unified movement, incorporating erudition with the language of polite society and bringing the philosophes together with scientists, aristocrats, and the upper bourgeoisie. The creation of the sovereign authority of public opinion also offered philosophes the prospect of exercising great influence for, as Duclos affirmed, "The man in power gives orders, but the intelligentsia govern because they in turn form public opinion which sooner or later subjugates or overthrows all forms of despotism."[9]

In his inaugural discourse to the Académie Française in 1767, Thomas argued that those who govern cannot at the same time enlighten. The state thus needed a class of men who would dedicate themselves to disseminating knowledge and purifying the morals and customs upon which all law depended. Men of letters who cultivated the ideals of the *honnête homme*—the decent, well-bred, reasonable man—or of the *homme de bien*—the compassionate, generous man who was as interested in the heart as the head—were the perfect choice to lead the nation morally.[10] Such men would move the people with a rhetoric so eloquent that their "hearts would throb, their facial expressions change, their tears flow. Their souls would be carried outside themselves, seeing, feeling, existing within the soul of the writer who animated them and who exercised a dominion over all their movements."[11]

The journals reported that Thomas's discourse was greeted enthusiastically, particularly by women, and lengthy extracts were printed in the *Journal des dames*. Women writers like Mme la Baronne Duplessy shared the philosophes' vision of merging science and sociability, engaging the heart as well as the mind, as an opportunity for bringing qualities traditionally identified narrowly with one or the other gender together in a fruitful interchange. In planning a series of lectures for the Musée des Dames, she observed that women brought a civilizing, pleasing air to men who, if left alone amid the sciences, would never be inspired to cultivate the sensibility and benevolence that lifted humanity above barbarism.[12]

Mme Necker continued along the same lines, observing that women who believed they had truly cultivated their spirit were mistaken if they had only a literary education. No, the pleasant would be incomplete without the useful: women needed to study history, hygiene, medicine, ethics, and physics as well as literature. Science, in turn, was enriched by joining imagination with reason. Necker believed that Newton's discoveries originated in an intuition of truths that he would later prove rationally.[13]

Duplessy and Necker were not theorizing in a void. Women's interest in science and medicine made them an eager audience for public lectures on natural history, anatomy, and botany; avid collectors of biological curiosities; and ready subscribers to a growing number of journals specializing in popular science. If they were not admitted to membership in the scientific academies, women would establish another academy, an academy of public opinion—the salon—where the philosophes' dream of making science and society more humane might be realized.[14] Reformers like La Condamine, who was shut out from presenting a memoir in favor of inoculation at the Royal Academy of Sciences in 1765, could find an audience here, as well as in journals like the *Journal encyclopédique* which circulated their views to a broader public.[15]

As strong a current as the Encyclopedists' conception of enlightened science was in the eighteenth century, however, it is important to note that it was running against another, equally forceful, current originating in the academies. In his opening address following the reorganization of the Royal Academy of Sciences in 1699, Bignon had made a point of contrasting the Academy of Sciences with the Académie Française. The Academy of Sciences, he asserted, does not seek to be *agréable*, but pursues the driest and most abstract truth. It is enough, he maintained, that the true be useful; it need not be pleasing. As Martha Ornstein has observed, Bignon's address separated science from other fields of inquiry in direct opposition to the Encyclopedists' efforts to link all forms of knowledge and make them accessible to the general public. It also hinted at the definition of an elite scientific community that, laying claim to superior authority by virtue of its superior insight into nature, would exclude amateurs and general philosophers.[16]

Bignon's address would serve as a touchstone for later academicians who opposed expansion in the membership of the academy, agreeing with Lavoisier that the academy was a working association, not a debating society or an oversized salon, and that it had to be protected from *"demi-savoir."*[17] In his *Essai sur la société des gens de lettres et des grands*, d'Alembert explicitly contrasted science with letters, arguing that the greater the value of a scientific work, the more independent it was of public opinion.[18]

Sharing d'Alembert's sense of the differences between science and letters, Condorcet pleaded for the authority and independence of science against the popularizers like Bernardin de Saint-Pierre, who declared, "Let Everyman be a scientist," and against the amateurs who rallied to Bernard in de Saint-Pierre's call for experimentation.[19] As secretary of the Royal Academy of Sciences, Condorcet parted company with philosophes like Jaucourt on the notion that public opinion should adjudicate questions of scientific merit. Equating science with reason itself, he placed its authority firmly in the academy. As Keith Baker has observed, a tension between scientific elitism and democratic liberalism lay at the heart of Condorcet's social science.[20] It emerges clearly here.

The reluctance of the Royal Academy of Sciences to follow the agenda set for science and society by the Encyclopedists was shared by individuals outside the academy. In 1768 Bachaumont's *Mémoires secrets* described the farce of commoners invading the Académie des Belles-Lettres and holding a mock meeting after the Swiss Guards had retired, and commented wryly that the entry of crowds of women into the Académie Française for the reception of the Abbé de Condillac had completely changed the tone of the meeting, bringing smiles to the most severe countenances.[21]

Fearing the encroachment of the salon's frivolity into all realms, critics of salon society like Rousseau were unlikely to have found women's forays into the academies amusing. To them, the salon atmosphere was antithetical to serious work, meditation, and the cultivation of genius. In the salons, people got together to please and to be pleased, and pleasure required decorum, conformity, and politeness—values that consigned all who observed them to mediocrity.[22] Concurring with Rousseau on this point, d'Alembert remarked, "In England it was enough that Newton was the greatest genius of his century; in France he would also have been expected to be likeable."[23]

In the salons, what counted was one's wit, all Voltaire's protestations to the contrary in his *Encyclopédie* article "Men of Letters" notwithstanding.[24] Remarking on the importance of the *bon mot* in polite society, Mme de Genlis reflected on Voltaire's celebrity: "I saw the women especially flutter, dream, and fret about framing a fine and spiritual response; the witticism uttered, they would part with the impression that upon leaving this salon, one carried away a portion of the glory and spirit of M. de Voltaire."[25]

Conservative critics shuddered to think of women dabbling in science, making claims to knowing everything without having learned anything, equating elegance of manner or expression with elegance of thought.[26] Thus in his *Correspondance secrète*, Métra made no effort to disguise his distaste for Valmont de Bomare, a popular writer and lecturer on natural history whose works, along with Buffon's, Plisson cited in her consultation on late births. Described by Métra as the focal point of all glances, the magnet that set the pace of all meetings, Valmont de Bomare was supposedly a master at winning over listeners with his fawning air, gutteral and honeyed voice, delicately shaded diction.[27] In Métra's characterization of Valmont de Bomare, the union of science and letters envisioned by Jaucourt and Thomas devolved into the charlatan described by Gouriet.

Although herself an intellectual woman of high social standing and thus potentially an object of attack from male critics of the feminization of culture, Mme Thiroux d'Arconville shared Métra's sense that the salon reinforced the habitual boredom that she considered the greatest source of women's suffering. Having been traumatically disfigured by smallpox at an early age, she withdrew from salon society and threw herself into her work, which she regarded as the universal remedy for all ills. After taking courses in anatomy at the Jardin Royal des Plantes, Thiroux d'Arconville retreated to her study to read works on physics, medicine, chemistry, and natural history and became the author of thirteen works, including histories, essays, a translation of an important anatomy text, and a novel.[28]

Thiroux d'Arconville differed from critics like Métra and Rousseau, however, in her refusal to see the controversy over locating science in the salons in gender terms. Métra and Rousseau worried that the integrity and independence of men of letters would be undermined in the salon and found the worst faults of dilettantism to which the Encyclopedists' emphasis on general knowledge was vulnerable concentrated in the women who ruled the salons. Unlike Thiroux d'Arconville, they expressed little concern with the deleterious effects that salon life might have on the work of women of letters.

The fact that women exercised such great and apparently capricious influence over kings, ministers, academies, and public opinion made them targets for liberal critics of absolutism as well as for conservative critics of the philosophes.[29] Sympathetic with the Encyclopedists' goal of having men of letters set the rules of taste and philosophy for the rest of the nation, if not with their predilection for the salon, d'Alembert urged the philosophes to eschew any appearance of charlatanry. Arguing that charlatanry degrades both spectator and actor, he predicted decadence in both letters and science if men of letters emulated the charlatans in their thirst for reputation and money.[30]

D'Alembert hoped for the introduction of a new value system that would end the subservience of men of talent to the hereditary nobility by placing nobility of thought and deed on the same level as nobility of birth. Such a value system would free scientists and men of letters from the lower ranks of society from pursuing fame and fortune as a means of compensating for ignoble birth. Insofar as it was itself the creation and reflection of a society that valued hierarchy by birth, the Royal Academy of Sciences advanced toward d'Alembert's ideal of meritocracy only slowly and amid considerable controversy.[31]

But even those who favored meritocracy were not convinced that it necessarily implied renunciation of fame and fortune. Differing with d'Alembert, the lawyer Linguet urged men of letters and the arts to cultivate celebrity as an alternative to nobility. In contrast to the nobility, who served the king as fighters, judges, or secretaries, men of letters should serve the public. Their most important *paternité* was *la voix publique*.[32] Linguet made no mention of *maternité*; such language would, no doubt, have been too divisive.

The authority to be accorded public opinion was thus an intensely debated issue, among reformers as well as between reformers and conservatives. The fact that women were thought to have a profound role in shaping public opinion further complicated matters, for even some of the most committed advocates of enlightenment balked at completely breaking down the distinctions between science and letters; reason and imagination; expert and amateur; learned and unlearned; male and female. Such thoroughgoing revision of the ideals of science and society involved much more than a challenge to traditional notions of hierarchy, privilege, and patriarchy. It represented the ultimate democratization, an end that was not to be attained even after the Revolution, when meritocracy of talent supposedly replaced hierarchy by birth, yet class and gender became even more accentuated differentiators of people.

Conflicting Visions of Medicine

Sociologists like Wolfgang Van den Daele and Joseph Ben-David have argued that the Enlightenment revived the Baconian program of social reform, but that its advancers were intellectuals, philosophes, and men of letters rather than men of science. Asserting that the philosophes were not scientists and that their community did not coincide with that of the scientists, they identify the eighteenth century as the point of irreversible demarcation between experimental philosophy and the movement for cultural and social emancipation.[33]

There are elements of truth to this argument, especially if one focuses on the programs enunciated by academies like the Royal Academy of

Sciences, which was established by the crown with a specific purpose in mind. Still, our survey of the debate over the values that should inform science and letters brings into question the notion of a strict demarcation between men of science and men and women of letters. Neither scientists nor philosophes were free from the attraction of the competing and sometimes conflicting values, perhaps because the institutions that sustained science and letters were not yet mutually exclusive. The Royal Academy of Sciences did not yet monopolize all serious scientific activity, nor were scientists entirely removed from salon society and the intellectual influence and companionship of women. Hence it would be impossible to strictly categorize either scientists or philosophes.

Nowhere was the force of competing values felt more intensely than by physicians and surgeons, who simultaneously emulated both scientists and philosophes and whose debates over professional ideals reveal the inconsistencies inherent in the socially constructed images of both the man of science and the man of letters. As our study of case histories in the debate over late births has revealed, the case history was considered the foundation of progressive medicine. Yet it was itself a hybrid of science and literature, mixing theory and observation with imaginative reconstruction of motives or events bound to elicit public interest. Because eminent Parisian physicians and surgeons associated simultaneously with a number of institutions including, but not limited to, the Faculty of Medicine, the Royal Society of Medicine, the Royal Academy of Sciences, the Royal Academy of Surgery, the Collège Royal, and the Jardin du Roi, their professional ideals could not be defined by a single institution, whether it be reputed to be a bastion of conservatism like the Faculty of Medicine or hailed like the Collège Royal and the Jardin du Roi for initiating a pedagogical revolution.[34]

Eschewing exams, diplomas, tuition, and even formal registration, the Jardin du Roi was especially notable for breaking down barriers between professionals and amateurs as it attracted physicians, surgeons, and pharmacists together with interested members of the general public to such novelties as a dissection of a woman who died with embryo intact or the autopsy of an elephant from the menagerie at Versailles. Intent on gaining as many direct and exotic observations as possible for his volumes on natural history, Buffon established an extensive correspondence network from the Jardin du Roi, rewarding savants and functionaries throughout the world with the title of correspondent of the Jardin or of the Cabinet du Roi.[35] Such precedents help explain why the debate over late births attracted such a broad and engaged audience.

Without a single institutional center, the medical community found it difficult to enforce consensus within the ranks. As Terry Parssinen has observed, the values and norms of the medical community were constantly

94

in flux. This was true in France as in England. The profession encompassed distinct, sometimes competing groups, each of which defined community standards differently.[36] There was room within the profession for those drawn to the purely scientific aspects of medicine as well as for those imbued with humanitarian impulses. Even the criteria for selecting the most celebrated physicians of the Faculty of Medicine of Paris were elastic and diverse. Hazon listed four groups worthy of inclusion in his 1778 review of famous physicians of the Faculty. Included were famous practitioners; savants who wrote; men of rare virtue; and finally those who, by their zeal, rendered important services to the Faculty and the public.[37]

Moreover, definition of the ideals and duties of the medical practitioner was not left solely to the medical community. Philosophes, government and church officials, and the general public—especially women—expressed their expectations of doctors and surgeons in society. The interaction between physicians and their clients made medicine especially susceptible to the influence of public opinion, pulling it in sometimes contradictory directions. Unlike men of science, physicians followed a well-defined career path that offered rich financial rewards to those who could attract a large clientele or hold various positions at institutions of learning, the court, and hospitals simultaneously.[38] Thus it was not surprising that, as Mme de Chastenay remarked, Fourcroy preferred the fortune of a fashionable doctor to the renown of an eloquent chemist.[39] The favor of women was considered crucial to such social and economic ascent because women were traditionally entrusted with the health care of their families and were reputed to influence institutional appointments.

Yet even as physicians were dependent on public esteem, they also exerted a good deal of influence over public opinion. After the Revolution, the duc de Lévis recalled the astonishing influence that a small number of eminent physicians exercised over their high-ranking patients, especially women, under the Ancien Régime.[40] De Chastenay, too, remembered that in those days, "Maman always believed she was sick, and I could not list all the famous doctors who came to the house." The importance of doctors could not be overemphasized: "they were sought out by the world of high society and they moved freely in it, without however being a part of it."[41] The advice of doctors was no less important to women of the bourgeoisie. Of Mme de Maraise, it is noted that "in the hierarchy of her preoccupations, health assuredly comes right after, if not before, the liquidity ratio."[42] De Maraise owned and consulted several books by doctors, including Tissot and Buchan.

Women were not, however, dependent on male medical practitioners for advice on matters of health, nor did they receive such counsel uncritically. The authors of *De l'éducation physique et morale des femmes,*

Riballier and Cosson, contended that it would be hard to assert the natural superiority of men over women because nature had given women, not men, the powers of self-sufficiency and self-preservation. It was from their mothers, after all, that women learned their knowledge of the simples.[43] De Maraise estimated her knowledge of medicine as highly as physicians' knowledge, telling friends that they could follow her advice as if it came from a doctor with the highest degree. Mme Roland found the articles on nursing in the *Encyclopédie* wanting, preferring the counsel of Petit but finding it necessary to correct Petit, too. She appealed to "honest women, tender mothers, not to believe deceptive art or blind sensibility, but to listen to and follow their hearts."[44] Similarly, Mlle de Malboissière disputed Bouvart's choice of remedies for her fiancé's scarlet measles and reproached him for his lack of sensibility.[45] Mme La Tour du Pin also expressed mistrust of celebrated physicians (this time, Barthez and Baudelocque) who gave her up for dead following the still-born birth of a daughter and the onset of scarlet fever. Hearing the doctors' pronouncement that La Tour du Pin would be dead within two hours, her maid sent for a surgeon who administered controversial remedies so forceful that the lady regained consciousness.[46]

The doctors and surgeons who wrote the most notable consultations on late births attracted public attention by writing, teaching, editing, and moving in elite social circles. They were just the sort of practitioners whom the duc de Lévis had in mind when he remarked on the astounding influence a few medical practitioners exercised, and anecdotes about them proliferated in journals like Grimm's *Correspondance littéraire* and Bachaumont's *Mémoires secrets* as well as in works like Sue's *Anecdotes historiques, littéraires et critiques sur la médecine, la chirurgie, et la pharmacie*. Collections of anecdotes like Sue's, which recounted amusing and incredible incidents occurring sometimes in the face of death, enjoyed a vogue in the late eighteenth century and were excerpted by various journals including the *Journal des dames* of 1766. Anecdotes about the physicians involved in the debate over late births later found a place in the memoirs and letters of people like Barbier, Brissot, Marmontel, the Marquis de Ferrières, Mme Suard, and Mlle de Malboissière as well as the duc de Lévis. By examining this literature alongside the official eulogies of the academies, we can explore the ways in which the personae of the figures in the debate were presented to the public and perceive how they contributed to the larger debate over the relationship between science and letters and the role of the physician in society.

While the consultations of physicians speak for themselves, a reading of contemporary journals gives us insight into how these reports and their authors were perceived by the public. Indeed, in the cases of Grimm's *Correspondance littéraire* and Bachaumont's *Mémoires secrets*, the authors' reputations influenced judgment of their work. Of the medical experts who wrote consultations on late births, Bouvart and Petit, who were best known to the public, embodied strikingly different images of the physician.

Both Bouvart and Petit were known for their rhetorical skill, but they seemed to use it for different purposes and with different effects. The *Correspondance littéraire* characterized Bouvart as a privileged butcher on the streets of Paris because of his penchant for slandering colleagues like Tronchin, Bordeau, and Petit.[47] Indeed, passions ran so hot in the debate over late births that the use of invective would itself become an issue. By 1769 the personal animosity between Bouvart and Petit had reached such a point that Petit complained to Sartine, the lieutenant general of police, about Bouvart's insults. Especially grievous was the fact that Bouvart had reproached Petit for his incorrect style, asserting slyly that Petit didn't know how to *coudre* (sew) his ideas together properly. The term *coudre* alluded to Petit's ignoble ancestry: he was the son of a tailor. Bouvart's use of the term, and the offense that Petit took at it, reveal that the tension in the Ancien Régime between the ideals of a meritocracy of talent and hierarchy by birth affected physicians as well as men of science and letters. D'Alembert's dream of ending the subservience of men of talent to the hereditary nobility had clearly not been realized.

While Bouvart was ennobled by the king in 1768, it was Petit who was hailed by the journals as the hero of the people. The *Correspondance littéraire* praised Petit's work for its logic, humor, integrity, and familiar style, while the *Mémoires secrets* credited Petit's eloquence with attracting large crowds to the Jardin du Roi. At the end of Petit's course, one student compared him to Jesus Christ. We are told that Petit responded to this outburst by shedding tears of joy, and all the spectators were moved by such a touching scene.[48]

As Anne Vincent-Buffault has observed, shedding tears in the late eighteenth century was a socially approved way of expressing sensibility. The most popular authors were not the philosophes like Voltaire or Diderot but novelists like Mme de Graffigny, Mme Riccobini, or Baculard d'Arnaud who made people cry. The experience of crying allowed readers to receive a moral lesson pleasurably and without the intervention of reason. Tears could engrave moral precepts on the soul and change a person's character without resort to philosophical speculation; rhetoricians who were able to move people to tears successfully fulfilled the Enlightenment principle of joining the useful to the agreeable. Cultivation of tears began in the salons and theaters but, as the scene described above implies, found a place in more academic realms like the Jardin du Roi as well and could transform a public gathering into a kind of political assembly.[49] Petit thus was an important figure in bridging the two spheres—science and culture—by bringing the values of culture to play within prestigious institutions of science.

Petit seemed not unwilling to cross the line distinguishing the professional from the charlatan if it were in a patient's interest for him to do so. Thus when a man, terrified by a charlatan's predictions that he would experience three attacks of convulsion, the last one fatal, appealed to Petit, Petit dressed up as a sorcerer and confirmed the charlatan's prognosis of convulsions, but concluded that the final attack would not be deadly. Petit spoke with such conviction that the patient's imagination was struck, and he was healed after following some simple remedies. The *Mémoires secrets* praised Petit for being more a philosophe than a doctor, in this case joining the talents of a consummate actor to extensive knowledge of anatomy, but noted that Petit was criticized by some doctors for degrading his profession.[50] Although Petit's ruse did not win widespread approval within the medical community in the 1760s, such strategems would later be endorsed by Pinel, a figure credited with introducing a revolution in the treatment of mental patients in the early nineteenth century.

The official eulogies composed for the academies echoed the images of Petit and Bouvart recorded in the journals. Following Petit's death in 1794, Latour, a doctor and *officier de santé*, composed a eulogy honoring Petit on the dedication of a bust of the deceased in the consulting room for the poor which Petit had endowed in Orléans. Latour praised Petit for his intellectual humility, sensibility, and compassionate concern for the fate of the individual and the good of society, as evidenced in his consultations on inoculation and late births. Especially praiseworthy was Petit's humanity in defending a virtuous woman and an innocent child.[51]

Petit's compassion for women and commitment to studying women's disorders did not, however, win him universal admiration, as the eulogy of the *officier de santé*, Tap, written in *an* III, reveals. Obstetrics and gynecology had traditionally been devalued by physicians who feared that their involvement in these matters would degrade the profession. Aspersions had been cast upon Petit's integrity, despite his prominence, as a result of his interest in women's health. Rejecting rumors spread by Deforges's *Femme jalouse* that Petit, a bachelor, was a true libertine,[52] Tap argued that there was nothing indecent in Petit's regard for women: no one cherished women more than Petit, nor had anyone rendered them such important services.[53] The fact that the issue of indecency was raised in the case of Petit, as it repeatedly was in attacks on charlatans including Mesmer, reveals the deep ambivalence of French society toward women's cultural influence. Defenders of what were characterized as "feminine values" could be discredited by insinuations that something more powerful than values (e.g., sexuality) motivated them.

The eulogy that Guenet offered to the Faculty of Medicine of Paris upon Bouvart's death in 1787 drew a very different portrait of how the exemplary doctor should treat patients and relate to women.[54] Guenet emphatically contrasted Bouvart's relationship to the public with those of the Swiss physician Tronchin and the numerous charlatans on the streets of Paris. Tronchin was physician to Diderot and d'Alembert; friend and confidant for a time to Rousseau; and an habitué of Mme Necker's salon. Whereas Tronchin and the charlatans gained public esteem through flattery and deception, Bouvart, Guenet maintained, owed his celebrity to an imperious tone emanating from unalterable convictions and unrelenting commitment to the truth.

Bouvart's enmity toward Tronchin had stemmed in part from the fact that Tronchin was not a member of the Faculty of Medicine of Paris and thus was not qualified to practice in Paris, despite the great popularity of his new methods of healing. But the conflict went further—to a fundamental difference in approach to patients. Bouvart, Guenet asserted, was no modish physician who, in order to gain popularity, would readily accede to someone else's ideas, amuse his patient, and confer momentary consolation in lieu of real, if painful, healing. He spoke with his patients very little and was convinced that they could not understand detailed explanations and that their fantasies regarding their diseases could provide him with little insight. Women, especially, Guenet tells us, were shocked by such treatment, but Bouvart was unrelenting, ferociously valuing candor and utility over sociability and sensibility.[55] Guenet thus drew a portrait of Bouvart the genius spending long hours alone at night in his study in pursuit of truths that could redeem humanity. It was an image that would, no doubt, have struck a responsive chord in Bignon as well as in later critics of salon society, including Poinsinet, whose play *Le Cercle ou la soirée à la mode* ridiculed the frivolity, intrigues, gallantry, ignorance, degradation, and unproductivity of salon society, including in scene 8 a compliant and silly physician. First performed at the Comédie Française in 1764, the play enjoyed such popular acclaim that it remained in the theater's repertory for seventy-six consecutive years.[56] Mercier's *Tableau de Paris* would present a similar portrait of physicians in 1781. Here the serious, pale, authoritative physician was contrasted with the agreeable, witty, ostentatious, incompetent fop.[57] Guenet's portrait of Bouvart was thus carefully constructed to present Bouvart as the antithesis of the salon doctor so well known to the theater-going public. In Guenet's eulogy, Bouvart's rigidity was seen as independence from the pressure of the people or the powerful and was regarded as the sign of a true savant.[58]

Condorcet, the other eulogizer of Bouvart, acknowledged that rigidity was one of Bouvart's defining characteristics but warned that superior intellect had to accompany such firmness; in mediocre men, intractability only amounted to stubbornness. He regarded Bouvart's early and unrelenting rejection of inoculation as a sign not of genius but of stubborn resistance to innovation. He found Bouvart's stubborn refusal to consult with physicians outside the Faculty of Medicine of Paris regrettable, noting that it would have barred him from discourse with some of the greatest physicians of the age, including Boerhaave, Sydenham, Stahl, and Morgagni, had they journeyed to France.[59]

Condorcet's eulogies are of special significance because, as secretary to the Royal Academy of Sciences and a prominent philosophe, he spoke for both organized science and the movement of enlightenment in France. The eulogies are all that Condorcet was able to accomplish of his goal of writing a history of the sciences; they provide glimpses of his vision of the direction the sciences and society should take. Framed to win the general public over to the cause of science and scientists, the eulogies were eagerly awaited and widely discussed by Condorcet's contemporaries outside the academy.[60] Those defining the exemplary physician bear a striking, if initially somewhat surprising, resemblance to the approaches taken toward nature and medicine by women like Mlle Plisson, Mme Necker, and Mme de Genlis.

At the beginning of his eulogy of Bouvart, Condorcet admitted that it was difficult to judge the work of physicians, for whom practice necessarily loomed larger than theory. No records were kept of the successes and failures of physicians, nor were detailed accounts of treatments published. As a result, the reputation of a physician was molded by public opinion or the claims of rivals, neither of which Condorcet considered reliable. That this should be so was, Condorcet inferred, evidence of the primitive state of medicine. He believed that medicine would be the last science to be perfected because simple, reliable medical facts and general and constant principles of medicine were difficult to establish.

As difficult as Condorcet said that it was to judge a physician, he proceeded to do just that, and the judgment was severe. Although Condorcet agreed with Bouvart that investigation of late births was difficult, particularly when the parties involved had an interest in obstructing truth, he rejected Bouvart's recommendation that an arbitrary limit to gestation be set. Given the uncertainty of science on the subject, Condorcet shared Plisson's belief that it was fairer and more reasonable to examine all the facts presented in each case, following the principle that the more an alleged fact goes against the common order of nature, the more it must be substantiated. Because a court decision would be based on medical judgements, the scientific evidence must be weighed all the more rigorously.[61]

Condorcet, like Guenet, contrasted Bouvart's treatment of patients

with Tronchin's, but with different effect. Bouvart, he noted, had a reputation for being more concerned with saving his patients than with
sparing them pain and did not hesitate to prescribe excruciating remedies
whose salutary effects were debatable. Condorcet interpreted Bouvart's
approach as based on a quest for mastery over nature and over his
patients. Bouvart expected his patients to submit to him entirely, an
approach that Condorcet found wanting, for it precluded attentiveness
to patients' suffering and responsiveness to their questions. On this point,
Condorcet's vision of the proper goals of medicine was closely aligned to
that of Necker. "The pretension of all the doctors," Necker observed, "is
to distinguish themselves from nature in order that their miracles not be
confused with hers. Their duty should be to join with her in such a manner
that it would be impossible to distinguish which of the two was at work."[62]

Tronchin's new method, which emphasized regime and consolation
over violent remedies, could not be reduced to a quest for mastery of
either nature or the patient.[63] Standing in fundamental opposition to the
norms of French medicine, his techniques had prompted a rethinking of
traditional treatments, particularly of women and children. Whereas Bouvart's aggressive approach worked with violent illnesses, Condorcet
believed that it was considerably less effective in chronic disorders. Tronchin focused on the moral dimensions of chronic illnesses, seeking to
discover his patients' sentiments by establishing a friendship with them.
Their confidence in-him enhanced his ability to heal even illnesses unrelated to the imagination. It was his patients' attachment to him that
distinguished Tronchin from his colleagues.[64]

Condorcet's approbation of Tronchin sounds very much like de Genlis's
praise of Tronchin's countryman, Michel Schuppach, a celebrated empiric
who lived on a mountaintop and, without any formal instruction, healed
nearly all those who sought his aid by focusing on regime and nutrition.
De Genlis admitted that some would call Schuppach a charlatan, but she
praised him for his spirit, sensibility, and agreeable conversation, pro-
nouncing him a doctor-philosopher.[65] Despite Condorcet's commitment
to protecting science from the onslaught of charlatanry, these were the
very qualities that he considered exemplary in a physician.

As the contrasting images of Bouvart and Petit presented in journals,
plays, and eulogies reveal, the values and norms of the medical community were in flux, and the questions that perplexed physicians regarding
their role in society paralleled those that preoccupied men of science and
of letters at the same time. Answers were shaped by the interaction of
the medical community with the Republic of Letters and would be revised
after the Revolution. Thus, although the major participants in the debates
were celebrated by their contemporaries and their busts or portraits displayed prominently in the halls of the Faculty of Medicine of Paris, later

critics would question the long-term significance of the debates and of the physicians who played such prominent roles in them. In the 1820s, the *Dictionnaire des sciences médicales* dismissed Bouvart as a man whose reputation depended more on his character than on his merit and, while initially declaring Petit one of the most accomplished practitioners and professors of the previous century, concluded that his works were few and unimportant, distinguished in neither content nor style.[66]

The presence of women was alluded to throughout the dialogue on science, medicine, and cultural authority, but the actual voices of women were often excluded from the press, to say nothing of the academies of science and medicine. For example, Mme Reffatin, the midwife who wrote to Le Bas on the subject of late births, was one of only two women to see her letters published in the *Journal de médecine, chirurgie, et pharmacie* in all its forty years of circulation. Another popular medical journal, the *Gazette de santé*, was blatantly misogynistic under all of its successive editors. Even dedicating one's book to one's wife, as Barbeu du Bourg did for his popular *Le Botaniste François*, was cause for comment, for it was envisioned by many as a notable, and not particularly desirable, deviation from custom.[67]

Because Reffatin and Plisson were not members of professional corps or prestigious academies, no official eulogies honored them after their deaths. In contrast to later commentators who singled out Plisson's essay on late births for its dispassionate analysis of the issues, contemporary commentators, including Sue, Louis's eulogist, denigrated her participation. He declared that Plisson's consultation amounted to a résumé of all the others. "Besides," he observed, "it does not seem that the reasoning and reflections of the author made much of an impression, since no one did her the honor of critiquing them. Perhaps this is the effect of French gallantry, which spares the writings of the fair sex; perhaps also our learned Naturalists have disdained entering the lists against a girl who had for her guide only nature and reason."[68]

Even journals that admired Plisson's work focused on her other writings. Thus the *Journal des dames* announced the publication of her odes in 1764, while *L'Année littéraire* enthusiastically endorsed her *Maximes morales d'un philosophe chrétien*, written in 1783, as a salutary alternative to modern philosophy.[69] Here Plisson asserted that evangelical ethics were completely in harmony with reason and that God had imposed an order on the universe that rational creatures were obliged to follow. Goodness consisted in conformity; evil, in deviation from order.[70] No mention was made of Plisson's earlier essay on late births which had acknowledged the possibility of aberrations from order in the natural world. Still, if women's voices were sometimes not given the courtesy of a reply or were subjected to severe sarcasm, they were not without influence. As a review of women's writings reveals, views were often strongly held; forthrightly expressed; and grudgingly, if indirectly, acknowledged. The confluence of the views of Condorcet—philosophe *and* man of science—with those of Mlle Plisson, Mme Necker, and Mme de Genlis bears testimony to this fact.

The themes of charlatanry, struggle for cultural authority, and quest for mastery over nature touched upon in the debate over late births would become ever more prominent by the 1780s. They would serve as a springboard for the controversy engulfing Mesmer, who seemed to some to be the century's consummate charlatan and to others to be the harbinger of a new regime for the body and for society itself. The next chapter will reveal how debate over the legitimacy of alternate modes of treatment and of the physician-patient relationship merged with reflections on the need to control bold and licentious women. Attacks on the feminization of culture would ultimately be transformed into conflicting accusations regarding who was responsible for the degeneracy and disorder sapping the vitality of the traditional institutions of the Ancien Régime. Radically different proposals for restoring the social body to health and harmony would emerge, but although the principles of hierarchy and privilege would be vigorously contested, commitment to patriarchy would be unanimous and would assume a sanctity unseen in the 1760s debate over late births.

CHAPTER FIVE

The Debate over Mesmerism,

1778–1787

Mesmer's Challenge

Approximately fifty years after François de Pâris was buried in the cemetery of St. Médard and twenty-five years after the collateral heirs challenged Renée's claim to a late birth, Franz Anton Mesmer arrived in Paris declaring himself the possessor of secrets that would transform medicine. He promised to heal those whom traditional medicine had failed to cure— the blind, deaf, epileptic, and paralytic victims of epidemics and smallpox as well as sufferers of cancer, gout, jaundice, ulcers, and hernias. Emphasizing the moral foundations of physical disorders, he eschewed the usual arsenal of remedies popularly rumored as likely to kill as to heal and focused instead on stimulating the sensibility of his patients in order to restore them to health.[1]

Mesmer not only offered a whole new cosmology by which to understand the causes of health and disease and bring patients into harmony with nature; he also provided a social milieu for healing that was vastly different from the somber, frightening, and incomprehensible private consultations offered by traditional doctors and surgeons. Challenging the conviction that the patient's only role was to obey, Mesmer encouraged his patients' active participation in their cure and devoted special care to establishing the right atmosphere for healing. As one contemporary observed,

> M. Mesmer's house is like a divine temple upon which all the social orders converge: abbés, marquises, grisettes, soldiers, doctors, young girls, accou-

cheurs, the dying, as well as the strong and vigorous—all drawn by an unknown power. There are magnetizing bars, closed tubs, wands, ropes, flowering shrubs, and musical instruments including the harmonica, whose piping excites laughter, tears, and transports of joy. Add to these objects the allegorical paintings, padded consulting rooms, special places designated for crises, a confused mixture of cries, hiccups, sighs, songs, shudders. One is forced to agree that this new form of spectacle is very tantalizing, requiring nothing less than the greatest genius to produce. So one finds at M. Mesmer's only creatures given over to pleasure or to hope.[2]

The wands, baths, mirrors, and musical instruments were theatrical elements to be sure, but all ostensibly employed for a higher medical purpose. They were the instruments of magnetization, intended to encourage crises of convulsions, expectorations, and evacuations. These crises were supposed to act upon the nervous system to restore the body's liquids and solids to their proper equilibrium.

This last notion of Mesmer's was not new; traditional doctors and surgeons employed an array of calmatives, evacuants, irritants, tonics, and baths to restore the body's equilibrium.[3] What was new was Mesmer's tactic of restoring this equilibrium not by physical remedies, but by bringing the action of a universal magnetic fluid to bear on obstructions within the nervous system. He taught that this universal fluid permeated all celestial bodies, the earth, and all sentient creatures. When its free circulation through the nervous system was obstructed, a person became ill. Health could be restored only by magnetization, which supposedly reestablished the mutual magnetic influence between celestial and human bodies, enabling the magnetic fluid to circulate freely again throughout the patient's body.[4]

Mesmer made immodest claims for his new method of healing. It could, he maintained, accurately diagnose the origin, nature, and progress of even the most complex diseases, halt their development, and restore the patient to health without exposing him or her to the dangerous repercussions characteristic of traditional physical remedies. Animal magnetism would, he proclaimed, bring the art of medicine to a point of perfection that had eluded traditional doctors and surgeons.[5] There was clearly no room in his epistemological universe for Hecquet's appreciation of the inscrutability of nature; for Bouvart's acknowledgment of the difficulty of interpreting the laws of nature; or for Petit's affirmation of the real, yet mysterious, causes of electricity and magnetism.

By devising a form of treatment that encompassed the old mystical tradition of healing by the touch of an exalted personage and the new mode of healing through nature's electrical impulses, Mesmer assured his theories a broad popular appeal. They were embraced by commoner and notable alike, though for quite different reasons. The theories enchanted the most superstitious and uneducated commoners, who remained convinced of the power of magic even in this age of Enlightenment. They proved no less fascinating to enlightened elites dabbling in what had become the most fashionable pastime of the day—popular science.

As increasingly larger crowds were drawn to Mesmer's healing spectacles, the crown began to wonder if the movement did not constitute the same kind of threat to public order and the authority of the state that the Convulsionary movement had been fifty years before. Once again, the crown appealed to the medical community for an assessment of the authenticity of such remarkable cures and the validity of the unorthodox doctrines associated with them. In 1784 it commissioned two inquiries into mesmerism, one to be conducted by a joint committee drawn from members of the Royal Academy of Sciences and the Faculty of Medicine of Paris, the other by members of the Royal Society of Medicine.

It should be noted, however, that the specific area of medical jurisprudence relevant to Mesmer's cures was different from that pertaining to the healings of the Convulsionaries of St. Médard. Whereas the medical experts in the earlier case had been asked to evaluate the validity of miracles, the commissioners in 1784 were to judge the legitimacy of an experimental method of healing. In the past, the medical community had proved most reluctant to endorse experimental or proprietary remedies because they represented an affront both to their understanding of nature and to their authority to regulate medical practice. Mesmer's case was thus bound to attract the interest of all who had attempted to gain recognition for unorthodox remedies as well as those who had benefited from them.

The Reports of the Academies

Both commissions challenged the legitimacy of the mesmerists' cures. The commissioners of the Royal Society of Medicine focused on the difficulty of proving the existence of an invisible fluid. They maintained that proof could be established only by the effects of the fluid in the form of internal sensations, healings, or convulsions. Yet internal sensations were often equivocal and illusory. Nor were healings demonstrable proof of the efficacy of animal magnetism because other factors such as exercise, the cessation of remedies, or hope could be responsible.[6] This was exactly the approach taken by Nigon de Berty in discrediting the healings of the Convulsionaries of St. Médard fifty years earlier and by Bouvart in rejecting Renée's claim to a late birth. Natural explanations were always preferable to miraculous or unorthodox ones. The commissioners of the Royal

Academy of Sciences and the Faculty of Medicine attended a number of lectures and healing sessions conducted by Deslon, Mesmer's most prominent disciple, and concluded that the crises characteristic of mesmerist cures could be attributed to three causes—touching, imagination, and imitation. Troubled by the spectacles attending mesmeric treatments, they urged that public treatments be discontinued.[7]

While the public reports of both commissions dismissed summarily and authoritatively the medical significance of animal magnetism, in secret the members expressed a deep anxiety over the threat of disruption the movement posed to the medical community and the social order. They worried whether traditional medicine could meet the standards of proof that they demanded of mesmerism. An extract of the registers of the Faculty of Medicine of Paris of December 1, 1784, reveals the extent to which mesmerism had aroused the concern of the Faculty. "The Faculty," the dean declared, "finds itself in a state of crisis that requires immediate help."[8]

Given the seriousness of the challenge facing the medical community, it was urgent that its members join together in asserting that "medicine is a real science, based on certain principles and on the experience of several centuries," contrasting it to magnetism, "a chimera that kills."[9] Identifying medicine as a "real" science along the model of physics was problematical, however, for as L. W. B. Brockliss has pointed out, eighteenth-century medicine lacked the mathematical base that invested physics with certainty and was stymied by problems of proof when it attempted to adopt the same evidential epistemology as physics.[10] It faced special hurdles when it came to nervous disorders, which were attributed to invisible and hence unquantifiable phenomena. The most perspicacious eighteenth-century inquirers into the mental origins of disorders thus tended not to be physicians, but novelists, correspondents, and memoir writers.[11]

Few members of the medical community felt comfortable with the alternative of judging the validity of medical science by the efficacy of its cures. The limitations of traditional medicine on this point were obvious, and even critics of Mesmer like M. A. Thouret, a commissioner for the Royal Society of Medicine, acknowledged that it was precisely in areas like nervous disorders that charlatans occasionally worked wonders.

Accordingly, the strategy the Faculty adopted for dealing with the mesmerist threat was to avoid plunging into the problem of epistemological certainty at any cost. Instead, it focused on public relations and prepared to wage a war of rhetoric unrivaled since the debate over late births in the 1760s. The dispute over prerogatives which had been waged for decades between doctors and surgeons would have to be stilled and more concerted efforts made to influence public opinion. It was suggested that playwrights, actors, and journalists be recompensed for attacks on mesmerism in the theater and the press and that books and articles investing mesmerism with the aura of enlightenment be removed from booksellers' shelves.

In addition to composing the much publicized report to the king, the commissions of the academy and the faculty submitted another report that they urged be kept secret. It expressed fully their fears of the threat that animal magnetism posed not to the physical health of its devotees but to the moral fabric of society. As such, the problem required a moral rather than medical solution. Like the medical consultants appointed by the government to investigate the Convulsionaries of St. Médard, the commissioners focused on the most radical, the most bizarre, and the most controversial aspects of mesmerism. Naturally, the preponderance of female proselytes attracted to the movement and their susceptibility to convulsions became foci of attack.

Like Hecquet, Astruc, and Bouvart before them, the commissioners argued that women were by nature more inclined to convulsions, just as they were more imaginative, emotional, and sensual. The relationship between the male magnetizer and his female patient, characterized as it was by touching and other forms of close physical contact, was in the commissioners' eyes fundamentally and dangerously erotic. They suggested that women, unreflective creatures after all, were stimulated by the emotions the magnetizers had aroused in them in the course of public treatments and sought to continue more advanced experiments in private—all, of course, in the name of medical science. "Exposed to this danger," they observed, "strong women draw away; the weak can lose their morals and sanity there."[12]

As in the case of the Convulsionaries, the social status of the female followers of mesmerism played an important role in determining the manner in which the medical community formulated its critique. Because these women came from a different stratum of society, though, their convulsions were diagnosed differently. The Convulsionaries generally came from the lower orders of society. Doctors had called into question the legitimacy of the illnesses and cures they experienced by alluding to their modest origins. Reasoning that women of their social status were peculiarly susceptible to vanity and greed, the doctors had discounted their testimony. In contrast, the women attracted to mesmerism came from families of considerable means or position and were more vulnerable to charges of frivolity or ennui than of deceit. "Most women who are drawn to magnetism," the commissioners declared, "are not really ill; many come either through idleness or for amusement."[13]

In an age in which salon society was coming increasingly under the influence of Rousseau's critique of culture, however, the charge of frivolity or idleness could seem as grave as that of fraud or deceit. Certainly a number of prominent women associated with the philosophes, including Suzanne Necker, Julie de Lespinasse, and Angélique Diderot, were known to have suffered nervous disorders and were suspected of using complaints about female troubles to assure that they would be the center of attention. Center stage was not, however, where the commissioners or Rousseau and his followers believed women should be.

In his *Letter to d'Alembert*, Rousseau had warned of the dangers the theater presented to corporative, patriarchal society: "See how this man [an actor], for the sake of multiplying his jokes, shakes the whole order of society; how scandalously he overturns all the most sacred relations on which it is founded; how ridiculous he makes the respectable rights of fathers over their children, of husbands over their wives, of masters over their servants!"[14] The threat posed by mesmerism might be seen as even more potent than theatrical performances, however, for the mesmerists had transferred the spectacle out of the salon, academy, and auditorium into the streets, transforming the whole city of Paris into a theater and its inhabitants into actors and spectators.

Attacks like Rousseau's on feminine frailties did not fail to gain public attention and sympathy. The public had already proven a ready audience for numerous treatises intended to transform the family and society by educating girls for their proper roles as wives and mothers.[15] Indeed, the composition of such a treatise was considered a first step for anyone with philosophic aspirations. These attacks on feminine frailties were aimed at individual girls or women and beyond them the larger issues already broached in the debate over late births: the seductive sway of aristocratic values and the feminization of culture.

Rousseau and his disciples evoked the fear that men were losing their natural virtue and culture its strength as men became increasingly like their inferiors, women, who were exercising an indirect, hence arbitrary, power over the appointments that men sought to academies and government offices. The abstraction, woman, thus became a symbol for the vanity, abuse of power, and degeneracy that seemed to characterize the later years of the Ancien Régime. Severe measures would have to be taken to end the domination of bold and licentious women and restore quality to the arts, letters, the social order, and the state.[16]

But the licentiousness imputed to women affected men in more than merely abstract terms. Susan Okin has noted that Rousseau returned again and again to the theme of establishing paternity. It appears not just in the *Discourse on Political Economy* and the first draft of the *Social Contract*, but also in *Letter to d'Alembert*, *Emile*, and *Emile and Sophie or the Solitaires*. She attributes Rousseau's obsession with the problem of establishing paternity to his exaggerated terror of contracting syphilis.[17]

In addition, as the debate over late births demonstrated, the threat that female promiscuity posed to a society preoccupied with the orderly transmission of property and status through inheritance can hardly be overemphasized. Thouret credited Maxwel, a famous charlatan whom he identified as Mesmer's prototype, with recognizing the taboo surrounding the topic of female promiscuity. "It is not prudent," said Maxwel, "to treat of such objects because of the dangers that can result. If one even spoke openly on this point, fathers could no longer be sure of their daughters, husbands of their wives, nor could women answer for themselves."[18] The controversy over the legitimacy of Renée's child reveals that the taboo alluded to by Maxwel was breaking down in the 1760s. By the 1780s, concern over the physical, moral, and social consequences of promiscuity would dominate public consciousness and spearhead movements for reform. Adultery was reputed to have sapped the vitality of the Ancien Régime, undermining the nobility's claim to superior virtue and the sacramental character of kingship.[19]

The commissioners closed their report by appealing to their sovereign's fear of social unrest. They warned that if the mesmerists' discontent were allowed to develop, it would grow beyond the capacity of any force to contain it. "Nothing," they warned the king, "prevents the convulsions from becoming habitual and from spreading in the cities into epidemics, extending to future generations."[20] This language was strongly reminiscent of that employed by Hecquet when speaking of the Convulsionaries fifty years earlier. The added allusion to a threat to future generations could only have heightened the concerns of officials who had become increasingly attuned to the connection between healthy citizens and a healthy economy and fearful that the sexual deviation associated with the aristocracy would lead to the suicide of the French race.

If the disorders for which Mesmer's followers sought cures were primarily moral, so too should be the cures. Commissioners and critics outside the medical community urged that the physical and social ills of society be treated by restoring and purifying the traditional values of hierarchy, privilege, and paternity. One writer, Devillers, objected to mesmerism because it challenged the notion that man was different from the rest of creation. Nature, he maintained, was the womb from which all things come, but without being brothers. Chastising the mesmerists, he exclaimed, "You would have vegetables enter our family; by this reasoning you would extend our lines of kinship to the mineral realm; for the rocks, the metals are, like us, the work of the Omnipotent. What a strange abuse of these words, "Nature is a common mother!"[21] Such reasoning had obvious social and political implications that gave traditionalists like Devillers pause: it would destroy any natural justification for hierarchy in society and the state.

Other writers attacked the mesmerists for promising miraculous cures or relief from suffering which were beyond human capacities to achieve. Suffering, they declared, could never be entirely obliterated, and the mesmerists did their patients and the medical profession a disservice by encouraging false hopes that it could. Particularly annoying to these critics was the notion that women might be able to escape the pain of childbirth through animal magnetism. Such a promise could not hope to be fulfilled, argued the most conservative critics, nor should it be, for according to Genesis, the labor of childbirth was inflicted upon women as a punishment for original sin. Forever after, "woman gives birth in pain."[22]

Just as childbirth was considered an intrinsic part of women's role, so too, increasingly, was breastfeeding. Nursing was seen by Rousseau and his followers as a way of demonstrating maternal commitment, of requiring women to focus their attention on something other than their own passing pleasures. It could serve as part of the cure for what Thouret believed was the cause of most of the nervous disorders troubling elite women. Deprived of any meaningful activity, these ladies sought relief from their "indolent and monotonous" existence in a rich fantasy life. Why not provide these women with some appropriate occupation, thus discouraging "lascivious ties and sensual reflections"?[23]

Numerous leaflets circulated at this time in support of nursing. They suggested that refusing to nurse was a sin against nature that violated sacred family bonds and endangered health. Most late-eighteenth-century advocates of maternal nursing refrained from arguing, as Hecquet had fifty years earlier, that nursing should be regarded as part of the punishment for sin. They did, however, agree with Hecquet that women who did not nurse were guilty of inhuman, impious, and adulterous conduct. A woman's infidelity in this case was not to her husband, but to her child. "Who does not see in this conduct a kind of infidelity in the woman?" Hecquet had exclaimed. "For if in ordinary adultery the woman gives her children a father who is someone other than her husband, in sending children out to nurse she gives the children of her husband a mother other than herself."[24]

In 1782 the surgeon Coupel wrote a letter to the *Affiches du Poitou* echoing Hecquet by alluding to the degeneration of family lines caused by adultery and vice. Coupel's approach differed from Hecquet's, however, in recognizing the devastating physical and moral impact on the family of male infidelity and the need for men to live up to the obligations their patriarchal authority entailed. Placing the mother who refused to nurse on the same level as the syphilitic father, Coupel declared, "If there is little difference between a wife who gives her children a father other than her husband and a barbarous woman who gives the children of her husband a mother other than herself, with what colors should we paint these indifferent, craven, or cruel men who strike a dagger into their sons' breasts and poison their spouses?"[25]

Not all proponents of maternal nursing, however, were necessarily advocates of a restoration of traditional values. Women supporters of maternal nursing spurned the adultery imagery of Hecquet and Coupel and propounded the sentimental rather than moral aspects of nursing. They focused on the enhanced relationship between mother and child that would result from maternal nursing rather than on the specter of marital infidelity and family deterioration in its absence. Thus the midwife Mme Le Rebours emphasized the rewards of nursing when she declared how sweet it was to have one's own children for friends. Following the Revolution, she would testify to her son's tender devotion, attributing it to maternal nursing and urging other women to follow her example.[26] Mme Roland's final words to her daughter in 1793 emphasized the special bond of intimacy that nursing had created, "Adieu, cherished child, you whom I have nursed with my milk and whom I would like all my sentiments to penetrate. I press you to my breast."[27]

Women also tended to be more frank and pragmatic in weighing the risks as well as the benefits of maternal nursing. They cited stories of infants contracting venereal disease from their hired nurses and of mothers suffering the ravages of milk fever, but also acknowledged the equally grave threats to which breastfeeding exposed women who insisted on nursing their children when they were ill or pregnant with another child.[28]

Given the intense rhetorical campaign in favor of maternal nursing, one is inclined to ask what sort of effect it had. Research indicates that despite the popularity of *Emile* and the wide circulation of literature in favor of maternal nursing, women's behavior across the social spectrum changed little during the late eighteenth century. In 1780 the lieutenant of police Lenoir estimated that of twenty-one thousand infants in Paris, only one thousand were being breastfed by their mothers.[29] Most aristocratic women continued to regard nursing as dangerous, animalistic, or an imposition. Bourgeois women, considering city air vicious, did not cease sending their young infants out to the countryside.[30] As Maurice Garden has documented in his study of Lyon, bourgeois women and well-paid working women were more likely to send children out to nurse than were poorly paid workers, even though the mortality rate of wet-nursed children was 50–66 percent.[31]

Garden has also demonstrated that among the working classes the practice of sending a child out to nurse was directly related to the work of the mother and the possibility of paying the child's *pension*. Wives working alongside their artisan husbands, silk workers, and women in the food trade thus were more likely to send their children out to nurse than were domestics, widows, hatters, and porters.[32] Contrasting the ideals of Rousseau which circulated widely among the provincial elite with the realities of working women's lives, Garden argues that administrators failed to grasp the social dimensions of the problem. The same may be said of physicians, who tended to attribute women's failure to nurse to their vanity and voluptuousness rather than to economic necessity.[33]

Still, some efforts were made to attack the problem on other than a moral level. The Royal Society of Medicine conducted experiments to find a safe alternative to mother's milk, but the project was doomed to failure until a process of sterilization could be perfected.[34] In Lyon, an Institut de Bienfaisance, financed by donations from private benefactors, was established for 112 working women who wished to nurse their children. Even as they tended to the economic needs of these women and children, however, the administrators emphasized the contribution they were making to public morality by requiring that the women it supported be married.[35]

The Mesmerists Respond

Mesmer and his supporters responded to their critics' attacks with a direct appeal to the people. Their strategy for attaining popular support was to expose their opponents' weaknesses while making themselves appear as unthreatening as possible. As a result, their perception of the epistemological limitations of medicine tended to be less penetrating and their vision of the proper constitution of the family more conservative than had been the case for some of the more radical supporters of late births in the 1760s. The cautiousness of the mesmerist camp can especially be seen in its discussions of the relationship between mind and matter, the phenomenon of convulsions, and women.

Although committed to radical reform of traditional medical theory and practice, Mesmer's disciples adamantly refused to concur with even the moderate critics that the basis of mesmerism's effectiveness lay in the imagination of the patient rather than in a magnetic fluid. Rather than articulating a new mental, emotional, or spiritual basis for health, the mesmerists insisted on meeting traditional medicine on its own terms by holding that all disorders, and all cures, had a physical basis. They did this because any challenge to the physical basis of a cure effectively brought into question the reality of the disorder itself.

Like the defenders of the Convulsionaries of St. Médard, Mesmer's disciples sought to deemphasize the importance of convulsions in healing and to downplay the presence of women in the public treatment rooms. Most healings, Deslon and Valleton de Boissière argued, took place without convulsions and involved "a crowd of sick people of all ages, sexes, social conditions afflicted with diverse disorders."[36] Those who insisted on grouping women together by gender without considering differences in their rank or personal qualities were chided for their lack of chivalry, for not being "more generous toward a sex on whom we confer no other arms than weakness."[37]

Mesmer's supporters seemed determined not to be drawn into a debate of the woman question. They did not relish being cast in the thankless role of defenders of women in an age in which misogynistic rhetoric still dominated both popular and enlightened literature.[38] It was safer to share their critics' distress over the degeneracy accompanying the feminization of culture. In contrast to their critics, though, the mesmerists held traditional medicine responsible for this degeneration and contended that animal magnetism alone could bring about the moral as well as physical regeneration of women. Even as Valleton de Boissière spoke of realizing women's potentialities, however, it is clear that he did not envision a broadening of their function. The value of animal magnetism lay in enabling women to give birth and to be beautiful, charming, and graceful by nature rather than art.[39]

Mesmer himself argued that animal magnetism, rather than dissolving social bonds, would reinforce the social order and enhance the authority of the fathers, mothers, and pastors to whom it was entrusted.[40] Rather than luring women away from the domestic circle, it would encourage them to fulfill their maternal roles by giving them the means to preserve the health and well-being of their families.

Mesmer's proposal of investing lay persons with the power of healing themselves resonated deeply among the public. During the eighteenth century, there was a pervasive feeling that the folk heritage of medicine, rooted in the notion that every man should be his own physician, was eroding. The loss of power the individual experienced over his or her health care paralleled and was linked to the loss of power local communities suffered as a result of the expanding state bureaucracy. A large medical self-help literature had grown up in opposition to the drive of professional doctors and surgeons, aided by the state and sometimes by the church, to take responsibility for community health care out of the hands of local empirics and of the people themselves. It is only within this context that the extraordinary appeal of Mesmer's attacks on tyrannical medicine, which he claimed seized man from the cradle and weighed on him like a religious prejudice, can be understood.[41]

Mesmer's challenge to the authority of traditional institutions would become more strident in his followers, who attacked both the conservatism of the medical elite and the ignorance of country surgeons, arguing that the medical community had fallen far short of Descartes's vision of what an enlightened science of medicine might accomplish. In the *Discourse on Method* (1637), Descartes had observed that all that men knew was almost nothing in comparison with what remained to be known and speculated that humanity could be free of an infinitude of maladies of mind and body if sufficient knowledge were gained of their causes and the remedies to be found in nature.[42]

What had gone wrong? Why had the progress Descartes envisioned not been realized? Like Tronchin, the physician who had gained the esteem of so many philosophes, including Diderot, d'Alembert, and Condorcet, the mesmerists contended that the medical community had erred by seeking to master rather than find guidance in the workings of nature. Paraphrasing what he imagined Nature would say to these overweening doctors and surgeons if she could talk, the lawyer Servan wrote,

> "Remember that for four thousand years you have not ceased to disturb, torment, shatter all my works in order to make by yourselves what you call an art. How much work and what effort! You have devastated the vegetables, cut the throats of animals, extracted minerals, dissected cadavers, penetrated the most hidden parts. Then you have boasted of your discoveries, the masterpieces of your imagination and industry, throughout the world. Be sincere and answer me: Have you lengthened the life of man? Have you healed any more ills than I have? Have you at least assuaged them? Have you not, on the contrary, augmented them?"[43]

One of the most eloquent defenders of mesmerism, Servan had served as *avocat général* at the Parlement of Grenoble, where he had taken on important and controversial cases. Although the specific points Servan argued varied according to the case, all his cases seem to have been precipitated when private interests like honor or love were violated or pitted against each other and became an object for public concern.[44] In 1765, Servan's address to the Parlement of Grenoble on the need for lawyers and judges to study philosophy had created a sensation. In law, he had argued, philosophy's love of humanity was put into action.[45] Servan's contribution to the controversy surrounding mesmerism reveals, however, that by the 1780s, arguments for reform were best advanced in another venue—the court of public opinion.

The forcefulness and popularity of Servan's critique provides an important qualification, at least in the domain of medicine, to Carolyn Merchant's searing portrait of the exploitation of nature and the domination of women which the rise of modern science entailed.[46] Merchant makes a convincing case for the invasive character of the language of early modern science, one that might equally well apply to medicine. Yet although twentieth-century scholars seem not to have noticed these characteristics before the publication of Merchant's book, one should not infer that the significance of this language went unnoticed or unchallenged in the eighteenth century. The debates over the role of the physician in society and over mesmerism gave expression to two competing and diametrically opposed approaches to nature and allowed the public to decide which should prevail. The fact that these debates were intense, prolonged, and far reaching indicates that the choice was not easy.

But the mesmerist supporters found fault with more than the traditional medical community's approach to nature. For them, an equally important factor in the lack of medical progress lay in corporative rivalries. Their attacks extended to corporative society as a whole. Identifying traditional corporative institutions as the source of all physical and moral ills, mesmerist supporters suggested that the medical community and the state had an interest in perpetuating the physical debility and moral decay of the people. The false needs and excessive desires stimulated by civilization had created the dependence essential to the functioning of the absolute state. Were these needs and desires to become less compelling, the bond of sociability would be lost, and the raison d'être of the state with it. Reform in people's enervated physical regime could precipitate a change in their temperament and lead to demands for freedom and equality. The more radical proponents of mesmerism suggested that the state had encouraged and profited from the lack of medical progress in the early modern period and was committed to preserving the status quo. As one Mandevillian writer observed, "Among us, the medical corporation is a political corporation whose destiny is linked with that of the state and whose existence is absolutely essential to the state's prosperity. Thus in the social order, we absolutely must have illness, drugs and laws, and the distributors of drugs and laws have perhaps as much influence on the customs of a nation as the trustees of its laws have."[47]

The Debate Moves to the Countryside

The tension created by corporative rivalries reflected in this mesmerist rhetoric found full expression in the provincial press and in Thouret's correspondence with provincial doctors and surgeons on the subject of magnetism. Thouret edited and published extracts of this correspondence in 1785, a year after his *Recherches et doutes sur le magnétisme animal* had been published and circulated in the provinces. On the basis of this correspondence, Thouret claimed that the appeal of animal magnetism was far from uniform. It seemed to arouse greater popular excitement in Guienne, Brittany, and Lyon than it did in Provence and Languedoc. University centers like Montpellier and Rennes proved less likely to succumb to the craze than uncultivated towns like Marseille and St. Malo. In Loudun, where the memory of Urbain Grandier and the nuns who had accused him of sorcery in the 1630s was still strong, mesmerism failed to take root at all.[48]

In his introduction to the *Recherches*, Thouret reiterated the medical arguments against animal magnetism and concluded smugly that no medical body in France had endorsed the new healing method. A study of the archives of the Royal Society of Medicine preserved in the Académie Nationale de Médecine in Paris reveals, however, that Thouret's extracts of letters from provincial correspondents were highly selective. The impression of consensus within the medical community conveyed by Thouret's survey is not borne out by an analysis of the letters themselves. This archival material throws into question Robert Darnton's characterization of the mesmerist controversy as a conflict between insiders and outsiders, professionals and nonprofessionals, those who had a stake in preserving corporative privilege and those who did not.

Although it is true that the doctors and surgeons who corresponded with Thouret supported the society's strong stand against animal magnetism, several mentioned that other doctors or surgeons practicing in their region had become devotees of mesmerism. Not only doctors and surgeons, but other prominent figures including curés, government functionaries, and military men had received instruction and begun practicing animal magnetism in the provinces. It is clear from this correspondence that traditional alliances between the state, church, and medical community were breaking down.[49]

Provincial doctors and surgeons who opposed mesmerism tended to interpret their colleagues' espousal of it as a personal affront and a betrayal of trust for the medical community at large. They regarded the mesmerists as simply the latest and most celebrated representatives of a large group of charlatans who competed with the professional medical community for a limited clientele. Declaring themselves *épiciers, herborists, oculists, botanists,* or *chymists,* these charlatans claimed to possess the secret remedy that could cure all ills. Sporting impressive but chimerical titles and bearing all the trappings of nobility, including servants and hunting steeds, they put on a fine performance intended to awe an impoverished and gullible public.

To critics like Maury, a doctor from Sezanne and editor of the *Journal de Nancy*, the people's fascination with such panaceas seemed to signal a regression of culture, for it bore an uncanny resemblance to the absorption in magic, rhabdomancy, and pyretomania a century earlier.[50] Although the provincial doctors and surgeons wrote numerous heated letters to the Royal Society of Medicine complaining about charlatans in the countryside, the society was ill equipped to offer them more than moral support.[51] The society's inability to act decisively reveals the limitations of authoritarian institutions in a supposedly absolutist state. Effec-

tive power was constantly undermined by the need to balance and manipulate different power groups.[52] Even after the commissioners had
denounced mesmerism, local journals continued to print testimonials from
curés who had employed animal magnetism to cure everything from tooth-
ache to hydropsy. Such endorsements, which appeared frequently in
advertisements, were considered more crucial to the popular acceptance
and commercial success of a remedy than the recommendation of any
scientific academy or faculty of medicine.[53]

The only recourse left to disgruntled doctors and surgeons was to enlist
the aid of the local prosecutor and lieutenant of police. Because doctors
and surgeons seldom succeeded in eliciting public support for such under-
takings, however, neither of these officials approached the task with great
alacrity.[54] In Nantes when the dean of the Faculty of Medicine, Bonamy,
complained to the lieutenant of police, the magnetizer Boissière simply
ceased public treatments and was allowed to continue his private cures
in secret undisturbed.[55] In Millau en Rouergue the local doctor, Pelet,
had no recourse at all, for he discovered that the local prosecutor had
himself become a member of the Society of Universal Harmony.[56]

The most effective means in the provinces of arousing public support
for action against the charlatans was the same one employed by the
medical bodies in Paris against the mesmerists: to focus on the moral
threat that charlatanry posed. Thus when Maury, a doctor practicing in
Sezanne, sought to discredit the claims to miraculous cures made by the
marchand épicier Le Blanc, he noted the opulent appearance that Le
Blanc had assumed in order to beguile the "little people." In addition,
he alluded to Le Blanc's illicit relationship with a young girl who gave
birth every year to a new infant who, curiously enough, died shortly after
birth.[57] Although some doctors, like Maury, only insinuated that charlatans were providing women with abortifacients, others like Robin de
Kiervalle, a doctor practicing at Josselin in Brittany,[58] and Doucet, the
surgeon of Frolois près Ste. Reine in Burgundy,[59] braved the demands of
delicacy to describe explicitly how charlatans in their communities
actually trafficked in abortions.

The demand for abortifacients was reputed to be so great that traffic
in them seemed a sure way to revive a languishing practice. Advertisements for such remedies appeared frequently in the provincial journals
and escaped censorship because they called the remedies "restoratives"
that would rid women of all manner of obstructions and restore order
and regularity to the menstrual cycle.[60] Baraillon, a Royal Society of Medicine correspondent practicing in Chambon en Combraille, described the
practice of one charlatan in this manner: "A would-be surgeon, left
ignored in his home village, proclaimed himself a man who *healed moth-*

erhood, treated the spleen, restored the disordered womb (sacred terms), and his house was immediately filled with patients."[61]

Allusions to charlatans trafficking in abortions were bound to reverberate in a Christian culture. They also served to demarcate professional doctors and surgeons, who were faithful to the Hippocratic oath, which specifically forbade abortions, from empirics and charlatans, who were not bound to it. In ancient Greece, the article prohibiting abortions had been important in distinguishing Hippocratic doctors, for the prohibition of abortions went against common medical practice. Hippocratic doctors prided themselves on adhering to a much stricter dogma than that embraced by most of their colleagues. Emphasizing purity and holiness, this dogma held that the embryo was animate from the time of conception and that sexual intercourse was acceptable only for the purpose of procreation. In the Christianization of Europe, the Hippocratic oath had served as a means of bridging the gulf between classical and Christian cultures.[62] Perhaps it could bolster the waning authority of the traditional values of hierarchy, privilege, and patriarchy in early modern Europe.

Women empirics were even more subject to insinuations about their dubious morality than men. A letter from a subdelegate to an intendant in Champagne regarding a woman's illegal medical practice typifies the reaction of authorities to women empirics. Marguerite Lany of Charny-le-Bachot had been arrested and convicted of illegally practicing medicine. After spending six months imprisoned in Troyes, she was released on condition that she not return to her village and that she refrain from practicing medicine. The pledge proved impossible for her to fulfill; not only did she return to Charny-le-Bachot, but she was besieged by people who came from as far as ten leagues away to seek her cure. Even the harshness of her remedies, which consisted primarily of bleedings and purging, did not daunt them. Appealing to the intendant for direction, the subdelegate remarked, "This woman has never had any smattering of medicine. She is subject to wine, was seduced as soon as her age and figure permitted, and prostituted her little girl who lived with her. Finally, sir, she is one of those detestable subjects whom it would be advantageous to purge from the country and even the realm, if possible."[63]

Dubious morality was attributed not just to empirics but to midwives as well and reflected the intensified campaign of church, state, and medical community to bring midwives under closer regulation and control. Cazabonnu, a surgeon practicing in Toulouse, observed that the midwives he knew were "very ignorant, knowing neither how to read, nor write. . . . Because they are called only by the women of the people, they earn very little. Almost all make up for this meager income by receiving every sort of creature and courtesan and continuing their trade in intrigue and prostitution, to the great scandal of their quarter."[64] The charge of prostitution was commonly levied against women empirics and midwives because midwives, like prostitutes, knew how to terminate, as well as advance, a pregnancy.

The knowledge that midwives derived from traditional sources was regarded with suspicion by the medical community and with apprehension by some members of the general public. This knowledge seemed to endow the women with a peculiar, even illicit power. As specialists in female beauty and the art of seduction, midwives were thought by the common people to hold the secret of the difference between the sexes, and it was believed that they could make women fertile or cause sterility.[65] They were also often the only recourse for young, unmarried girls who found themselves pregnant. The midwives would typically keep the pregnancy secret but, in accordance with the Edict of Henri II, could attest that the birth was not accomplished clandestinely. Once an infant was born, the midwives would take it to be baptized and discreetly place it with a nurse or in a foundling home.[66]

Unfortunately, the anger vented by members of the medical community against charlatans often played itself out on their patients as well. Pujol, a Royal Society of Medicine correspondent practicing in Castres, prided himself on his Enlightenment credentials and wrote with dismay that his town had entirely lost its senses and was possessed by the demon of magnetism.[67] Finding it impossible to convert his patients to his viewpoint, Pujol found himself in extreme cases compelled to manipulate their superstitions in order to effect healings. On one occasion, Pujol admitted that he had been afraid to administer febrifuges to a woman who was six months pregnant and in danger of miscarrying as a result of a double tertian fever. "I thus made the most of the circumstances," he confessed: "a sorcerer did his work; my imbecilic patient was healed suddenly and without remedy by the very fact of her stupidity."[68]

Pujol was unusual in meeting the public at its own level by resorting to a sorcerer's aid in his treatment. More typically, doctors in the countryside would angrily abandon their benighted patients to their own devices and feel vindicated if the patient became worse or died, as they were sure he or she must. The superior moral tone affected by many provincial doctors and surgeons is epitomized in a case history detailed by Meillardet, a doctor practicing at the military hospital in the town of Gray: "Here is something singular and amazing at the same time. A poor girl took it into her head to profit from a contagion of dysentery and to pass off an abortion and its effects for dysentery. But was this unfortunate girl mistaken! Because the treatment for the one is very different from that for the other, she was not long in becoming the victim of her bad faith in declaring her state. She was dead in a very few days."[69]

The Ambivalence of the Provincial Press

The determined opposition to mesmerism of medical practitioners like Pujol and Meillardet stands in striking contrast to the lay public's ambivalence to the phenomenon reflected in the coverage of the provincial journals.[70] The attitude of the editors of these journals toward mesmerism was much the same as their attitude toward any other kind of medicine practiced by empirics. Even as they wrote editorials deploring the ill effects of the empirics' remedies and printed the letters of doctors and surgeons denouncing the empirics, they felt no compunction about printing advertisements praising these same remedies and giving instructions about how to obtain them.[71] Perceiving the news value of mesmerism, whether as a milestone in the history of medicine or simply in the history of the human spirit,[72] the editors printed long excerpts of the reports of the commissioners denouncing mesmerism alongside equally long excerpts of Mesmer's appeal to the Parlement of Paris attacking the commissioners and the elite bodies they represented for their despotism.

In addition to the commissioners' reports and Mesmer's letters, the two writings on mesmerism which appeared most frequently in the provincial journals were extracts of Thouret's *Recherches* (1784) and a work by Paulet entitled *Mesmer justifié* (1784). *Mesmer justifié* opened with an elaborate depiction of the scenes typifying mesmerism's public treatments and was followed by an equally detailed description of Mesmer's theories. It then attacked the Society of Universal Harmony for charging all those interested in mesmerism or seeking healing an entry fee of one hundred louis, hinted at the lasciviousness underlying the cures, and described the violence of the crises and the death of one of the movement's most prominent disciples, M. Court de Gebelin, a few paces from the mesmerist tubs. All this was done tongue-in-cheek, under the pretense of defending the movement.[73]

Rather than printing extracts of the body of the work, however, most provincial editors printed only the opening paragraphs, which likened Mesmer's house to a temple to which people of all estates were drawn with the happy confidence that they would be healed. The music and laughter characterizing Mesmer's public treatments were placed in stark contrast to the fearful silence and painful remedies that marked the private consultations of traditional doctors with their patients. This contrast was followed by a long description of the magnetizer's techniques, which amounted to a guide for simulating Mesmer's treatments oneself. Although the descriptions of the public treatments and techniques were followed by caveats about the fatuous or untested nature of animal magnetism, these disclaimers had little force against the seductive power of the paragraphs preceding them. For all the editors' claims of impartiality, the effect of their editing strategies was to weight the dispute as much as possible in Mesmer's favor without provoking the ire of the commissioners or the censors.[74]

Although the provincial journals published the rulings of the commissioners on mesmerism and on other new medical techniques like medical electricity and natural magnets, even they had begun to grow weary of the unwillingness of the medical community to approve any of these remedies. Thus the editors of the *Affiches du Dauphiné* shared the frustration of the editors of the *Journal de Paris* when they remarked that the spirit of skepticism, having become so fashionable, had perhaps gone too far.[75] Were not, for example, the testimonies of hundreds of patients and twenty celebrated doctors adequate to convince the enlightened medical community of the benefits of medical electricity? By the 1780s, it was enough for the ordinary lay person to observe the successful cure of a neighbor through animal magnetism in order to be convinced of its benefits, all the scholarly reports of government commissions to the contrary notwithstanding.[76] Public opinion had effectively become the final court of appeal, surpassing the authority of church, state, and academy more so than in the 1730s or even the 1760s.

Conclusion

As the medical community found its competence and authority challenged in the controversy over mesmerism, it derived little support from its traditional alliance with the church. In their efforts to establish an enlightened science of medicine, many doctors had made a point of dissociating medicine from its theoretical and administrative links to theology. Unlike Hecquet, enlightened doctors in the 1780s sought not to admire but to control nature. The fact that this goal eluded them gave rise to anxiety over the limitations of man rather than admiration of the majesty of God. In addition, reports that local curés were as likely to side with the magnetizers as with the correspondents of the Royal Society of Medicine reveal that the traditionally close cooperation between the medical community and the church was breaking down.

Increasingly unsure of its own power base, the monarchy did not dare attempt to end the mesmerist controversy through an act of authority, as it had when it closed the cemetery of St. Médard on the Convulsionaries in the 1730s. This is not to say that the crown was not worried over the mesmerists' threat to the principles of hierarchy and privilege. It feared, however, that any autocratic attempt to stifle the movement would only stir the fires of discontent among moderates. In the more authoritarian regime of Saint-Domingue, which was dominated by the younger sons of noble families seeking political and administrative authority denied them in France, the crown did not hesitate to proscribe the practice of animal magnetism among blacks in 1786.[77]

Finding themselves unexpectedly on trial, the commissions appointed to investigate mesmerism attempted to mitigate the appeal of the movement by focusing on its most radical and controversial aspects, and this is where the issue of women became pivotal. Mesmer's critics sought to undermine the authenticity of the mesmerist cures by questioning the reality of the *maladies des femmes* they were employed to heal. In cases where they could not discredit the movement by demonstrating the ineffective or dangerous nature of its cures, they hinted at the threat to public morality which the supposedly illicit relationship between the practitioner and his female patient posed.

The allusions these critics made to the mesmerists' moral irregularities provided an opportunity to broaden the debate considerably and to raise issues regarding salon society which had already been touched upon in the debate over late births. Women's influence on culture was linked to the abuse of privilege which seemed to be responsible for the degeneracy of the Ancien Régime. If women were made to submit to patriarchal authority, quality could be restored to the arts and letter, virtue to society, vitality to the race, and stability to the state. Such a course aimed at renovating, rather than eradicating, traditional values of hierarchy, privilege, and patriarchy.

The mesmerists, however, even as they challenged the principles of hierarchy and privilege, remained committed to the restoration of patriarchy. On this point, they proved more conservative than the most visionary supporters of late births like Le Bas in the 1760s. Accusing the medical community of contributing to the decline in public morality, mesmerists promised to bring human laws back into harmony with the laws of nature. Duty and authority would be fused. The obedience of children would be transformed into the obedience of subjects, the union of brothers into the union of citizens, the love of family into the love of country.[78] Such a restoration depended on the restoration of the patriarchal family, with women ministering to the needs of their husbands, children, and country. On that point, both sides could agree.

How do we account for the mesmerists' separation of patriarchy from hierarchy and privilege? If it seems logically inconsistent, it was nevertheless politically astute. This same separation occurred during the Revolution, when political radicalism was often accompanied by socially conservative attitudes toward the family. As François Furet and Denis Richet have observed, the "Revolution was not caused only by economic and social conditions, but also by anecdotes, scandals, and accidents exposing the licentiousness of the elite."[79] Moral reform was regarded as the necessary precondition of social and political reform. One might say that the inflammatory rhetoric generated by eighteenth-century medical causes célèbres reached its height in the mesmerist controversy, furthering certain Enlightenment goals for reform even as it undermined others.

CHAPTER SIX

Ignorant and Superstitious or Overly Refined? The Convulsive Female in Physicians' Critiques of Culture

The debates over the Convulsionaries, late births, and mesmerism reveal how sexual symbolism was employed by opposing sides either to maintain the social order or to promote change. Issues of gender and social condition merged in the scrutiny of traditional values of hierarchy, privilege, and patriarchy. At a certain point, however, advocates of the Convulsionaries as well as of mesmerism abandoned the traditional association of patriarchy with hierarchy and privilege. They fervently disputed the legitimacy of organizing society and the state on the basis of hierarchy and privilege but ultimately disavowed radical reform of gender roles or of family structure. In the 1780s, Mesmer reaffirmed the Jansenists' endorsement of patriarchy of the 1730s, though he cast it in a more modern light, under the guise of the cult of domesticity. Only in the 1760s debate over late births do we see a thoroughgoing reappraisal of women's role, but even then women were readily associated with spectacle and charlatanry in order to discredit the philosophes. A serious reappraisal of the ideal of patriarchy entailed hazards for even the most committed reformers.

The debates over medical causes célèbres involving *maladies des femmes* illuminate larger social and political tensions, but the questions of how these tensions affected the actual medical treatment of women and of why women were drawn to unorthodox cures of the sort promised by the Convulsionaries or mesmerists remain unanswered by the causes célèbres literature. To understand the impact of ideology on the quality of health care afforded women in the eighteenth century, we need to shift our focus from the general to the highly particular and examine some of the many case histories concerning convulsions in the medical archives.

It should be noted that although the term *convulsions* was used in the medical *causes célèbres* literature to describe the spectacular crises that attended Convulsionary and mesmerist cures, it had a much broader meaning in the eighteenth century. The terms *convulsions, vapors,* and *hysterical affections* were commonly applied interchangeably to countless illnesses with similar symptoms, illustrating the lack of precision with which nervous disorders were diagnosed, if they were diagnosed at all. Over the course of the century, more than one hundred scholarly books were written on the subject, and advertisements for empirical remedies for nervous disorders appeared frequently in the provinical journals and almanacs.[1] But in 1782 the Royal Society of Medicine acknowledged that doctors could not agree on the causes of these disorders, much less on appropriate cures, and admitted that nervous illnesses were clouded in obscurity. As the celebrated physician Robert Whytt had commented in 1766, some doctors called any malady they did not understand a nervous disorder.[2]

Still, as L. J. Jordanova has observed, the importance of the nervous system could not be overemphasized. Because it linked the physical with the mental, it was believed to express the total state of the individual and to serve as a barometer of the impact of social change.[3] In his *Eléments de physiologie*, Diderot argued that most disorders stemmed from the nervous system and used his understanding of nervous disorders to inform his philosophical studies and arguments for reform.[4]

The representatives of the Faculty of Medicine and of the Royal Society of Medicine identified mesmerism with the cure of nervous disorders in an effort to undermine its appeal and significance. Physicians generally regarded such illnesses, as well as unorthodox methods of treating them, as frivolous if not illusory. It could be argued, though, that the very fact that mesmerism was associated with convulsions broadened its significance, for the problem of convulsions was more serious and pervasive than the reports issued by the Faculty of Medicine and the Royal Society of Medicine on the mesmerist cures would have one believe.

The medical critics of the Convulsionaries and mesmerism might well have emphasized the sexual overtones of the convulsions to discredit the movements and to divert public attention from their political significance. This emphasis, however, also indicates the suspicion and impatience with which many doctors regarded all nervous disorders, including convulsions. Nervous disorders had proved singularly unresponsive to the medical community's arsenal of physical remedies. Many doctors feared that unorthodox experiments like those of the mesmerists would undermine efforts to establish an enlightened science of medicine free from the superstitions of their rivals, the empirics.

Even as it accumulated information on the conditions that bred epidemics and epizootics, however, the Royal Society of Medicine was receiving numerous letters from provincial doctors who noted the widespread occurrences of convulsions in the countryside and asked for advice in treating them. The situation was becoming so critical that convulsions had been likened by one correspondent to a perpetual epidemic.[5] The Royal Society of Medicine finally responded to the pressure of this correspondence. Observing that "nervous disorders are very widespread, and have never been more common in the two sexes," the editors of the SRM *Histoire* announced a competition in 1782–83 for the best essay on their nature, causes, and cures.[6]

The fact that the Royal Society of Medicine solicited essays on the subject of convulsions in 1782 does not mean that speculation about them had been absent before then. By the 1760s, an Enlightenment model of the typically convulsive patient had gained credence among a broad segment of the enlightened medical community and the educated public. This model was presented in some detail in the *Encyclopédie* article entitled "Vapeurs."[7] The common conception of vapors was that gases emanating from the womb in women and the hypochondria (upper abdomen) in men rose to the brain and filled it with strange and extravagant ideas that provoked bizarre behavior. More sophisticated writers, who denied the existence of such gases, attributed the convulsions commonly associated with "vapors" to irritations rising from the nervous fibers of the lower abdomen to the brain.

Although these convulsions afflicted both sexes, women were thought to be more susceptible to them than men, the number of hysterical women seeming to exceed by far the number of hypochondriacal men. Urban aristocratic and bourgeois women were believed to be particularly prone by nature and emotional condition to convulsions. Strong uncontrolled emotions like anger, sorrow, fear, and disappointment were thought to provoke convulsions, as was unrestrained or overly repressed sexuality. Since the potential virulence of women's emotions and sexuality had been imaged in popular and scholarly literature alike throughout the early modern period, the notion that it should manifest itself in convulsions was readily received.[8]

If convulsions were rooted in woman's nature alone, their frequency should remain constant throughout history. Many enlightened writers, however, were convinced that the occurrence of convulsions, far from remaining constant, had increased dramatically over the course of the eighteenth century. They attributed this proliferation to the efforts of increasing numbers of bourgeois women to emulate the leisured, luxurious life-style of aristocratic ladies. It seemed as if, little by little, the fashions, language, and values of the nobility were being assimilated by the bourgeoisie. As the Goncourts note, "Every day there is a new elevation, a satisfaction of vanity, a usurpation. At the end of the century, one can scarcely distinguish the bourgeois woman from the great lady. The bourgeoise has the same coiffeur, the same tailor, the same accoucheur. What remains of the simplicity of bourgeois life . . . the intimacy of households? Everywhere one finds the usage of separate beds, which formerly signified a quarrel, a rupture, presaging litigation for separation.[9]

To the extent that the education of girls was blamed for reinforcing the ideal of the leisured lady, it was regarded as vicious and in need of reform. The increase in female literacy was viewed with mixed emotions by many writers who believed that the physical, mental, and moral health of women had been seriously impaired by their infatuation, borne of idleness and boredom, with vapid novels. As one contributor to the *Gazette salutaire* commented, "A girl who, at age 19 reads rather than runs, should be a vaporous woman by age 20 and not at all a good nurse."[10] Social commentators reasoned that the problem of convulsions in women would be substantially mitigated if girls were raised with the expectations and provided with the skills to fulfill their proper roles as wives and mothers.

The campaign for domesticity was waged on the artistic plane as well, as engravings of the works of Greuze and Moreau le Jeune circulated widely in books and almanacs from the 1760s onward. Texts including the *Encyclopédie*, Buffon's natural history, La Fontaine's tales, and Rousseau's *Emile* and *La Nouvelle Héloïse* were all lavishly adorned with Moreau le Jeune's engravings, which were analyzed in detail and often profusely praised in journals like *L'Avantcoureur*, *Mémoires secrets*, *Correspondance littéraire*, and *Journal des dames*. Capturing sentimental moments in family life, these engravings celebrated filial piety, love, and marriage and proved to be especially appealing to the bourgeoisie and the common people. They constituted a style of engraving termed "la gravure vertueuse," which stood in distinct contrast to "la gravure gallante," which tended to be more risqué and was reserved for the nobility. Lavreince was the most important representative of the second style. Not all artists were identified with only one style: on the eve of the Revolution, Debucourt worked simultaneously in both styles.[11]

Aristocratic and bourgeois women writers including Mme de Miremont, Mme Cosson, Mme Thiroux d'Arconville, Mme de Genlis, Mme Duplessy, Mme d'Epinay, and Mlle d'Espinassy[12] joined the men in excoriating the ignorance, timidity, idleness, and vanity traditionally bred in young girls by a convent education and arguing for the urgency of educational reform. They agreed that boredom was the greatest enemy of virtue and emphasized the importance for women of devotion to duty and commitment to work.

Thiroux de'Arconville, de Genlis, de Miremont, and Cosson saw education as a means of providing women with a greater measure of autonomy. Although most of these writers believed that increased autonomy could enhance the position of women in marriage, there was room for some skepticism. Thiroux d'Arconville was the most forthright in expressing doubts about the effects of marriage on women when she asserted that it was suitable only to a phlegmatic character. While fulfilling all the duties of wife and mother herself, she believed that marriage and dependence were inseparable; only with the death of her husband could a woman gain freedom.[13] Her ambivalence toward marriage was shared by Mlle de Malboissière, whom Alain Decaux characterizes as an exemplary young woman of the Enlightenment because of her impressive scholarly achievements. Despite a romantic sensibility, de Malboissière viewed marriage as a risk to happiness and liberty and commented that it was wise to marry women off young; otherwise, they wouldn't marry at all.[14] The reservations of women like Thiroux d'Arconville and de Malboissière had little impact, however, on physicians' treatment of women and did not lead to a new position for women in the social structure.

Social commentators linked convulsions in men, as in women, to a certain degree of alienation or maladaptation. Scholars and clerics who maintained a distance from society, preferring to spend their time thinking and dreaming, were thought to be particularly susceptible to convulsions. Ambitious men whose social advancement had been blocked were also considered prime candidates for convulsions.

The political explosiveness of the discontent manifested by convulsive men and women had been recognized by the editors of the *Encyclopédie* as well as by the critics of the Convulsionaries and of the mesmerists. Focusing on the psychological rather than the physiological bases of convulsions, the editors recommended employing the whole arsenal of traditional remedies as a last resort. First, the patient's regime should be simplified and purified, and his or her expectations of life brought into conformity with social reality. Rather than challenging the principles of social and sexual hierarchy upon which the Ancien Régime was based, the editors advised that "to form a true idea of one's meager knowledge and little merit, to believe oneself always favored, whether by fortune, the prince, or nature, beyond one's talents, to listen to reason and act in accordance with good manners, are the best means of protection against vapors."[15]

Although the Enlightenment model of convulsions articulated in the *Encyclopédie* was widely accepted by Parisian and provincial doctors alike, the correspondence that provincial doctors directed to the Royal Society of Medicine presented a very different picture. Having attempted to apply the Enlightenment model and found it wanting, provincial doctors began to formulate an alternative model that reflected the different environmental conditions, social tensions, and cultural configurations of the countryside.

If they differed dramatically from their urban colleagues in their analysis of the causes of convulsions, however, provincial practitioners agreed that domesticity was the proper cure. Here, as in the debates over the Convulsionaries and mesmerism, larger cultural critiques might vary, but in each, the principle of patriarchy was consistently reaffirmed. The models of convulsions advanced by urban and provincial physicians differed in the way they linked issues of gender and social condition. Like the critiques of mesmerism, the Enlightenment model of convulsions extended attacks on women to censure of a degenerate elite. In contrast, the provincial practitioners' model resembled critiques of the Convulsionaries by fusing distrust of women with fear of the ignorance and presumption of the lower social orders.

Only when confronted with the divergent models of convulsions offered by Parisian and provincial practitioners, did the Royal Society of Medicine begin to recognize the limitations of each. What had originated as supposedly objective diagnoses of disease had evolved into cultural critiques that proved to be of limited utility. By announcing its essay competition in 1782–83, the Royal Society of Medicine finally officially acknowledged the seriousness and pervasiveness of the problem of convulsions and recognized the need to devise better strategies for understanding and treating convulsive patients. That the problem was too complex for doctors alone to solve would become increasingly evident as the days of Revolution drew nearer.

This chapter examines the diverging models of convulsions that reflect the tensions of French society in the century of Enlightenment. First, it explores the broader question of the frequency with which convulsions were reported and the possible connections between stress and convulsions. Then it looks closely at case histories of convulsions occurring at specific phases of the female life cycle in order to test the prevailing wisdom that marriage was the most effective antidote to convulsions.

The Enlightenment Model versus the Reality of Convulsions in the Countryside

In the countryside, convulsions were reported as frequently and as routinely as fevers. The nosologic observations of Charmeil, chief surgeon of the military hospital at Montdauphin in the Hautes-Alpes, were typical of observations made by provincial doctors throughout France. In his report to the Royal Society of Medicine, Charmeil observed that "the acute rheumatism, angina, and inflammation of the lungs have continued to prevail without being unyielding. During these months there have been apoplexies and sudden deaths. The convulsive illnesses familiar to this region have been more violent than normal. Some verminous fevers have also appeared and have yielded to the appropriate remedies."[16]

Despite their frequency, the etiology of convulsions remained obscure. Spielman of Strasbourg believed they were hereditary and therefore incurable, while Terrède of L'Aigle focused on their sexual basis and treated his patients with camphor, bleedings, and cold baths. Serrez of Cologne prescribed poultices for two cases of convulsions which manifested very different symptoms—the first, severe infection; the second, a tumor. Oberlin of Strasbourg and others regarded convulsions not as a disorder per se, but as simply a symptom of fever.[17]

Many doctors, like Dablaing of Douai, and surgeons, like Borde of Thiers,[18] appealed in desperation to the Royal Society of Medicine for aid in diagnosing and treating convulsions that had stubbornly resisted a cure. Publicly, however, most doctors preferred to adopt a tone of confidence in their treatments. They tended to follow the pattern of Gallot, a doctor of St. Maurice-le-Girard who, publishing his nosologic observations in the *Affiches du Poitou*, remarked upon the stubbornness with which nervous disorders resisted treatment but refused to endorse the popular view that they were incurable. Seeking the most innovative medical education possible, Gallot had attended Antoine Petit's courses at the Jardin du Roi in 1764, taken his degree a year later at Montpellier, and returned to practice in Poitou. He was associated with more than eleven learned societies and was a frequent contributor to medical journals, to which he sent numerous letters at the expense of the intendant and under his countersignature. "Devoured by a fever for letter writing," he corresponded with Mme Necker about the possibility of establishing a network of small rural hospitals for chronic and incurable diseases, women in labor, and indigents and was one of the first persons in the Fontenay region to subscribe to the *Encyclopédie*. He was one of very few provincial physicians to be elevated from the rank of correspondent to provincial associate of the Royal Society of Medicine.[19]

With great self-assurance, Gallot proclaimed that nervous disorders could be cured by his herbal treatments and attributed the inefficacy of most cures to patients' procrastination in seeking treatment and carelessness in following prescriptions. In private, however, Gallot's hopes for his convulsive patients were considerably less sanguine. In a letter to the Royal Society of Medicine dated a year after the publication of his nosologic observations, he described the seemingly incurable case of a girl suffering from four distinct maladies, including nervous symptoms, after a fall. Like his colleagues, Gallot admitted that he was at a loss as to what remedy to employ and appealed to the Royal Society of Medicine for advice.[20]

Considering their own limited understanding of convulsions, doctors showed remarkably little forbearance with the failings of their patients. To the popular mind, vapors and convulsions had an aura of mystery, and charlatans frequently based their cures of convulsions on popular superstitions. As with mesmerism, some doctors used the issue of convulsions to attack the charlatans and berated the public, especially women, for ignorance and passivity in accepting the excuses of charlatans who sought to hide their incompetence by attributing the deaths of their patients to vapors.

In 1774 M. Nicolas, president of the college of doctors of Nancy, submitted a letter to the *Affiches du Dauphiné* in which he told how an empiric had induced horrible convulsions in a sixty-five-year-old woman suffering from an acute fever by subjecting her to thirty-two purgations in as many days. "The Medicaster," he remarked, "who knew only about Manna and Senna, was at the limit of his Latin; and taking care not to call a doctor whom the patient requested, he gravely assured some stupid little woman that she had hysterical vapors: a burlesque pronouncement, worthy of an exemplary and degrading punishment."[21]

Other doctors used the provincial press to publish their discoveries of successful, if unorthodox, cures. Often, however, one doctor's theory contradicted another's, as when Ingen-Housz announced in the *Affiches de Toulouse* that convulsions were provoked by flowers while Dufresnoy, practicing in Valenciennes, Flanders, attributed the cure of convulsions in one of his patients to the salubrious odor of narcissuses. The editors of the *Journal de Troyes* were skeptical of Dufresnoy's claims of having made an important medical breakthough by extracting the sap of the flowers and administering it to his convulsive patients. They concluded their coverage of the subject with the simple observation, "This plant is a poison."[22]

The consultants of the Royal Society of Medicine responded conservatively to their provincial colleagues' appeals for advice. They enumerated the available physical remedies while remaining noncommittal on the question of psychological dimensions that treatments might assume when physical remedies had been exhausted. When Boucher, a doctor from Grenoble, asked for advice on a case of convulsions that had not responded to diluents, purgatives, cold baths, and bleedings, the society's advisers Tessier and Neauroi recommended only a slight variation in treatment. They suggested mineral water, laxatives, warm baths, and bleedings. However, after itemizing the physical remedies that might be employed, they observed that the patient's ailments might have a moral rather than a physical cause, in which case their remedies would be useless. How to proceed from there was left to Boucher's discretion.[23]

Although there was still a strong sentiment within the enlightened medical community that convulsions, associated as they were with the life-style, sexuality, or emotional intensity of women, did not constitute a serious or even real medical problem, the provincial doctors' letters to the Royal Society of Medicine reveal that the effects of convulsions were not to be taken lightly. While their causes might be considered frivolous, the emotional and physical toll the convulsions took on women were not.

To the historian, the incidence of convulsions might be seen as an indicator of the emotional strain women suffered. Grief and fear, provoked by the fragility of life and the insecurity of existence, were recognized to be major sources of convulsions in the countryside. Although sudden and unexpected death was an everpresent fact of life in the eighteenth century, the insecurity of existence was not necessarily accepted with equanimity. Chifoliau, a doctor practicing in St. Malo, demonstrated what dire effects the news of a loved one's death could have on a young woman with the case of a twenty-two-year-old girl who was thrown into a deep melancholy and fits of convulsions upon learning of her fiancé's death. The girl's abdomen swelled; menstruation ceased. The local surgeon told the girl's parents that she was suffering from hydropsy, but rumor had it that she was pregnant with an illegitimate child. Chifoliau gave her tonics to induce evacuation of the water to no avail; the girl died. In his autopsy, Chifoliau discovered a monstrous tumor of the ovary. He had no doubt that it was a direct consequence of the trauma the girl had suffered.[24]

Examples of the havoc that fear could wreak on the nervous system were reported in the provincial papers and documented in the letters of provincial doctors to the Royal Society of Medicine. The *Affiches pour les Trois Evêchés et la Lorraine* in 1780 reported the story of a woman who dropped dead in horror at the sight of two neighbors being burned alive.[25] Taranget, a doctor practicing in the town of Douay and outlying villages, described the case of a young girl entering adolescence who was thrown into severe convulsions by a clap of thunder that came too close for comfort. Although Taranget employed the usual arsenal of remedies, including antispasmodics, baths, and bleedings, he was unable to break the girl's delirium. She died on the thirty-seventh day of treatment.[26]

Men were not exempt from emotional upsets, either. The *Affiches pour les Trois Evêchés et la Lorraine* reported that a twenty-year-old peasant lost the faculty of speech after receiving some bad news. Isuard, surgeon of Embrun, had trouble treating a thirty-five-year-old artisan who became feverish and indulged in obscene posturings and discourses after his parents opposed his remarriage.[27]

Epidemics were an even greater source of emotional stress. Many doctors believed in the existence of a vicious cycle of epidemics and anxiety: epidemics provoked emotional stress, which in turn precipitated more epidemics. As Bonhomme, a doctor from Avignon, observed in a letter to the Royal Society of Medicine: "Some moments of dread and fright have produced in Avignon, especially among the women, illnesses that are still occupying us. There are the putrid or bilious fevers, the crushing apoplexies, the comatose affections. The women have suffered suppressions that have been more or less dangerous. These indispositions have been followed by hysterical vapors, hemoptysis, mental derangement; and several of these illnesses have resisted the best recommended remedies."[28]

Ripert, a doctor from Apt, reported that collective convulsions occurred immediately after the sudden death, through indigestion, of someone in the village. People were frightened by sudden, seemingly fortuitous deaths and manifested their fear in convulsions. The more frequently they occurred, the more dangerous the convulsions became. Ripert recounted the story of a wig maker named Bernard who was so afraid of dying in an accident that his fear was realized, and of a Mlle Cayre who suffered the same fate. Ripert believed that the most effective way of combatting the fear that generated collective convulsions was to educate people about the physical causes of and means of preventing accidental deaths and recommended that the municipality assign a doctor and a surgeon specifically to this task.[29] Another doctor, Revoltat, described vividly the kind of panic that sudden, unexpected death provoked in the inhabitants of Vienne in Dauphiné in 1778: "There were during this time two sudden deaths: two women, one a nun about 42 years old, stout, fresh, fleshy as a result of little exercise. The other was 45 years old, unmarried, subject to fluxions of the eyes. Both died within an hour or two. In a small city all these events are known in an instant, the alarm carries the news to all corners, fear takes hold of all spirits, Pandora's box is open."[30]

Such panic and collective convulsions were only a prelude, however, to what the Revolution would provoke. Bonhomme held the terror inspired by the Revolution responsible for an unprecedented increase in both physical and psychological disorders, including fevers, liver complaints, apoplexy, and hysteria. Although he had employed sedatives to mitigate these disorders, Bonhomme believed that only the reestablishment of political stability could bring convulsions under control. His sentiments were echoed in an observation made in the *Almanach sous verre* of 1792 regarding the maladies occasioned by the Revolution: "The Doctors remark that there are people who, having unexpectedly encountered cadavers and bloody heads while walking down the street, have suffered palpitations, distressing insomnia, terrible dreams. Others have been frightened to the point of losing their head. In Paris alone, they add, there are 800 more insane people than ordinarily."[31]

Emotional stress was a natural consequence of the precarious conditions of existence in eighteenth-century France, but stress was not generated by external circumstance alone. Sexuality also seemed to be a source of considerable anxiety for early modern women. Enlightenment writers perceived a connection between sexuality and convulsions and advocated marriage as the most appropriate antidote to convulsions. According to the Enlightenment model of convulsions, sexual intercourse purified the body of humors that, if not discharged, could have a corrosive impact on the mind. Although sexual intercourse was thought salubrious for both men and women, it was considered essential for men because "men, freer, less restrained, are apt to be less upset by sex than women; it is rare that their spirit is disturbed by it."[32]

In an age in which sexual excess was equated with the moral and physical degeneration of the race, Enlightenment writers did not advocate complete sexual abandon. Instead, they urged moderation, and to encourage restraint, they reminded their readers that "although excretion of the retained semen can be harmful, an immoderate amount of semen can at the same time become the source of very serious illnesses."[33] Nor did Enlightenment writers countenance sexual expression outside marriage. The number of books written on the subject suggests that the medical community's concern with eliminating masturbation in men was matched only by its preoccupation with quelling convulsions in women.[34] The parallel between masturbation in men and convulsions in women was drawn frequently; both were regarded as symptoms of deleterious sexual excess.[35]

Adhering to the Enlightenment model of convulsions, provincial doctors routinely recommended marriage as an antidote to convulsions. Their correspondence reveals, however, that marriage and motherhood were as likely to cause as to cure convulsions. Just as frightening to women as epidemics was the prospect of childbirth which marriage inevitably brought with it. Childbirth raised the possibility of death, the likelihood of permanent infirmities like prolapsed uteruses, and the promise of complications like hemorrhaging and fevers.

The provincial physicians' observations on the effects of marriage on women, while diverging from the Enlightenment model, are confirmed by the correspondence of aristocratic and bourgeois women. Mlle de Malboissière's letters are punctuated with references to friends like Mme de Meulan, who had experienced a difficult birth; Mme de Pomery, whose four-year-old son, always ill, had just died; and Mme de La Fortelle, who died of smallpox when she was six months pregnant and requested that her body be opened after her death so that the baby could be baptized.

Even women who gave birth easily to healthy children were not freed of anxiety. De Malboissière goes on to mention Mme de Saint Maure, who was as distraught over giving birth as Mme de Meulan, though for different reasons. Desiring to bear a boy as a means of enhancing her status within the family, de Saint Maure was disturbed to learn that she had instead given birth to her fourth daughter.[36]

Despite the ideology that defined maternity as a woman's unique vocation, advocated that all the education of a girl be directed toward maternity, and linked childbearing with improvement of a woman's health, some women revealed their ambivalence about childbearing in their letters. In her survey of eleven hundred letters written by the nobility from 1700 to 1860, Marie-Claire Grassi provides an evocative example of a woman who, expecting her fourth child, called the emphasis on maternity into question: "I am very angry that men do not give birth. I believe that they would receive the advice to start again very badly. I have never had a love of posterity and I have never believed that my children could contribute to the happiness of my life either in the present or in the future . . . Even if I had the health of a porter, I would nevertheless consider it a misfortune to have a large number of children; the last one was already too much."[37]

According to the provincial doctors' correspondence, convulsions were, to be sure, related to sexuality, but not in the manner the Enlightenment model suggested. The effects of repressed or unbridled sexuality troubled women less than anxiety over sexuality itself. This anxiety afflicted women throughout their lives: adolescent girls coming to sexuality; young women approaching the time for consummating their marriages; new mothers immediately before childbirth and during nursing; and older women facing the end of their fertile years. The typical manifestation of anxiety—convulsions—remained constant throughout all stages of sexual development. While feminist historians have noted the panic with which eighteenth-century physicians responded to the sexuality of women, little has been said about the discomfort with which the women regarded their own sexuality. The excerpts from the provincial doctors' correspondence that follow reveal the extent to which this discomfort went unrecognized by doctors and unarticulated by female patients. This correspondence lends weight to Giordana Charuty's interpretation of hysteria in the nineteenth century as a manifestation of women's rejection of their sexual identity and difficulty in coming to terms with particular phases of the life cycle. According to Charuty, hysteria typically troubled pregnant women in conflict over the prospect of maternity; mothers of families dreaming of their lost virginity; and women approaching menopause yet longing to remain fertile.[38] But let us look closely at the evidence from the letters of provincial practitioners indicating that convulsions seemed to accompany every phase of the female life cycle, from adolescence through marriage, pregnancy, and childbirth.

Convulsions in adolescent girls were occasionally the result of sexual teasing or assault but more often were a manifestation of anxiety at approaching sexual maturity. Incidents in which adolescent girls or young unmarried women had suffered convulsions and deliria as a result of being sexually teased or assaulted were reported both in medical journals like the *Gazette salutaire* and in provincial journals like the *Affiches du Dauphiné*. Acknowledging how tempting it was to tease young girls, the editors of the *Gazette salutaire* hoped to lessen the charm a bit by documenting the case of a twenty-year-old girl who was so frightened by the teasing of a group of soldiers that she lost her sanity. Alternately laughing and crying, she was unable to put together a coherent sentence or to care for herself.[39] A sixteen-year-old peasant girl suffered a similar mental alienation after being raped by a stranger. The incident had made such an impression upon her that she relived it in nightmares for several months, went into fits of convulsions, and appeared to have gone mad. Entrusted to the care of enlightened surgeons, the girls eventually recovered after rigorous treatments consisting of bleedings, emetics, purgatives, and laxatives. The *Affiches du Dauphiné* recounted the sad story of a young girl who suffered a different fate as a result of a similar experience: she became hydropic and died shortly thereafter.[40] The publication of such stories indicates a significant shift in mentality from the times in which rape was, if not officially sanctioned, at least seen as a necessary release for social tension.[41]

But young women did not have to be molested to feel anxious about their sexuality. Convulsions commonly occurred in adolescent girls just coming to sexual maturity. The disorder could last several weeks, months, even years, and was often accompanied by an aversion to food and to the evacuations that food consumption entailed. Many girls, although exhausted by the physical toll their convulsions took, refused to eat anything solid and were kept alive on liquids alone. A number of doctors, including Maret of Dijon, Maury of Sezanne, Marx of Hanover, and Peraud de Laurignai of Noirmoutier, sent letters to the Royal Society of Medicine describing the convulsive adolescents they had treated.[42]

The provincial doctors directed the society's attention to these cases because although virtually every weapon in the arsenal of remedies had been employed, cures were slow and faltering at best. Every case was different: where bleedings, emetics, purgatives, and baths worked in some, they were ineffective in others, and more exotic drugs like opium and cinchona were administered. Although the girls usually recovered, one wonders whether the treatments they received had any salutary effect. It seems likely that the treatments simply exhausted the girls' physical strength to the point where they were unable to continue expressing their anxieties through convulsions.

A detailed description of the rigorous treatments to which convulsive girls and women were subjected can be found in an article submitted to the *Gazette salutaire* by Mercadier, a surgeon practicing in Paris. Mercadier's patient, a young unmarried woman of twenty-three, was described as being melancholic by nature and leading too sedentary an existence. In December of 1759, she appeared to have contracted what Mercadier diagnosed as some kind of imbecility, for she spent several days crying continually and refusing to eat or drink. Learning that the woman's menstruation had stopped, Mercadier induced it by giving her an injection of saffron. The patient seemed to have returned to normal until the onset of her next menstrual period, when she again fell into a fit of tears and became delirious. The delirium gave way to a sluggishness in which normal body functions came to a standstill. The patient stopped eating, evacuating, and menstruating; her tears ceased, as did her speech. A doctor advised bleeding, but Mercadier believed the woman was too weak to undergo even a light bleeding and prescribed laxatives, purgatives, and baths instead.

After six weeks without improvement in her condition, the woman was admitted to the Hôtel-Dieu, where she was bled at the arm, the foot, and the jugular for two months, all to no avail. Finally her doctors discovered that their patient had a fear of cold water and plunged her into a frigid bath. When even this method seemed ineffective, her head was held under a faucet of cold water. The woman was released from the Hôtel-Dieu in June, seemingly cured of her disorder but having contracted a severe skin infection. Nevertheless, Mercadier concluded triumphantly that "since this time, she has been very well, has been married for two years, and enjoys perfect health."[43]

Mercadier indicated that he adhered to the Enlightenment model of convulsions. While this woman's case was too severe to make her a likely prospect for marriage immediately, the very fact that she was married soon after her recovery and remained healthy thereafter seemed to confirm what many enlightened doctors and surgeons already believed—that marriage was a powerful antidote to nervous disorders in women. As the correspondence of provincial doctors to the Royal Society of Medicine reveals, however, many women's convulsions began, rather than ended, with marriage and the anxieties it brought over sexual intercourse and childbirth.

Like Mercadier, most provincial doctors tended to adhere uncritically to the Enlightenment model linking convulsions to extremes of sexual behavior even when another explanation, such as women's fear of their own sexuality, might have been more revealing. One doctor, Ardent, practicing in Gap, reported the case of a woman who had been married only three or four days when she had a fit of convulsions. Since the woman was married, sexual repression could hardly have been the source. Ardent decided the cause must, therefore, lie in sexual license.

The woman's family initially consulted their local surgeon. This surgeon, characterized by Ardent as incapable of reflection, believed in allowing nature to take its course. He was confident that the woman's troubles would come to an end of their own accord. He did, however, send Ardent a letter describing the woman's condition. Ardent took an interest in the case and decided to pay the woman a visit. Making no effort to disguise his repugnance, he described her as

> a woman twenty-five or thirty years old, with a hot and bilious temper, sunken eyes with a menacing look, her upper lip and chin filled with long hairs of more than an inch. She had disagreeable features, a black rheum held the eyelashes together and the lips were full of this same humor. I would have immediately ordered a bleeding, but because she was subject to continual movements, I assuaged her by warm baths and a sedating infusion I made with tamarin. To achieve this effect I kept her in the bath for four hours, during which I saw a pubis darkened by a forest of black and very long hair, which confirmed to me the irritability of her temperament.[44]

The baths were followed by bleedings and more baths, and the woman seemed to have recovered within a few days. Ardent entrusted her to her husband's care with the advice that in the interests of preserving his wife's health, he moderate his sexual desires awhile. The cure was not, however, an unqualified success, for the woman went into convulsions again six months later. Her surgeon believed her condition was hereditary, while Ardent remained convinced that "this woman was too ugly ever to have been courted by a young man. Ignorant of all the liberties that marriage gives, she then gave in to all the desires of a strong and robust peasant husband. These pleasures so greatly disturbed the patient that she was assailed by all the symptoms described above."[45]

Ardent believed that ignorance was the only explanation for the surgeon's reluctance or refusal to adopt a radically interventionist cure. Unlike his surgeon, Ardent was unwilling to acknowledge the limited resources of medicine in the face of nature gone awry; he insisted that he could cure the woman. The surgeon, in contrast, had believed that the woman would be cured, not through his resources, but through the regenerative powers of nature. As my earlier discussion of Guenet's and Condorcet's portraits of Tronchin indicated, this polarization of attitudes regarding the roles of medicine and nature in the healing process was typical of the eighteenth century. In time, both sides would moderate their positions a bit, and recognize the necessity of appealing to both medicine and nature to obtain a cure.

After reading Ardent's description of his cure, one wonders if the woman suffered more from the surgeon's neglect or from the rigorous assaults Ardent made on her constitution. Clearly, Ardent's disdain and repugnance toward her limited his ability to address the psychological roots of her disorder. Rather than sympathizing with her difficulties in adjusting to the sexual demands of married life, Ardent was appalled at what he believed to be her sexual insatiability. It was clear that she did not measure up to his ideal of femininity and that he measured the success of his treatment in part by the degree to which he could bring her into conformity with this ideal.

An article by Marie-Claude Phan and Jean-Louis Flandrin on changes in the ideal of feminine beauty sheds some light on Ardent's response to his patient. They have found that notions of beauty and ugliness were inseparable from considerations of social status. Thus leisured women were much more likely than working women to have the pale complexion so greatly admired from the Middle Ages through the seventeenth century.[46] Nor was Ardent the only doctor to impose an ideal of feminine beauty on women, as the work of Alison Lingo on Liébault and H. G. Ibels on Tronchin makes clear.[47]

While the phenomenon of convulsions among young unmarried and newly married women was frequently recorded, convulsions either before or just after childbirth were just as commonplace. As Duvernin, a doctor from Clermont-Ferrand, had observed in his memoir to the Royal Society of Medicine in 1777, the prospect and actual experience of childbirth filled many young women with fears rendering them especially vulnerable to convulsions associated with the fevers that often followed childbirth.[48] Such fear was understandable since, according to Claude Grimmer, in the countryside and small towns, one of every eighty births involved the death of the mother or infant; one out of ten married women died in childbirth; and one out of ten infants was born dead.[49]

Hysterical convulsions that might normally disturb only the health or equanimity of a woman became life threatening during pregnancy. Tavernier, a doctor practicing in Pontcartier, warned of the devastating effects of anger on the constitution of a pregnant woman. He reported that a young woman of twenty-five, pregnant with her second child, became hysterical over a dispute with her mother-in-law. Her convulsions brought on hemorrhaging, and the woman died soon after.[50]

Doctors and surgeons had to proceed cautiously in treating convulsions in pregnant women. Although the convulsions could, as in the case described by Tavernier, induce miscarriages and the death of both mother and child, remedies could have an equally dire effect. Confronted with a convulsive woman named Marguerite Fortin, who told him she thought she was two or three months pregnant, Hardouineau, a doctor practicing at the Hôtel-Dieu of Orléans, administered laxatives, bleedings, and cold baths in order to calm the woman. The remedies brought an end to the convulsions but provoked an abortion and brought the woman so near death that last rites were administered. Marguerite Fortin was luckier, though, than others, for she managed to pull through the ordeal and was able to leave the Hôtel-Dieu fifteen days later.[51]

Depression and hysteria frequently afflicted women immediately after childbirth, and the usual remedies—bleedings, purgatives, laxatives, and baths—were used to combat them.[52] Some doctors, like Aublet of St. Jean-d'Angély, embracing the Enlightenment exaltation of motherhood, urged new mothers to combat convulsions by nursing their children.[53] Other doctors warned against nursing. Indeed, some convulsive mothers were physically unable to nurse their children. Analyzing the cases he had superintended, Planchon observed that women whose breasts filled with blood instead of milk the first day after childbirth generally became manic by the fourth day and died by the seventh day. He believed that nursing was probably the worst thing to recommend in such cases, even when the usual remedies were ineffective. Whatever the treatment, death seemed inevitable.[54]

Women's Work and the Problem of Convulsions

Although convulsions were typically associated with extremes in sexual behavior and marriage was recommended as the most appropriate antidote, certain environmental factors were acknowledged to play a role in stimulating convulsions. The Enlightenment model ascribed the increase in convulsions noted by many eighteenth-century physicians to the luxury that rendered work obsolete for many women. This model was formulated by Parisian doctors, and it may have described their patients perfectly. It was not, however, universally valid.

Provincial doctors had prescribed the antidote of marriage with only limited success. In its identification of environmental factors, the Enlightenment model seemed even farther removed from the reality of provincial medical practices. Provincial doctors observed increases in convulsions in small towns and villages and among working women. Clearly, an alternative model of convulsions had to be formulated. Few provincial doctors were ready to devise a comprehensive model, but many offered reflections on possible environmental sources of convulsions.

La Brossière, a doctor practicing in St. Malo, remarked upon the disposition toward melancholy evidenced by young and old, male and female alike, in his practice. He offered two different hypotheses to account for the high number of nervous disorders afflicting the people of St. Malo. The first was that the disorders were hereditary, passed from sailors, whose travels exposed them to venereal diseases, to their wives and children in the form of convulsions. The second was that the peculiar geography of St. Malo in terms of temperature, altitude, and humidity was responsible for the melancholy, nervous symptoms, and spasms of its people.[55]

La Brossière was not alone in attributing the prevalence of nervous disorders in his region to environmental factors. Didelot, a surgeon practicing in Remirement in Lorraine, remarked in a letter to the Royal Society of Medicine on the impact of rarefied mountain air on the nervous disposition, especially of newcomers. Yet the number of nervous disorders seemed to have increased dramatically over the course of a single generation. Didelot believed that a visible degeneration in the physical constitution of workers could be traced to the radical change in working conditions brought about by the transformation of the economy. Lumbering, the manufacture of wood products, and salt mining had all given way to textile manufacturing as the chief industry in the region. Condemning this unnaturally sedentary occupation, Didelot exclaimed, "How the current generation seems less strong and vigorous than the preceding one! Firm health, intact temperaments, and steadfast nerves can be found only among aged persons now."[56]

Didelot's concern over the deleterious effects of the conditions of labor on workers' health was novel but not unique. The *médecine du travail*, or occupational medicine, was just emerging as a subject of some interest to doctors and significance to the state in the late eighteenth century. Occupational medicine can be seen as a natural extension of medical topographies, the purpose of which was to discover causal links between environmental factors and disease. Doctors' interest in occupational medicine paralleled that of the editors of the *Encyclopédie*, who linked development of the crafts with improvement of the conditions of labor. On his voyage to Holland, Diderot was struck by the number and diversity of disorders that afflicted artisans. Observing "a multitude of unhealthy arts," Diderot wrote, "Painters, varnishers, pewterers, gilders almost all have chest and eye ailments; nearly all the journeymen printers perish by accidents to their limbs,"[57] and concluded that a good treatise on occupational illnesses needed to be written. His observations call into question the assertion by Claudine Herzlich and Janine Pierret that the public lagged behind doctors in perceiving the need for occupational medicine until the nineteenth century, which brought industrialization and the struggle for social justice.[58] Still, because the philosophes seemed not to recognize the economic need for women of modest means to work, they devoted little attention to the impact of the conditions of labor on their health.[59]

Until occupational medicine was established as a discipline in its own right, doctors specializing in the *maladies des femmes* rarely discussed the maladies of working women, which did not figure in the Enlightenment model of convulsions. As studies in occupational medicine progressed, however, it became apparent that the model was in serious need of revision. The model attributed convulsions to excesses associated with the life-style of the leisured classes and saw productive labor as one of the most effective antidotes. The letters of provincial doctors to the Royal Society of Medicine challenged such simple equations, for they revealed that a large number of female artisans and workers were also peculiarly prone to convulsions.

Provincial doctors contributed to the development of occupational medicine by submitting reports on health problems associated with specific trades. In 1781 Achard, the son of a paper maker who became a doctor in Marseille, sent the Royal Society of Medicine an essay on hatters' illnesses in which he attributed the violent headaches, hemoptysis, edema, and menstrual irregularities suffered by female hatters to the conditions of their labor. Men, he added, were not free from work-related disorders either. Achard believed that heavy exposure to mercury was responsible for the inordinate number and variety of nervous disorders, including trembling, convulsions, paralysis, and apoplexy.[60]

Although doctors ministering to aristocratic and bourgeois women had written long treatises on the deleterious effects of idleness and luxury, those who studied the health problems of working women were not so sure that work—at least work undertaken outside the household—was the cure for convulsions in women. Ramel observed that women spinners were much more likely than women of the leisured classes to suffer from both menstrual irregularities and convulsions.[61] Another doctor, Aublet, agreed with Ramel that women artisans were more likely to suffer from menstrual irregularities, but added that they were more fecund and were able to give birth with greater facility.[62] The evidence on the subject was inconsistent and inconclusive. Flangergues, a doctor practicing in Viviers, disagreed with both Aublet and Ramel. He reported several cases of women spinners whose menstrual irregularities ceased once they began working. These women seemed, however, to suffer more than their share of miscarriages, and Flangergues urged them to stop working during pregnancy.[63]

Another issue regarding the employment of women in workshops was whether or not the convulsions to which they seemed prone threatened to disrupt production. Surely this threat, were it genuine, would be sufficient grounds for removing women from the workplace. Cases of contagious convulsions culminating in miscarriage had been recorded by Desmery, a celebrated doctor practicing in Amiens.[64] Also inserted into the Royal Society of Medicine archives was an extract from the *English Chronicle* detailing a case of convulsions affecting a young woman in otherwise good health and communicated to seven other women who worked near her in a cotton mill. All work came to a halt for more than twenty-four hours as the women gnawed their flesh, pulled out their hair, knocked their heads against the walls. As reports of these seemingly contagious convulsions spread, it was feared that raw cotton had carried the plague into the community. The diagnosis of the doctor who examined the women was not nearly so alarming. He attributed the convulsions of his first patient to fright at having a mouse thrown in her face and those of her co-workers to the terror the first woman's convulsions inspired. After being separated and given various antispasmodics, the women seemed to recover and were able to return to work.[65] This incident was not unlike Boerhaave's case history of hysteria among women in a workshop in Leyden, which Diderot included in his observations on physiology.[66]

Doctors were concerned about the deleterious effects of working conditions on the moral as well as physical health of women. It was, indeed, on morality that Flangergues believed workshops in Viviers had had their greatest impact. He had ambivalent feelings about the workshops, which, although they had banished laziness, had also inspired a love of luxury hitherto unknown to Viviers. Flangergues feared that the close association between the sexes which the production of wool required would inspire sexual license and exploitation. Observing that workshop supervisors were usually male and their subordinates female, he feared that supervisors would use their authority to seduce the young women. Too many women, he noted, had been led to vice by being persuaded to exchange sexual favors for advancement in the workplace.[67]

Alain Lottin's study of illegitimate births and unwed mothers in Lille demonstrates that Flangergue's fears were not unfounded. Lottin discovered that unwed mothers tended to come from families in which the father was deceased and the mother worked full-time. Young girls in such circumstances did not enjoy the same protection as girls whose families remained intact. The largest number of unwed mothers came from the ranks of textile workers—especially those working in lace—and domestic servants.[68]

In attempting to account for his findings, Lottin reasoned that the direct and constraining relationship between the master of the workshop and the female workers sometimes extended to the sexual realm. The pressure to comply was in addition to whatever physical or sentimental attraction might develop as a result of close interaction between the sexes. The power dynamics within the workshop described by Lottin closely resemble those within the household depicted by Sarah Maza in her study of servants and masters in eighteenth-century France.[69] It thus hardly seems surprising that the rates of illegitimacy should be highest among workshop employees and household servants. Léon Abensour adds that couturiers and domestic servants earned insufficient wages to support themselves and needed some additional means of support, which in some cases they found in a sexual liaison.[70]

The conditions of labor varied greatly from workshop to workshop and region to region. Some areas, anticipating Flangergues's specter of vice, integrated religious instruction into the routine of workshop life. In Le Puy, for example, assemblies of women were held every winter. Although the principal object of these assemblies was to impart religious instruction, the women attending them made lace while they learned their catechism. This juxtaposition of religious instruction with work proved very successful. A significant portion of the female population was drawn to the assemblies, and lace making became an important source of commerce within the region.[71] In the late eighteenth and early nineteenth centuries, inculcation of the Christian virtues of submission and obedience contributed to the development of a docile work force in Le Puy and throughout France. Odile Arnold notes a striking case of a workshop in Saint-Vallier which was ruled exactly like a monastery, with hours of meditation, canticles, and silence before bedtime. Accommodations for young female workers adjoined the living quarters of nuns.[72]

Once work-related disorders were addressed, the question of how they could be reduced or eliminated had to be resolved. Some doctors believed it was the function of the occupational medicine practitioner to harmonize the seemingly conflicting interests of industrial development and workers' health.[73] Others, however, assumed a very uncompromising stance on the subject. Beerenbrock, a doctor practicing in Montpellier, outlined the nervous disorders to which gilders were exposed and suggested that these workers could preserve their health only by quitting their trade entirely. For those who refused to take his advice, Beerenbrock had little sympathy, regarding them as irremediably poor or avaricious.[74]

Although doctors were willing to tolerate daughters of artisans and laborers working as long as they remained single, they looked askance at women who continued to work after marriage, especially after they had become mothers. Some doctors attributed the high rate of mortality to the fact that working women either had to neglect children or send them out to nurse. Morgue de Montredum even drew correlations between peak production periods in Montpellier and upswings in infant mortality.[75] Later historians of the impact of industrialization on demography have confirmed these correlations.[76]

Martin, a doctor associated with the Hôtel-Dieu in Narbonne, Languedoc, submitted a study to the Royal Society of Medicine in which he linked the convulsions of children to the conditions of their mother's work. His prescription for a three-year-old child who tossed his head back and forth habitually and seemingly involuntarily was to remove the child from the room in which his mother, a spinner, worked. Martin had hypothesized that the movements of the child's head were stimulated by the movement of the spinning wheel. And he may have been correct, for when the child was removed from the workplace, the movements stopped. Another woman, who earned her living staging dog shows, consulted Martin about her eight-year-old son who had been tormented with convulsions for two months. Rather than agreeing with the mother that the child's convulsions were due to a cold, Martin noted a similarity between the child's trembling and that of the dogs he tended. In this instance also, Martin urged that the child be removed from the workplace.[77]

We can see from their treatments of convulsions in working women and their children that few doctors advocated fundamental change in the social or economic order. If the conditions of labor promoted convulsions and other maladies in women, the solution was for women to withdraw from the work force. No one argued that the conditions of labor should be transformed or that the survival of many a family depended on women's labor.

Nor did doctors seem attuned to *intendants'* campaigns to expand rural industry or seem cognizant of the extent to which such expansion depended on a ready supply of women and children workers. In his study of rural industry in early modern France, Eugenii Tarlé notes that officials in Limousin worked actively to develop domestic industry, distributing more than fifteen hundred spinning wheels to poor female spinners between 1760 and 1775.[78]

Tarlé also observes that in the canton of Quesnay, cloth manufacture and sale were the only occupations of poor families. In the countryside, women and children dedicated themselves to these pursuits for eight months of the year, while in the cities they spent the whole year working in textiles. In Limoges and its environs, women and children were solely concerned with spinning.[79] Tarlé's statistics for cotton production at Saint-Dyé near Blois are significant. Of 2,100 workers employed, there were 1,800 women spinners, 180 women winders, and only 70 male weavers and 50 male dressers.[80] Employment of women and children made economic sense. Tarlé notes that the wages for male weavers, though hardly high (six livres per week), were twice that for female spinners, whose wages he terms completely insignificant.[81]

Given their commitment to economic development, intendants sometimes displayed more perspicacity regarding the need to transform working conditions than did doctors. Thus Alain Decaux quotes the intendant Bouillon, who in 1765 became alarmed at the frightening lot of women pullers in the weaving industry: "I am told that for modest gains they work for eighteen hours a day and end by catching considerable illnesses that sooner or later render them unable to work and they die in misery." Bouillon concluded that it would not be a bad idea to accept the offer of an inventor which would make the work at the loom easier: "He would thus save the Hôtel-Dieu sixty to eighty beds that the pullers occupy presently with illness coming from the weight of the pull."[82]

Most of the hygienic literature directed toward women mirrored the class bias evident in the Enlightenment model of convulsions. As often as not, though, the assumptions made in this literature went unexamined. For example, a book addressed to reducing infant mortality written by Jacques Ballexserd and awarded a prize by the Academy of Mantua gave a detailed regime to be followed by the pregnant woman. She should avoid fatiguing herself unduly or becoming idle. She was advised to occupy herself agreeably, interspersing hours of repose with short walks in which she would take care not to expose herself to great wind or humidity. If her home was in the city, it should be located on a spacious street, far removed from sewers, cemeteries, hospitals, tanneries, and laundries. If it was in the countryside, it should be on a dry plain, away from stagnant marshes and rivers that might overflow. No advice was offered to those who were not in a position to choose where they might live or whether they would work. As the editors of the *Affiches pour les Trois Evêchés et la Lorraine* observed after printing excerpts from Ballexserd's book, "These observations, excellent in themselves, are suitable only to well-to-do people."[83] Those who were not well off were left to their own resources. One wonders how effectively such a book could combat infant mortality, whose toll was much more devastating on the children of the poor than those of the rich.

The picture that Yvonne Knibiehler and Catherine Fouquet present of the condition of women workers in the nineteenth century is not reassuring. They conclude that "the working mother is a bad reproducer (she conceives many children, but few are viable and all are stunted). She can neither nurse them nor care for them herself, and sometimes she abandons them. She is never their educator; it is at the nursery, the day shelter, and before long the factory that they will learn to live. The transmission of domestic knowledge is not possible in these conditions; the mother teaches her daughter nothing except suffering, resignation, sometimes revolt."[84]

Models of Convulsions as Cultural Critiques: The Provincial Practitioners' Critique

Although the correspondence that provincial doctors submitted to the Royal Society of Medicine revealed the inadequacies of the Enlightenment model of the convulsive patient, the doctors made few alterations in this model. Provincial doctors studying convulsions in working women did not concur with their Parisian colleagues that convulsions were bred of boredom and debauchery, but they did join them in intimating that women's physical and mental health would benefit if they devoted themselves to their proper roles as wives and mothers. The typically bourgeois image of women as mothers immersed in the concerns of managing their households and nurturing their children became an ideal that all women— working, bourgeois, and aristocratic alike—were encouraged to emulate.

Even though the provincial case histories as well as some of the writings of aristocratic and bourgeois women disclosed that marriage was as much a cause as a cure of anxieties and convulsions, the enlightened literature continued to portray marriage as the ideal state for women. Those women who, whether through inclination or necessity, did not adhere to this ideal were chastised and made to feel guilty. The parameters of socially acceptable activity for women, already rather limited during the Ancien Régime, became even more constricted as the ideal of domesticity and the sentimentalization of the family took hold over ever-widening sectors of society and women lost their foothold in the workplace.

Doctors lent impetus to this trend by suggesting that women could best preserve their own and their children's health by assuming tasks such as breastfeeding and rearing small children, which had traditionally been relegated to people outside the family. The strengthening of the bond between mother and child when women assumed increased responsibilities within the family thus entailed the weakening of the bonds linking women to the outside community.

However imperfect a reflection of reality it presented, the image of the convulsive female which appeared in the enlightened literature thus served an important ideological function. It was used by proponents of bourgeois culture to undermine the appeal of aristocratic culture and to provide women with new role models. To the extent that education was responsible for perpetuating the old aristocratic ideal of the leisured lady and the nervous disorders associated with it, enlightened writers urged its reform. Enlightenment, they suggested, had been carried too far in the case of aristocratic and socially ambitious bourgeois women. The reforms they advocated focused on developing domestic skills rather than abstract reasoning or social graces in girls. Women were to find fulfillment in managing their households efficiently rather than in dazzling onlookers in the salons or at court. Only then could the problem of nervous disorders be resolved.

Provincial doctors and surgeons approached the problem quite differently. They envisioned the wives and daughters of peasants and artisans whom they treated not as the products of a decadent, overenlightened culture, but as the victims of ancient superstitious beliefs that had been preserved within popular culture. The traditional medicine of their rivals, the empirics, was rooted in this popular culture. As the guardians of popular culture, women were the most prominent purveyors and recipients of its remedies and beliefs. In contrast to their Parisian colleagues, provincial doctors and surgeons believed that the solution to the problem of nervous disorders lay in the greater dissemination of enlightenment to women rather than its circumscription.

In both cases, the image of the convulsive female served as the basis for a critique of culture. Both Parisian and provincial doctors were guided by a bourgeois ethic exalting enlightenment, work, and domesticity—all in proper moderation and due proportion. Whereas, however, Parisian doctors used the image of the convulsive woman to attack the distorted values of an aristocratic culture they were intent on reforming, their provincial colleagues regarded the convulsive woman as a symbol of the erroneous beliefs underlying a popular culture they were bent on uprooting.

Many of the superstitions provincial doctors hoped to eradicate had religious roots. Not only were overly religious women thought to be particularly susceptible to convulsions, but women tended to turn to religion as a means of understanding their convulsions and making them acceptable to themselves and society at large. In a religious context, the ravings and apparently bizarre behavior of hysterical women took on a new light. Women who might otherwise have been dismissed as mentally unbalanced were embraced as saints who had experienced or performed miracles. The emotions of melancholy and fear which rigorous religious instruction was believed to inspire were the very emotions thought to give rise to convulsions. Thus it was not unusual for Barthez, chancellor of the Faculty of Medicine of Montpellier, royal censor, and contributor to the *Encyclopédie*, to urge a woman to avoid emotional upset and to refrain from long religious meditations as part of a strategy for recovering from epilepsy thought induced by menstrual irregularities.[85] Ayrau, a doctor practicing in Mirabeau, held a melancholy brought on by long meditations on the mysteries of religion responsible for a case of hysteria degenerating into madness in a twenty-two-year-old woman.[86] In like manner, Meglin reported a number of cases of convulsions that seemed to have been passed on from mothers to daughters in Guebevillier, a small town in the Haute-Alsace. He linked convulsions to extremes of virtue and vice in women, adverting to the hazards of a sedentary, contemplative, overly mystical existence as well as its opposite.[87]

Collective convulsions among young girls occurred frequently in churches. Whereas some doctors, like Ripert of Apt, attributed the convulsions to fear inspired by overly zealous preachers,[88] others like Meglin and Cornefroy attributed them to the cold, humid atmosphere of the churches or to the unhealthy fumes emitted by the poorly constructed tombs beneath or adjacent to many church edifices.[89]

The frequency of convulsions in the provinces as well as in Paris broadens the significance of the debates over the Convulsionaries and mesmerism. Skepticism marked treatment of individual cases as well as of cases of collective convulsions. Like their Parisian colleagues, provincial doctors questioned the reality of convulsions and the judgment of those who believed in them. In order to be taken seriously, convulsive women had first to overcome suspicions of ignorance or deceit. Well-publicized inquiries into convulsions were made frequently in the countryside.

Cases of convulsive women who evacuated foreign objects occurred periodically and never failed to pique the public's curiosity. Several were noted by Diderot in his study of flukes of nature and women's nervous disorders.[90] In 1754 the bishop of Langres sent the Faculty of Medicine of Paris an assortment of rocks in various sizes and shapes reputed to have been evacuated by a young girl of his diocese. The faculty appointed a committee of three doctors, Malouin, Guettard, and Morand, to examine the rocks and give an opinion on their nature and origin. On the basis of the committee's report, the faculty ruled that the rocks were composed of mineral rather than animal matter and did not originate in the girl's body. It suggested that the girl had introduced the rocks into her stools and vomit in order to deceive the public, and closed the case with the time-honored explanation that "thus throughout history hysterical girls have been known to dream up different strategies for seducing gullible spirits, putting on a spectacle, and attracting respect or alms."[91]

Other cases that caused a stir involved convulsive women or girls who took to their beds, refusing to eat or drink and thus supposedly freeing themselves from the needs to urinate, defecate, and menstruate. One such case was described in a letter from Brittany addressed to the editors of the *Gazette salutaire*. A young woman aged twenty-four had become famous throughout the region by refusing to eat or drink for two years. Although she had grown steadily weaker and more emaciated, she had managed to remain conscious and was capable of responding to the inquiries of her many visitors. Lest readers of the journal be skeptical of the veracity of his report, the author observed that "many honorable people who have come expressly to be eye witnesses of an extraordinary fact can attest to its truth."[92]

A similar, though more prolonged and dramatic, case of convulsive abstinence came to the attention of the Royal Society of Medicine in 1784. St. André, a doctor practicing in Tarascon, chronicled his encounters over fourteen years with a woman named Marie Malepeyré, who reputedly refused to eat or drink, yet maintained normal body weight and color. A devout Catholic, Mlle Malepeyré was the daughter of a poor miner in the village of Olbie. At the age of seventeen she was afflicted with an unquenchable thirst. She gradually stopped eating, sleeping, and evacuating and seemed to derive religious satisfaction from the facts that she did not dirty her linen and could not bear to be touched.

Although Malepeyré was lucid most of the time, she occasionally lapsed into a religious ecstasy in which, she said, the gates of heaven lay open before her and she could communicate with the souls of the dead. Such an occurrence in a village of poor, ignorant people was, St. André observed, bound to create a sensation: "The wonder was announced everywhere; all the people ran to see the miracle and revere the saint; all the faithful were eager for her to accept their presents."[93] They came to her seeking to confess and to receive communion. Since she had a gift for prophecy, they sought her advice in their temporal affairs and asked her to reveal and intervene in the fates of their dead ancestors.

Once the pilgrimages had begun, the local magistrate started to worry that the girl might be swindling the public and kept her under surveillance for eleven days, after which three doctors issued a *procès-verbal* recording Malepeyré's testimony and that of her guards. The report certified that she experienced great difficulty swallowing; just the sight of a spoonful of water was enough to throw her into convulsions. This report evidently satisfied the civil authorities, but St. André continued to wonder whether the condition was real or simulated. Since, however, Malepeyré had refused his request to examine her, he lacked the evidence to challenge her testimony directly.

As the years passed, St. André continued to hear about marvels surrounding this woman. Fourteen years after the onset of the illness, Malepeyré allowed St. André to visit her and revealed something she had not mentioned in the first inquiry: she had vomited blood periodically since the onset of her illness. Her attendants informed St. André that Malepeyré had for several years had a wound, which they had never seen, in the lumbar region but that it seemed to cause her very little pain. St. André was convinced that the blood found in Malepeyré's linen was menstrual fluid, for it was inconceivable that a wound in a region that supported the weight of the body would not cause pain.

St. André urged another inquiry, this time by persons whose judgment could not easily be swayed. If the new inquiry found that Malepeyré were misrepresenting her condition, then the public would be disabused and Malepeyré would be shamed. If, on the other hand, the physical evidence corroborated her testimony, the medical community would be able to formulate an etiology of her disorder and devise a cure. St. André could envision no middle ground between exposure of deception and discovery of a disorder, however rare. Either way Malepeyré was bound to lose her religious status. Although St. André had made the connection between Malepeyré's revulsion from her menstrual cycles and her obsession with fasting, he had failed to explore the cultural and psychological dimensions of the woman's condition. He was thus unable to understand the horrible dilemma his solution posed for her, much less restore her to health.

In attempting to understand Malepeyré's behavior, historians can draw upon the insights of Patricia Crawford's article defining the cultural links between menstruation and defilement, profanation, and sin.[94] Erna Hellerstein notes that even in the mid–nineteenth century Joan of Arc's energy and courage were attributed to the fact that she did not menstruate.[95] Medieval historians Caroline Walker Bynum and Rudolf Bell have argued that women's refusal to eat and other acts of extreme self-denial represented efforts to assert personal autonomy against a dominant patriarchal culture.[96] Whether refusal to eat in the Middle Ages can be equated with anorexia and interpreted in the same light through the eighteenth century to the present or whether each case can be understood only within its specific cultural context is a matter on which Bell and Bynum disagree. Given the long cultural tradition in France associating suspension of menstruation and refusal to eat with spiritual purity—indeed, sainthood—it seems reasonable to infer that these medieval precedents may have informed Malepeyré's actions.

In the eyes of many provincial doctors and surgeons, religion was inextricably linked to popular superstition, and superstition was responsible for the majority of convulsions in women. Women were typically portrayed as victims first and foremost of their own ignorance and then of empirics who preyed upon their superstitions. For this reason, many doctors envisioned themselves as health missionaries[97] entrusted with the responsibility of altering belief structures and dissuading patients from seeking the dubious resources of the empirics. Convulsions were so common in Poitou that a group of empirics calling themselves *rabaisseurs du mal de mère* ("manipulators of dislocated wombs") had set themselves up as specialists in treating just such disorders. They were, as one correspondent to the Royal Society of Medicine observed, much more dangerous and yet less maligned than their less exotic colleagues, the itinerant charlatans, women, and empirics who made a business of reciting popular medical adages and selling secret remedies. The methods employed by these *rabaisseurs* were so unorthodox that the correspondent thought it appropriate to describe them in some detail to his Parisian associates: "If a woman has hysterical suffocations, people rush to find a *rabaisseur*. He begins to tread with the hand, then with the knees, the contracted and convulsive abdomen of the hysteric until it turns black. I have seen a pregnant woman abort as a result of this operation, die almost without sacraments and her child without baptism. Other women have been victims of this extreme cruelty. How many have perished without my knowledge?"[98]

Despite the obscurity of many empiric cures for convulsions, not all of them went unnoticed by professional doctors or the provincial press. Those cases that were publicized became causes célèbres used by editors of provincial journals to demonstrate the necessity of instructing the people. The *Journal de Troyes* in 1783 reported a dramatic example of the tragedy, bred of ignorance and superstition, that could befall convulsive women and their families.[99] It involved a middle-aged woman named Marie Semaine, wife of a laborer named Fraudin, who lived in Cerisiers-en-Othe, a small village southwest of Troyes. Mme Fraudin suffered from hysterical convulsions that had failed to respond to any of the usual remedies. She became convinced that an evil spell had been cast upon her and that only a sorcerer could counter the spell and restore her to health.

Jean Gallifier, an aged man with a frightening demeanor who was known throughout the canton as a redoubtable sorcerer, was asked to reverse the evil spell. Assuring Fraudin of a quick healing, Gallifier advised her to say some masses in preparation for the evening when he would come to reverse the spell. When Gallifier arrived at the Fraudin home, he locked himself in a room with the patient, her husband, one of their daughters, and a son-in-law. All the openings to the room were closed in order to keep the devil out. Gallifier then lit a fire and began grilling a cow's heart that had been pierced with ninety-five nails. No one left the room that night. When the Fraudins' other daughter came to the house the next morning, she was unable to rouse anyone and had to summon a locksmith to open the door. Inside, they encountered an overpowering stench and the dead bodies of all the participants in the spell.

Rather than reflecting upon the tragic effects of ignorance and superstition in the Fraudin misfortune, as the editors of the *Journal de Troyes* did, Fraudins' neighbors drew a rather different moral from the story.

Whereas the editors believed that the Fraudins died of asphyxiation, the neighbors were convinced that these deaths were the work of the devil. They reasoned that Gallifier had provoked the devil's wrath by failing to adhere exactly to the intricate forms prescribed for conducting a spell. For them, the lesson to be drawn was not to play games with the devil, whose power on earth remained a threat to mankind's health and security.

Recognizing the religious roots of many superstitions and the considerable influence that curés exerted on public opinion, provincial doctors and surgeons hoped to enlist the aid of the curés in their campaign to eradicate error. To their dismay, they discovered that local curés often proved as gullible as the people when bizarre illnesses or miraculous healings were reported. One well-publicized debate in which a provincial curé and doctor found themselves at odds concerned a young woman, Marguerite Fontenet, the wife of a weaver. Cormont, the curé of Trémilly, submitted a letter to the *Journal politique* recounting the story Mme Fontenet told him and the local court regarding the secret birth and mysterious disappearance of her three children.[100]

Cormont reported that Fontenet had experienced an extremely difficult pregnancy beginning in October and almost ending in miscarriage or premature birth six months later. A surgeon was called when Fontenet seemed to be going into labor but instead had fallen into hysterical convulsions that endangered her life. The surgeon saved her by administering bleedings and emetics, and Fontenet was restored to health. Her pregnancy continued. By June, her abdomen had become so swollen that her neighbors thought she must be ready to give birth.

At this point, according to Fontenet's deposition to the court, disaster struck. Returning home around 8:30 the evening of June 17, she noticed a man with a threatening demeanor standing near the house. Her husband reassured her that her fears of the stranger were groundless, and the matter was dropped. The next morning, the same man entered the house and, finding Fontenet alone, proposed to assist her at the birth of her child. He promised that it could be accomplished without pain to Fontenet or the child. Fontenet, frightened, sent the man away and went to tell her neighbor of the encounter. When she returned that afternoon, she found herself again alone in the house and saw the same man enter and close the door.

Fontenet testified that upon seeing him again, she was so frightened that she fainted. The man laid Fontenet in her bed, tied her hands behind her back, and gagged her, declaring that the birth would proceed. He put a candle between Fontenet's legs and seemed to deliver a child without touching Fontenet. The child was followed by another and yet another— the first, a blond; the second, a brunette; and the third, a redhead. The third had only one leg. After placing the three infants on a nightshirt, the stranger told Fontenet to look at them but not to touch them. He removed three bloddy masses, presumably the placentas, staunched the bleeding, and declared, "There you are, just as if you were a young girl again; the surgeon who will heal you will be very skillful." After tossing the placentas into the fire, the stranger wrapped the infants in a blanket, placed them in a pocket of his frockcoat, and departed.

Fontenet's husband returned seven and a half hours later to find his wife covered with blood and in a state of shock. In response to the husband's cry of fright, neighbors came running, cut the cord tying Fontenet, and sent for a surgeon. The surgeons revived Fontenet, examined her, and found her abdomen completely flat. The only evidence of a birth was the blood on Fontenet's legs and on the nightshirt where she said the infants had been placed. When Fontenet regained consciousness, she demanded to see her infants. Lest she become too agitated, she was told that they had been sent out to nurse.

The next day two doctors, Maignot and Barbolain, examined Fontenet. They could not be convinced that she had in fact given birth, for irritation of the womb and lactation were absent. Cormont remained steadfast in his belief of Fontenet's story. He felt vindicated when the signs the doctors had been seeking appeared four days later and were verified by these doctors and five surgeons. Cormont submitted his letter to the *Journal politique* in hopes, he said, of giving the medical community cause for reflection. Perhaps they might learn from this incident how to deliver children painlessly and how to restore women who had given birth to their virginal integrity. He also hoped the *Journal politique* would circulate the description of the stranger broadly so that he could be apprehended.

The editors of the *Journal politique* printed Cormont's letter in their August 1779 issue and the next month quoted from a letter they had received from the doctor, Maigrot, disavowing the blind and weak credulity that Cormont had attributed to him.[101] Maigrot maintained that he had always contended that Fontenet had never been pregnant or given birth. He attributed the swelling of her abdomen to an accumulation of blood, water, and gas that erupted in a moment of fright or insult. Although a white fluid had been secreted from Fontenet's breasts, Maigrot believed it was much too viscous to be milk. In light of the inconclusiveness of the physical evidence, the veracity of Fontenet's story depended on her word alone. Maigrot believed she had dreamed up the whole incident, but rather than accusing her of deception, he regarded her as the victim of an abused imagination.

If the strange man really did exist, Maigrot suggested that he was a seducer who had hidden his designs under the pretext of being an accoucheur. All the sensations Fontenet thought she had experienced in giving birth could, he maintained, equally have been experienced in intercourse. If the strange man did not exist, Maigrot believed that Fontenet, who had been subject to hysterical convulsions for some time, was capable of inventing him. That she should have invented the entire story seemed credible enough, for Fontenet had repeatedly promised her husband that she would give birth to three children resembling those in a portrait of St. Nicholas which hung in the church of Trémilly. Fontenet often visited the church to gaze at the portrait. In this painting, the three children were seated on a bench; the leg of the third child, a redhead, was obscured behind the bench. The similarities between the children in Fontenet's story and those in the portrait were unmistakable.

Maigrot's discussion of the case displayed an unusual concern with the psychological state of his patient, but even his analysis left the question of motivation unanswered. Although he linked Fontenet's story to her concern with having children, Maigrot never explained why she should have felt impelled, albeit unconsciously, to invent such a story. The modern reader is tempted to infer that instead of hazarding the pains of childbirth, which she evidently feared, Fontenet had evaded the burden of motherhood by giving birth to this fantasy. In this instance, as in many similar but less dramatic cases, hysterical convulsions can be seen to have been linked to women's fear of childbirth. Unfortunately, this fear went unrecognized or misunderstood by doctors and surgeons.

Because Trémilly was located near Bar-sur-Aube in the diocese of Troyes, Fontenet's story naturally attracted the attention of the editors of the *Almanach de la ville et du diocèse de Troyes*. The editors of this local almanac were not inclined to present the story as impartially as their colleagues from Bouillon had. They maintained that Fontenet's story could only be the work of an unrestrained imagination or of a deceitful mind and wondered if Fontenet had not felt the need to mask some indiscretion. In any case, they made it clear from the outset that they had no patience with superstitious folk who might be inclined to take Fontenet at her word. Nor did they feel it necessary to await the judicial inquiry before castigating the curé's guillibility and praising the doctor's judiciousness in the affair.

The editors of the almanac considered the Fontenet affair one more-skirmish in the continual battle to bring enlightenment to the countryside. Such incidents only served to remind them of the perpetual backsliding that marred whatever progress had been made. As if to shame their readers into acquiescence, they couched their discussion of the Fontenet story in these terms: "On reading this strange story, one feels immediately taken back to those centuries where wonders could be born merely if there were an imposter to publish them and an ignorant person to accept them. But in this time of light, where is the just spirit, the man the most modestly instructed in the operations of nature and of art who can see anything here other than a fable without truth, a tale that carries the characters of the most evident untruth?"[102]

They concluded their brief discussion of the incident with a remark that betrays their impatience with those who did not share their "rational" perspective. It was futile, they asserted, to reason with such people, who were hopelessly beyond the pale of enlightenment: "One could, in a longer discussion, refute all the accessory plausibilities that make up this edifice of lies; but it is necessary only to present the truth to educated people for them to see all its parts. Idiots and superficial spirits that feed on chimeras have even less need of discussions, because they are useless to them, and we do not doubt that all the efforts of reason are often obliged to yield to the torrent of prejudices."[103] This skirmish for enlightenment had little room for the subtlety or humor associated with the more renowned and effective advocates of the Enlightenment.

Conclusion: Convulsions, Cultural Critiques, and Revolution

Convulsions seemed pervasive in late eighteenth-century France, afflicting people of both sexes and all walks of life. The Enlightenment model of convulsions, focusing as it did on urban aristocratic and bourgeois women, presented a limited, even distorted picture of the problem of convulsions afflicting French society, as did the debate over mesmerism. The image of the convulsive female, however inadequately it might reflect the health problems of women, did, however, serve an important ideological function. To the minds of many enlightened writers, it effectively embodied everything that had gone wrong with an increasingly sophisticated, even decadent culture. To the historian, it reflects the tensions of an increasingly bourgeois society struggling to free itself from the sway of what it regarded as outmoded, but nonetheless seductive, aristocratic values.

An analysis of the correspondence on convulsions which provincial doctors addressed to the Royal Society of Medicine reveals that they accepted uncritically the model of convulsions formulated by their Parisian colleagues. Gradually, however, the dissonance between the social reality that provincial doctors encountered in their practices and the Parisian model became so intense that some other model was necessary. The patients the provinicial doctors treated were not idle aristrocratic or bourgeois women, but the working wives and daughters of artisans and peasants. Yet they were afflicted by convulsions, too.

Like their Parisian colleagues, provincial doctors sought an explanation for convulsions in environmental factors. The circumstances of working women were, however, quite different from those of aristocratic and bourgeois women and a new model of convulsions would have to reflect this difference. Provincial doctors identified labor rather than idleness, and ignorance rather than overrefinement, as the sources of convulsions in working women. The new model was thus an inversion of the old. It served as a critique of culture, too, but the object of attack was popular culture rather than aristocratic culture.

Although they attributed convulsions to different causes and their case histories revealed that marriage was the source of great anxiety and physical trauma for many women, provincial doctors upheld the Enlightenment model's prescription of marriage as the ideal state for women. Both Parisian and provincial doctors reinforced the bourgeois ideals of enlightenment, work, and domesticity by warning that women who deviated from their natural roles as wives and mothers risked endangering their own health and sanity and the welfare of their families.

The *Encyclopédie* article on convulsions, which linked convulsions in men to frustrated social advancement, advised men to form a more realistic notion of their place in society in order to cure their convulsions. Convulsive women, too, had to be put in their place, but a woman's place was determined by sex rather than by social condition. A study of medical correspondence, the learned journals, and the provincial press during the last two decades of the Ancien Régime reveals a growing concern with convulsions and the social and political discontent associated with convulsive behavior. Discontent among men of the lower orders of society and women of all orders seemed to be reaching a crisis point.

The literature's depiction of a phenomenal rise in convulsions on the eve of the Revolution may or may not be accurate. It does, in any case, convey the growing fear of the bourgeoisie that discontent would result in violent social upheaval rather than reform, jeopardizing the project of enlightenment, which aimed at transferring social and political authority from the traditional elite to an informed and rational public. The *Encyclopédie*'s advice to people suffering from convulsions was not, it should be remembered, to change society, but rather to bring their expectations into conformity with social reality. It was the purpose of the models of convulsions, formulated by physicians and infused with the ascendant bourgeois ethic, to do just that.

As the Ancien Régime drew to a close, the social value of the models of convulsions was reaffirmed, but their medical inadequacies were becoming ever more apparent. The prescription of enlightenment, work, and domesticity proved wanting even for women who seemed most to embody the bourgeois ethic, as Mme Necker's complaints of continual suffering from nervous disorders reveal.[104] Furthermore, medical diagnoses that functioned as cultural critiques obstructed formulation of alternative hypotheses and modes of treatment.

Still, because medical discourse and cultural constructs have been inextricably intertwined throughout Western history, it seems unlikely that attempts to solve medical problems through cultural critiques based on stereotypes of gender or class will ever be entirely abandoned. Social stereotyping certainly continued to inform discourse on disease in the nineteenth and twentieth centuries. As Herzlich and Pierret note, in the nineteenth century tuberculosis was simultaneously held to be an illness of the rich and a disease of the working class, the connotations evoked by the disease varying dramatically according to class: "Tuberculosis thus became bound up in two successive chains of signifiers: passion, the idleness and luxury of the sanatorium, and a pleasure-filled life "apart" on the one hand; the bacillus, the dank and airless slum, and exhaustion leading to an atrocious agony on the other. The disease therefore gave rise to a twofold discourse that both celebrated the consumptive and stigmatized the germ-carrier."[105] As carriers of both disease and revolution, laborers came to seem increasingly threatening during the nineteenth century, and discourse on disease served to propel a vast campaign aimed at making the working class virtuous and docile.

Examining stereotypes of sexuality, race, and madness employed in the nineteenth and twentieth centuries, Sander Gilman asserts that science creates fictions in order to explain facts. He sees no end to stereotyping, arguing that we need stereotypes in order to structure the world and to overcome our anxieties about lives that threaten to go out of control. The important task, then, is not to reform science or medicine; this would be impossible. Instead, we must understand the ideology behind the stereotyping.[106] By pushing the analysis of stereotyping back into the early modern period, we perceive how persistent, resilient, and subtle ideological themes pertaining to women, illness, and sexuality have been.

The Legacy of the Enlightenment

In recent years, two contradictory images of Enlightenment science and medicine have emerged. On the one hand, Daniel Roche portrays early eighteenth-century provincial academies as too often acceding to visions of nature as marvelous and mysterious and monstrous. Anatomy and zoology, in particular, offered scientists and the lay public a fantastic gallery of horrors and chimeras—of grotesquely deformed fetuses, animals, and plants; of fish-dogs, horses overrun with polyps, and sheep without heads. Roche argues, however, that by the 1760s, the true science had triumphed on all fronts by a series of ruptures. The ideas of Newton, Lavoisier, and the proponents of inoculation reigned supreme. Everywhere, the primacy of method prevailed: system builders were in disrepute; theories had to be proved by experimentation and observation. A true inventory of natural phenomena was assembled in order to conquer the power of the imagination.[1]

Roche describes the struggle for authority between the professional medical community and empirics or charlatans as the combat between reason and prejudice. There is no question of who should have won: while reason liberates the spirit, Roche declares, prejudice, insofar as it feeds on beliefs in the fantastic, imprisons it.[2] The rhetoric employed here is taken directly from the memoirs and proceedings of eighteenth-century scientific academies and societies of medicine. This was the way scientists and the professional medical community wanted science and medicine to be; the rhetoric offers no insight into the difficulty of achieving such an ideal. As our study of eighteenth-century medicine reveals, however, the struggle for enlightenment was by no means won by the 1760s or even the 1780s.

Carolyn Merchant's interpretation of early modern science is much darker. She finds the core of Enlightenment thought on science in the writings of Francis Bacon. In his own time, Bacon was considered the greatest propagandist for the new science, and his vision of science would later inform the ideals and work of the Encyclopedists. But what was the science Bacon envisioned? According to Merchant, human domination of nature was the primary theme of Baconian science. This theme was echoed in Descartes's desire for knowledge in the crafts in order that we might "render ourselves masters and possessors of nature."[3]

The language Bacon used was gender specific: scientists were male, and they consistently spoke of the nature they wished to transform as female. Nature had to be "bound into service," made a "slave," put "in constraint," and "molded" by the mechanical arts. Merchant argues that "Melding together a new philosophy based on natural magic as a technique for manipulating nature, the technologies of mining and metallurgy, the emerging concept of progress and a patriarchal structure of family and state, Bacon fashioned a new ethic sanctioning the exploitation of nature."[4] Bacon's vision of nature was informed by his vision of society; his devaluation of nature was directly connected to his disregard for women and thereby obtained social legitimacy. Merchant finds the legacy of "enlightened" values in the continued domination of women and nature; alternative visions of Enlightenment values, such as those we have explored in the debates over late births, the Convulsionaries, and mesmerism, are not discussed.

Sustained study of medical causes célèbres involving *maladies des femmes* reveals that there was no consensus during the Enlightenment about how science should be conducted or how society should be structured. We do not see in these debates, as Londa Schiebinger sees in eighteenth-century anatomy texts,[5] the propensity of elite European men with common interests and backgrounds to promote a particular view of women by stifling all dissent. On the contrary, in the debates examined here, all ideas were open to challenge and questioning. Various eighteenth-century writers, both within the professional scientific and medical communities and among the lay public, were as aware of the dangers of Bacon's and Descartes's dream of order and domination as they were of the promises it might hold. Ardent defenders and equally forceful critics of women both were given an opportunity to have their arguments weighed in the court of public opinion.

The debate over late births reveals how all the standard criteria of proof—the authority of the ancients, the universal laws of nature, observation and experience—were called into question and found wanting.

Medicine simply wasn't able to provide the definitive answers that society and the state demanded. The critiques of medical consultations about the Convulsionaries similarly demonstrate how fragile medical judgments were. Over the course of the eighteenth century, the medical community became increasingly troubled by the vulnerability of its judgment to dispute, especially as it found its professional authority challenged ever more stridently by empirics and charlatans.

Individual responses within the medical community to the challenges to epistemological certainty and professional authority were quite varied; they reflect the diverse approaches toward nature and society within the broader movement toward enlightenment. As Thomas Hankins has observed, although the Enlightenment exalted science, it would be a mistake to assume that the philosophes agreed with one another in their approach to nature or scientific method. Although Diderot, d'Alembert, Condillac, and Rousseau had been close friends in Paris, each went his own way by 1760. Whereas d'Alembert and Condillac remained loyal to a science built on mathematics, Diderot moved toward dynamic materialism and Rousseau inaugurated romanticism. "Nevertheless," Hankins continues, "there were certain common characteristics in their thought. Most particularly they believed that human actions should be regulated by nature and not by precepts taken from the Bible, and they believed that natural science gave insights into the workings of human nature."[6]

The debate over late births reveals, however, that even those elements of Enlightenment thought which Hankins identifies as fundamental were being called into question in medicine by the 1760s. Did natural science, indeed, provide insight into human nature and offer a model of the sort of society to which reformers should aspire? If so, what picture of nature did science disclose? Was nature inherently orderly or chaotic? Although d'Alembert, Condillac and Condorcet, like Louis, Bouvart, and Petit, believed in the existence of universal, immutable laws of nature, more skeptical philosophes such as Diderot and surgeons such as Le Bas challenged even this notion. The consequences of such a challenge are extremely significant. As Haydn Mason explains in his analysis of Diderot's *D'Alembert's Dream*, "this vision of a world where no rules of conduct apply except those imposed by society must be disturbing. Alone with his thoughts, Diderot has taken them to their extreme conclusions; it is not the moment for setting up philosophical safeguards. Yet the *Rêve* demonstrates, on the moral and social plane, the problem of a man-made society acting without reference to transcendental principles."[7]

In addition to challenging the epistemological authority of science and medicine, Diderot questioned the legitimacy of its corporative structure. The desire of a part of the medical community to establish consensus on the questions of late births and mesmerism stemmed from their conviction that enlightened medicine was inseparable from professional medicine. They believed that in order to dispel fantastic and absurd ideas from medicine, it was necessary to cut any ties between professional medicine and the ideas of empirics and charlatans. As such, their program was fundamentally at odds with Diderot's vision of how scientific research should be organized. In his article entitled "Encyclopedia," Diderot contrasted the attitudes of artisans and scientists toward knowledge. Although both groups identified knowledge with power, artisans had traditionally sought to restrict access to knowledge in order to compete more effectively in the marketplace, while scientists believed that scientific advances depended on the broad dissemination of ideas. The Encyclopedists favored the scientists and hoped to advance the mechanical arts by applying the method of the natural sciences to them. Above all, dissemination of ideas and the debate that would naturally arise from it were essential for progress. Thus, Diderot declared, "Learned men discuss things with each other, they write, they call attention to their discoveries, they contradict one another and are contradicted. . . Craftsmen, by contrast, live isolated, obscure lives."[8] Although most physicians and surgeons aspired to be scientists, many remained committed to institutional forms that Diderot associated with the crafts.

The debates over the Convulsionaries, late births, and mesmerism reveal the ambivalence some members of the community felt about entering a public arena, in which little distinction was made between the ideas of a medical professional and those of a learned or even just interested layperson. Enlightenment leaders like Voltaire presumed to speak authoritatively about medicine, but Voltaire's ideas were hardly unbiased: they were grounded in an inveterate hypochondria and an abiding suspicion of physicians. Voltaire embraced some of the superstitions regarding aberrations of nature which the medical community was intent on eradicating and exploited medicine's lack of certainty to challenge some of the most progressive ideas of science and medicine.[9] Given these tensions among those who claimed to be committed to the cause of enlightenment, how, then, was enlightenment to be defined, much less achieved?

The debates that we have explored are important precisely because Diderot's vision of the free circulation of ideas came close to being realized in them. The issues they raised about nature, medicine, and society were of such great interest to the lay public that they could not be contained within the walls of the faculties of medicine. Historians of science and medicine have too often listened only to voices coming from the faculties or government and have missed the full range of scientific and medical discourse, its complexity and its connections to larger cultural currents.

The issue of women figured prominently in all of the debates and is to be understood on many levels. For physicians and surgeons, the first level was that of medical theory and practice. Women were typically entrusted with the health care of their families. They frequently offered alternative visions of medical practice. Insofar as women were identified with superstition and charlatanry, their ideas about medicine were viewed with suspicion and their practice of medicine was seen as a threat to professional authority. The fact that women in elite circles were rumored to exert inappropriate influence on appointments to the academies only increased the tension.

But the debates over the Convulsionaries, late births, and mesmerism were not just testing medicine's limits of certainty, nor can they be reduced to quarrels over professional authority. Much more was at stake. The legitimacy of hierarchy, privilege, and patriarchy—the fundamental principles of early modern society—was itself on trial, and the language in which the trial was conducted was gender specific. Critics of aristocratic culture like Rousseau argued that the decadence of their age was to be attributed to the influence of women. Even Enlightenment figures like Diderot, who were especially sensitive to the unjust constraints the family-state compact had placed on women, were troubled by the specter of disorder that memories of the Convulsionaries provoked. How could authority be transferred from the king and his ministers to the court of public opinion if the women who figured so prominently both on the stage and in the audience of the causes célèbres were driven by irrational forces or were inclined to deceive?

Once the notion of an inherent natural order had been called into question, fears of disorder resonated with ever greater power throughout eighteenth-century society. As Sander Gilman has observed, what we really fear when the specter of disorder is raised is the irrationality of our own nature, but we tend to dissociate ourselves from this side of our nature by projecting it onto another.[10] The other on whom fears of disorder were placed in the eighteenth-century debates over the Convulsionaries, late births, and mesmerism might vary by social condition, but not by gender. The irrational other was always female.

Defenders and critics of mesmerism both argued that social ills would be alleviated if women were confined to the domestic sphere. In like manner, even as prominent philosophes feared the potential for charlatanry if women held sway over the court of public opinion, their critics identified the philosophes' movement itself with charlatanry. In the minds of the critics, the link between philosophes and charlatans was obvious and damning: both were inclined to the theatrical and tainted by their deference to the whims of women, whose taste ruled the theater and the salon.[11] The rhetoric of gender was thus used effectively and repeatedly by opposing sides, however different their social and political outlooks, were otherwise to discredit each other.[12]

Nor did such rhetoric play itself out during the Ancien Régime. As Joan Landes has demonstrated, the same language would be used by revolutionaries to remove women from the public sphere. Thus she notes that during the October Days,

"the unknown author of a polemic, *Les héroïnes de Paris*, ascribed to the marchers a sophisticated political objective to return the king to Paris where he would live under a permanent people's surveillance. But this same author spoke of channeling and reining in the women, warning that they must not model themselves after charlatans, street players, jugglers, magicians, and other uncontrollable popular entertainers. He would restrict them to guarding the tollgates into Paris to prevent the importation of spoiled grains and fruit; in short, he would make them into *bonnes bourgeoises*."[13]

Following the Revolution, the quest for medical certainty would be renewed. We see signs of it in Cabanis's *Du degré de certitude de la médecine*, which proposed to examine whether the principles of medicine have a solid basis or whether several philosophers were justified in reproaching medical science with uncertainty.[14] Whatever Cabanis's resolution of the question, however, the framers of the Napoleonic Code would not call upon medical experts to lay the foundation of a new social order. The new juridical order did not presume to adhere to universal laws of nature. The debates of the eighteenth century had demonstrated that such laws, if they existed at all, could not be proven. Another basis for authority would have to be forged, and it was found in Roman law.

Roman law placed greater restrictions on women than had either the customary laws of France or enlightened reformers of the early modern period. As Ian Maclean has observed, Roman law was itself part of a synthesis that presumed that nature, convention, and divine and human law all predisposed man rather than woman to govern. This point of view had been supported by theological, medical, ethical, and economic authority. It defined medieval views on women and continued to inform the Renaissance notion of woman, even though the authority of Aristotle, whose ideas lay at the basis of this synthesis, was under assault.[15] In like manner, although the authority of the ancients in science and medicine had been thoroughly challenged by the beginning of the nineteenth century, classical ideas regarding gender roles and the need for separating public and private spheres lay at the very base of the Napoleonic Code. They would shape attitudes and social practices pertaining to gender for the next two centuries.[16]

Feminist scholars have debated whether grounding social theory on natural law liberates or imprisons women.[17] Certainly Enlightenment views of women could be restrictive, but the debate over late births revealed that nature and science offered no indisputable authority for the subjection of women. It is regrettable that this legacy of the Enlightenment does not seem to have been preserved, for if it had been, it is questionable that social Darwinism and sociobiology would have enjoyed the vogues they have had in the nineteenth and twentieth centuries.[18]

This study has probed the ideology and practice of medicine in the eighteenth century and has demonstrated the close connection between medical causes célèbres and larger cultural concerns. Considerable effort has been made herein to rescue from oblivion the voices of little known female medical practitioners and writers. By integrating women's voices into the historical record in this manner, we see how important women's contributions were to medical debates and the formation of public opinion. By exploring medical case histories drawn from the farthest corners of France, we gain insight into women's experience with medicine and into the larger social relations that conditioned that experience.[19]

Still, a number of questions remain unanswered and perhaps unanswerable. Whom do we believe in the controversies engulfing women like Marie Mossaron, Renée, Catherine Berna, Elisabeth Sirven, Thérèse Ismère Famin, Mlle Granger, Marie Malepeyré, and Marguerite Fontenet, and how can we begin to understand these women? Were they telling the truth? Did they *believe* they were telling the truth? Or were they, as their critics maintained, guilty of falsehoods capable of undermining the whole social and political order? If we dispute assumptions like Hecquet's and Astruc's that it is woman's nature to err and deceive, might we nonetheless wonder if social conditions were such that deception was sometimes a necessary tool of survival? In the struggles over authenticity and legitimacy, recourse to seemingly miraculous cures or flukes of nature offered women in danger of being ostracized a measure of respectability.[20] Indeed, the institutions of corporative society and the terms of the family-state compact were such that it was only in areas of religion and medicine, which defied certitude, that women could find some small space in which to maneuver. How much use they made of such opportunities remains unclear.

This analysis of causes célèbres involving *maladies des femmes*, insofar as it has focused on the larger cultural concerns and ideological stakes involved, has only hinted at the ways in which women's experience of illness could transform their sense of identity and alter relationships of power and dependence within the family.[21] Firsthand accounts of women's affliction with smallpox and their terror of being rendered physically loathsome are available, as are accounts of how the experience of illness could provoke girls to challenge paternal authority and precipitate a reordering of family relationships. By examining women's letters and memoirs on matters of sickness and health, we can do much to unravel the complicated reality underlying the dominant images of women conveyed in the causes célèbres explored here. But this is another, long overdue study, as is systematic analysis of the diversity and significance of women's medical activity as bonesetters, charitable healers, dentists, empirics, folk healers, oculists, remedy vendors, surgeons, witches, midwives, and healing sisters.[22] It is my hope that these other aspects of the relationship between women and medicine in the Ancien Régime will soon become the subjects of full-scale historical inquiries.

NOTES

Introduction: Women's History and the Social History of Medicine

1. Michel Foucault, *Madness and Civilization: A History of Insanity in the Age of Reason* (New York, 1965), *The Birth of the Clinic: An Archaeology of Medical Perception* (New York, 1973), and *Histoire de la sexualité: La Volonté de savoir* (Paris, 1976).

2. See, for example, Jean-Pierre Peter, "Le Corps du délit," *Nouvelle revue de psychanalyse* 3 (1971): 99–108 and "Le Grand Rêve de l'ordre médical en 1770 et aujourd'hui," *Autrement* 4 (1975): 183–92.

3. Dorinda Outram, *The Body and the French Revolution. Sex, Class and Political Culture* (New Haven, 1989).

4. Claudine Herzlich and Janine Pierret, *Illness and Self in Society*, trans. Elborg Forster (Baltimore, 1987). Sander Gilman, *Difference and Pathology: Stereotypes of Sexuality, Race and Madness* (Ithaca, 1985). Bruno Latour, *The Pasteurization of France* (Cambridge, Mass., 1988). Robert Proctor, *Racial Hygiene: Medicine under the Nazis* (Cambridge, Mass., 1988). William Coleman, *Death Is a Social Disease* (Madison, 1982).

5. Peter Gay, "Enlightenment: Medicine and Cure," in *The Enlightenment: An Interpretation*, vol. 2, *The Science of Freedom* (New York, 1977), 12–23. In *The Role of Scientific Societies in the Seventeenth Century* (Chicago, 1928), 48, Martha Ornstein argues that Descartes was neither an anatomist nor a physiologist, but studied both sciences in order "to construct out of the current knowledge a physical basis for his philosophical views"—namely, that man and the universe were subject to the exact laws of mathematics and physics. Patrick Romanell, *John Locke and Medicine. A New Key to Locke* (New York, 1984), 9–10, advances the thesis that Locke's philosophical method and his focus on the limited scope of human understanding were grounded in his experience as a physician. Kathleen Wellman continues this theme in "Medicine as a Key to Defining Enlightenment Issues: The Case of Julien Offray de la Mettrie," in *Studies in Eighteenth-Century Culture*, ed. John Yolton and Leslie Brown (East Lansing, 1987), 17:75–89, arguing that La Mettrie's interest in medicine was the source both of his materialism and of his commitment to social reform.

6. Jean Meyer, *Diderot, homme de science* (Rennes, 1959), 361.

7. Ibid. Pierre Astruc, "Les Sciences médicales et leurs représentants dans l'*Encyclopédie*," *Revue d'histoire des sciences et de leurs applications* 4, nos. 3, 4 (1951): 359–68, and Maxime Laignel-Lavastine, "Les Médecins collaborateurs de l'*Encyclopédie*," ibid., 353–58. Also see Henri Zeiler, *Les Collaborateurs médicaux de l'Encyclopédie de Diderot et d'Alembert* (Paris, 1934), Richard N. Schwab, "The Chevalier de Jaucourt, Physician and Encyclopedist," *Journal of the History of Medicine and Allied Sciences* 13 (April 1958): 256–59 and "The History of Medicine in Diderot's *Encyclopédie*," *Bulletin of the History of Medicine* 32 (1958): 216–23.

8. Montesquieu, "Le Spicilège: 561," in *Oeuvres complètes*, ed. André Masson, 3 vols. (Paris, 1955), 2:847–48. Renée Waldinger, "Voltaire and Medicine," in *Studies on Voltaire and the Eighteenth Century*, ed. Theodore Besterman (Geneva, 1967), 58:1791.

9. Suzanne Doublet, "La Médecine dans les oeuvres de Diderot" (thèse, Bordeaux, 1933–34), 3. Daniel Mornet, *Les Sciences de la nature en France, au XVIIIe siècle: Un Chapitre de l'histoire des idées* (Paris, 1911), viii–2.

10. Robert James, *Dictionnaire universel de médecine, de chirurgie, de chymie, de botanique, d'anatomie, de pharmacie, d'histoire naturelle, etc.*, trans. Diderot, Eidous and Toussaint, 6 vols. (Paris, 1746–), 1: "Avertissement de l'éditeur."

11. Charles Paul, *Science and Immortality: The Eloges of the Paris Academy of Sciences (1699–1791)* (Berkeley, 1980), 12, 28, 99.

12. *Mémoires de l'Académie des sciences, des lettres et des arts d'Amiens*, 46 (Amiens, 1899/1900): 295.

13. Daniel Roche, *Le Siècle des Lumières en province: Académies et académiciens provinciaux, 1680–1789* (Paris, 1978), 1:235–45, 351–55.

14. Paul Delaunay, *Le Monde médical parisien au dix-huitième siècle* (Paris, 1906).

15. Michel Vovelle, *Piété baroque et déchristianisation en Provence au XVIIIe siècle: Les Attitudes devant la mort d'après les clauses des testaments (Paris, 1973)*. William Sewell, *Work and Revolution in France. The Language of Labor from the Old Regime to 1848* (Cambridge, 1981).

16. James McClellan, *Science Reorganized: Scientific Societies in the Eighteenth Century* (New York, 1985), xvii, 26. Roger Hahn, *The Anatomy of a Scientific Institution: The Paris Academy of Sciences, 1666–1803* (Berkeley, 1971), 155–58. Keith Baker, *Condorcet, From Natural Philosophy to Social Mathematics* (Chicago, 1975), 76–80.

17. Paul Delaunay, *Le Monde* and "L'Evolution médicale du XVIe au XXe siècles," *Bulletin de la Société française d'histoire de la médecine*," 22, nos. 1, 2 (1928): 28–29. Also see Toby Gelfand, *Professionalizing Modern Medicine. Paris Surgeons and Medical Science and Institutions in the Eighteenth Century* (Westport, Conn., 1980). Also Matthew Ramsey, *Professional and Popular Medicine in France, 1770–1830. The Social World of Medical Practice* (Cambridge, 1988).

18. For more on these earlier conflicts, see Terence Murphy, "Medical Culture under the Old Regime," *Historical Reflections/Réflexions Historiques* 16, nos. 2, 3 (1989): 307–50.

19. François Lebrun, *Les Hommes et la mort en Anjou aux XVIIe et XVIIIe siècle: Essai de démographie et psychologie historiques* (Paris, 1971), 284, 491–92.

20. Jacques Léonard, *Les Médecins de l'Ouest au XIXe siècle* (Paris, 1978), 1285.

21. François Lebrun, *Les Hommes*, 60–61.

22. Robert Muchembled, *Culture populaire et culture des élites dans la France moderne (XVe–XVIIIe siécles)* (Paris, 1978), 80, 204–26. For an analysis of physicians' attacks on charlatanry in the late sixteenth century, see Alison Lingo, "Empirics and Charlatans in Early Modern France: The Genesis of the Classi-

fication of the 'Other' in Medical Practice," *Journal of Social History* 19 (summer 1986): 583–604.

23. See Matthew Ramsey, *Professional and Popular Medicine*, 2–4, 314–16, for a useful description and bibliography of this sociological literature.

24. Ramsey, *Professional and Popular Medicine*; Gelfand, *Professionalizing Modern Medicine*. Recent British studies in the history of science have switched from analyzing sociopolitical influences on scientific ideas to studying the appropriation and transformation of scientific ideas by nonscientists. In "Prosopography as a Research Tool," *History of Science* 12 (1974): 21, Steven Shapin and Arnold Thackray assess

> the ways in which natural knowledge served as a key ingredient in a deep transformation of British thought, society and culture. Regarded as the exclusive preserve of expert scientists, it has indeed proved very difficult to see how enquiry into natural phenomena could have played such a role. Historiographically, we have been accustomed to disregard science as it percolates from men of science to the generally literate. It has either been dismissed as non-science, scientism (hence, irrelevant or pernicious), misunderstood science (hence, error), or popularized science (hence, trivial). In point of fact, science *as people think of it and as they use it* is every bit as historically important as science as scientists conceive of it.

Also see Adrian Desmond, "Artisan Resistance and Evolution in Britain, 1819–1848," *Osiris*, 2d ser., 3 (1987): 77–110.

25. For a survey of this growing body of literature, see Benjamin Nathans's review article, "Habermas's 'Public Sphere' in the Era of the French Revolution," *French Historical Studies* 16, no. 3 (1990): 620–44. Also see Keith Baker, "Politics and Public Opinion," in Jack Censer and Jeremy Popkin, eds., *Press and Politics in Pre-Revolutionary France* (Berkeley, 1987), 204–46 and "Politique et opinion publique sous l'Ancien Régime," *Annales. Economies, Sociétés, Civilisations* 42, no. 1 (1987): 3–25. And see Thomas Kaiser, "This Strange Offspring of *Philosphie*: Recent Historiographical Problems in Relating the Enlightenment to the French Revolution," *French Historical Studies* 15, no. 3 (1988): 556; Sarah Maza, "Le Tribunal de la nation: Les Mémoires judiciaires et l'opinion publique à la fin de l'Ancien Régime," *Annales. Economies, Sociétés, Civilisations* 42, no. 1 (1987): 73–90; and Dena Goodman, *Criticism in Action: Enlightenment Experiments in Political Writing* (Ithaca, 1989). Herbert Dieckmann emphasizes the importance the philosophes placed on shaping public opinion in "Themes and Structure of the Enlightenment" and "The Concept of Knowledge in the *Encyclopédie*," in *Essays in Comparative Literature* (St. Louis, 1961), 41–107. John Lough explores the intersecting worlds of writers—whether they be philosophes, playwrights, or journalists—publishers, and readers in *Writer and Public in France from the Middle Ages to the Present Day* (Oxford, 1978), 164–274.

26. Jean Ehrard and Jacques Roger, "Deux périodiques français du XVIII⁰ siècle: *Le Journal des savants et les Mémoires de Trévoux*," in *Livre et société dans la France du XVIII⁰ siècle*, ed. François Furet, 2 vols. (Paris, 1975 and 1980), 1:33–57.

27. Jeremy Popkin, "Introduction," in Censer and Popkin, *Press and Politics*, 11–19. Students of the press caution against using letters to the editors of journals as a sure means of gauging public opinion because many such letters were generated in-house and were not authentic. I would assume that this caution applies more to anonymous letters than to those signed by physicians, surgeons, and curés who can be identified.

28. Jean Lecuir, "La Médicalisation de la société française dans la deuxième moitié du XVIIIe siècle en France: Aux Origines des premiers traités de médecine légale," *Annales de Bretagne* 86, no. 2 (1979): 231–50 offers a good introduction and bibliography to the literature on medical jurisprudence. For more on specific primary texts, see chapter 3 herein. Not much research has been done on actual cases of medical jurisprudence in France or Europe, but Dr. A. Guisan surveys specific cases of paternity suits, hysteria, rape, and infanticide and notes the influence of French laws, especially the Edict of Henri II, on Swiss courts in "La Médecine judiciaire au 18e siècle, d'après les procédures criminelles vaudoises," *Revue suisse de médecine, ou Schweizerische Rundschau für Medizin*, no. 10 (1913), 421–32 and no. 16 (1913), 672–82.

29. Lecuir, "La Médicalisation," 240.

30. Ibid., 240–41.

31. Robert Kreiser, *Miracles, Convulsions, and Ecclesiastical Politics in Early Eighteenth-Century Paris* (Princeton, 1978) offers a fine analysis of the Convulsionary movement, but it does not focus on the role of medical experts in adjudicating the debates, nor does it pursue women's involvement in the movement in depth.

32. Sarah Hanley, "Engendering the State: Family Formation and State Building in Early Modern France," *French Historical Studies* 16, no. 1 (1989): 4–27 and "Family and State in Early Modern France: The Marriage Pact," in *Connecting Spheres: Women in the Western World, 1500 to the Present*, ed. Marilyn Boxer and Jean Quaetart (Oxford, 1987), 53–63.

33. Robert Darnton, *Mesmerism and the End of the Enlightenment in France* (New York, 1968).

34. See, for example, the 30 August, 1786 letter of Collomb and Coindre, physicians of Lyons, to the Société Royale de Médecine (SRM), SRM Archives, Académie Nationale de Médecine, Paris, carton 139, and the *Gazette salutaire* of 7 December 1769.

35. Renate Blumenfeld-Kosinski, *Not of Woman Born. Representations of Caesarean Birth in Medieval and Renaissance Culture* (Ithaca, 1990), 105–17, explores these themes for an earlier period, that of the witch-hunts. For a comprehensive treatment of the role of the midwife in eighteenth-century society, see Jacques Gélis, *La Sage-femme ou le médecin. Une Nouvelle Conception de la vie* (Paris, 1988). On p. 21, Gélis assesses the ambiguous position held by the midwife, who could either be an abortionist or denounce women seeking abortions, be an accomplice in infanticide or aid in its repression, be a facilitator in parents' abandonment of their children or assist authorities seeking to determine the identity of such parents. Presumably, the nursing sisters who staffed so many of the hospitals in the Ancien Régime presented no such ambiguity, but as Colin Jones notes in *The Charitable Imperative. Hospitals and Nursing in Ancien Régime and*

Revolutionary France (London, 1989), orders like the Daughters of Charity in the Montpellier Hôtel-Dieu were specifically prohibited from treating "femmes de mauvaise vie" or women in childbirth. On p. 143, Jones speculates that the latter prohibition may have been based on the assumption that women who gave birth in hospitals were inevitably women of ill repute, possibly infected with venereal disease.

36. *Parole de dieu et révolution. Les Sermons d'un curé angevin avant et pendant la guerre de Vendée*, présenté par François Lebrun (Toulouse, 1979), 86–89. Also see the abbé Dinouart's *Abrégé de l'embryologie sacrée, ou Traité des devoirs des prêtres, des médecins, des chirurgiens et des sages-femmes envers les enfants qui sont dans le sein de leurs mères* (Paris, 1775). Governmental surveys of the state of midwifery in the 1780s can be found in cartons 85–87 of the SRM Archives.

37. Colm Kiernan, *The Enlightenment and Science in Eighteenth-Century France*, vol. 59A of *Studies on Voltaire and the Eighteenth Century*, ed. T. Besterman (Oxfordshire, 1973), 86; Haydn Mason, *French Writers and Their Society* (London, 1982), 182–96; and Jacques Roger, *Les Sciences de la vie dans la pensée française du XVIIIe siècle: La Génération des animaux de Descartes à l'Encyclopédie* (Paris, 1963).

38. Joan Scott, "Survey Articles, Women in History II: The Modern Period," *Past and Present*, no. 101 (November 1983), 141–57.

39. Ian Maclean, *The Renaissance Notion of Woman: A Study in the Fortunes of Scholasticism and Medical Science in European Intellectual Life* (Cambridge, 1980). Maclean's description of Renaissance critiques of court ladies who deviated from the strictures imposed by the medieval synthesis bears a striking similarity to the rhetoric employed in the eighteenth-century medical causes célèbres. Thus Maclean notes on p. 64:

> The *taciturnitas* for which the domestic woman is praised is abandoned; her private exclusive relationship to a dominating husband is replaced by a public, promiscuous, social role in which, by convention, she is the dominant partner; she is splendidly arrayed, in spite of moralists' warnings about the feminine weakness for vanity, ornament, extravagance and luxury; she enjoys the delights of food, music and dancing despite her supposed propensity to sensuality.
>
> This mode of life conflicts not only with ancient prescriptions but also with Christian moral teaching. It raises to some degree the question of the double standard of morality, which relates most obviously to adultery but also is implicit in social freedom. It is to be expected that moralists in a patrilinear and patriarchal society would recommend a private and domestic role for women as wives, and reject social and marital liberty for both sexes except in the case of courtesans.

The exception accorded by Renaissance theorists, however, was no longer countenanced by critics of Ancien Régime society, whose numbers were rising steadily in the late eighteenth century. These critics equated women engaged prominently in the public sphere with courtesans and urged that a more rigorous standard of morality be applied to women and men from even the highest orders of society, whose deviance had previously escaped censure.

40. Ibid., 82.

41. See Cynthia Koepp's article on the *Encyclopédie* in *Work in France. Representations, Meaning, Organization, and Practice*, ed. Koepp and Steven Kaplan (Ithaca, 1986).

42. In *Women and the Public Sphere in the Age of the French Revolution* (Ithaca, 1988), Joan Landes surveys critiques of women's influence on public opinion, but the extent of that influence and the means by which it was exercised require further analysis. As the session on "Reassessing Habermas: The Cultural Construction of the Public Sphere in Eighteenth-Century France" held at the Annual Meeting of the Society for French Historical Studies in March 1991 made apparent, the conflicting currents in perceptions of women's involvement in the public sphere during the Enlightenment need to be sorted out much more systematically.

43. See chapter 5 herein. In *La Sage-femme ou le médecin*, 112–13, Jacques Gélis explores the ambiguous role of Mme du Coudray, whose late eighteenth-century courses in accouchement increased midwives' knowledge and presumably saved lives but also subordinated them to surgeons for good. Jean-Pierre Peter, "Les Médecins et les femmes," in *Misérable et glorieuse: La Femme du XIXᵉ siècle*, ed. Jean-Paul Aron, (Paris, 1980), 90, argues that women were crucial allies in nineteenth-century physicians' efforts to improve the physical and moral health of the poor, the aged, the morally deviant. Social control was an equal part of the agenda. "On va ensemble," he writes, "redresser, sauver, marier, assainir."

Chapter One. The Debate over the Convulsionaries of St. Médard, 1727–1765

1. Robert Kreiser, *Miracles, Convulsions, and Ecclesiastical Politics in Early Eighteenth-Century Paris* (Princeton, 1978), 153. Also see Robert Kreiser, "Religious Enthusiasm in Early Eighteenth-Century Paris: The Convulsionaries of Saint-Médard," *Catholic Historical Review* 61, no. 3 (1975): 364.

2. Catherine-Laurence Maire. *Les Convulsionnaires de Saint-Médard. Miracles, convulsions et prophéties à Paris au XVIIIᵉ siècle* (Paris, 1985), 13.

3. Ibid., 123, 219.

4. Ibid., 24. Also see Léon Abensour, *La Femme et le féminisme avant la Révolution* (Paris, 1923), 286–92.

5. *Consultation sur les convulsions* (Paris, 1735), 28.

6. Odile Arnold, *Le Corps et l'âme. La Vie des religieuses au XIXᵉ siècle* (Paris, 1984), 85–88.

7. *Consultation sur les convulsions*, 19.

8. *Exposition du sentiment de plusieurs théologiens défenseurs légitimes de l'oeuvre des convulsions et des miracles au sujet de la consultation des docteurs, du 7 janvier 1735* (n.p., 18 February 1735), 19. Also see Sauveur-François Morand, *Opuscules de chirurgie* (Paris, 1768–72), 297.

9. Rigault, "Lettre," Recueil de discours de différens convulsionnaires (1732–33), 276. Manuscript, Newberry Library, Chicago.

10. *Entretiens sur les miracles des derniers temps, ou Les Lettres de M. le chevalier——* (n.p., 1732), 7.

11. *Lettre à un confesseur touchant le devoir des médecins et chirurgiens: Au Sujet des miracles et des convulsions (n.p.,* 23 March 1733), 4.

12. Ibid.

13. Paul Delaunay, *Le Monde médical parisien au 18ème siècle* (Paris, 1906), 41. François Quesnay, a physician and critic of the Royal Academy of Surgery, noted yet another dimension to the close ties between the church and the medical community: "physicians, bound by their ecclesiastical background, had a horror of blood, women, and sex" (*Recherches critiques et historiques sur l'origine, sur les divers états et sur les progrès de la recherche de la chirurgie en France* [Paris, 1744], 27, paraphrased by Terence Murphy in "The Transformation of Traditional Medical Culture under the Old Regime," *Historical Reflections/Réflexions Historiques*, 16, nos. 2, 3 [1989]: 341).

14. Claude Joseph Prévost, *Principes de jurisprudence sur les visites et rapports judiciaires des médecins, chirurgiens, apothicaires, et sages-femmes* (Paris, 1753), 231–93.

15. *Procès-verbaux de plusieurs médecins et chirurgiens, dressés par ordre de Sa Majesté, au sujet de quelques personnes soi-disantes agitées de convulsions* (Paris, 1732), 2, 4, 7, 9, 11, 13, 15, 16.

16. *Réflexions sur l'ordonnance du Roy en date du 27 janvier 1732 qui ordonne que la porte du petit cimetière de la paroisse de St. Médard sera et demeura fermée, etc. Sur les procès-verbaux de plusieurs médecins et chirurgiens qui sont le fondement de cette ordonnance. Et sur les événemens dont l'exercise de l'ordonnance a été suivie* (n.p., 27 January 1732), 46–53. Also see Kreiser, *Miracles*, 211–213.

17. *Réflexions sur l'ordonnance du Roy*, 38.

18. Louis-Basile Carré de Montgeron, *La Vérité des miracles opérés à l'intercession de M. de Pâris et autres appellans, démontrée contre M. l'Archevêque de Sens* (Utrecht, 1737).

19. Louis Nigon de Berty, *Requête du Promoteur Général de l'Archevêque de Paris* (Paris, 1735), 19.

20. Ibid., 63.

21. Ibid., 58, 64.

22. Ibid., 67.

23. Ibid., 19. Also see Sauveur-François Morand, *Opuscules de chirurgie* (Paris, 1768–72), 297.

24. Le Vasseur et Clerambourg, *Lettre* (n.p., 1735), 3.

25. Louis Jean Le Thieullier, *Lettre à M.L.N.* (n.p., 27 December 1735), 3.

26. Marie Mossaron, *Lettre à Monseigneur l'Archevêque de Paris, au sujet de ce qui est dit dans son Ordonnance du 8 novembre 1735, contre le miracle de sa guérison. . .* (n.p., 1735), 15.

27. Ibid., 51.

28. Ibid., 56–69.

29. *Consultation sur les convulsions*, 23, 29. Nigon de Berty, *Requête*, 69.

30. Charles Hugues Le Fevre de Saint Marc, *La Vie de M. Hecquet, Dr. Régent et ancien doyen de la Faculté de Médecine de Paris. Contenant un catalogue raisonné de ses ouvrages* (Paris, 1740), 78.

31. Félix Vicq d'Azyr, ed., *Encyclopédie méthodique, ou par ordre des matières. Médecine* (Paris, 1792), 7:77–90. Among Hecquet's works on other topics were: *Divers ouvrages sur la petite vérole* (Paris, 1722) and *La Médecine, la chirurgie et la pharmacie des pauvres*, 3 vols. (Paris, 1740).

32. Le Fevre de Saint Marc, *La Vie*, 78.

33. Michel Foucault, *Folie et déraison* (Paris, 1961), 666–70. This is in contrast to Jan Goldstein's assertion of the novelty of Hecquet's approach in " 'Moral Contagion': A Professional Ideology of Medicine and Psychiatry in Eighteenth-and Nineteenth-Century France," in *Professions and the French State, 1700–1900*, ed. Gerald Geison (Philadelphia, 1984).

34. Susanna Barrows, *Distorting Mirrors: Visions of the Crowd in Late Nineteenth-Century France* (New Haven, 1981), 45. My analysis of the Convulsionary and mesmerist movements of the eighteenth century undermines Barrows's assertion that women were seen by many in the Third Republic as more dangerous and more problematical than ever before.

35. Philippe Hecquet, *Réponse à la "Lettre à un confesseur touchant le devoir des médecins et des chirurgiens, au sujet des miracles des convulsions"* (Paris, 1733), 12.

The notion that sexuality pervaded the whole being of women and not of men influenced the manner in which cases of impotence were adjudicated during the Ancien Régime. Cases challenging the fertility of women were seldom heard, for infertility was thought to be a consequence of frigidity—a temporary phenomenon. Also, the physical signs of impotence were more easily discernible in men than in women. See Nicolas Desessarts, *Causes célèbres*, 2 (1775): cause 5; 9 (1775): cause 20; 13 (1776): cause 32; 91 (1782): cause 279; 171 (1789): cause 561. Also see Jean Baptiste Denisart, *Dictionnaire* 2 (1771): 700–705 and Pierre Darmon, *Le Tribunal d'impuissance. Virilité et défaillances conjugales dans l'ancienne France* (Paris, 1979). In his article on impotence, *Dictionnaire philosophique, Oeuvres complètes*, 1:471–72, Voltaire deplored efforts to determine whether or not a marriage had been consummated as inconclusive and an unconscionable assault on privacy, noting that it was only the Christian religion that had established tribunals to adjudicate quarrels between brazen wives and shameful husbands.

36. Philippe Hecquet, *Le Naturalisme des convulsions dans les maladies de l'épidémie convulsionnaire* (Soleure, 1733), [1st part], 64.

37. Ibid., 181.

38. Philippe Hecquet, *Le Naturalisme des convulsions démontré par le physique, par l'histoire naturelle, et par les événemens de cette oeuvre, et démontrant l'impossibilité du divin qu'on lui attribue dans une lettre sur les secours meurtriers* (Soleure, 1733), 2d part, 99–101.

39. Hecquet, *Le Naturalisme*, [1st part], 168.

40. Ibid., 152.

41. Hecquet, *Le Naturalisme*, 2d part, 105.

42. Ibid., 107.

43. Hecquet, *Réponse*, 7–8.

44. Ibid., 9–10. Also see Hecquet, *Le Naturalisme*, [1st part], 18, 34, 141, 146.

45. Hecquet, *Le Naturalisme*, 2d part, 112.

46. Ibid., 28.

47. Philippe Hecquet, *La Médecine théologique, ou La Médecine créée, telle qu'elle se fait voir ici, sortie des mains de Dieu, créateur de la nature, et régie par ses loix* (Paris, 1733), 1st part, 542–43.

48. Le Fevre de Saint Marc, *La Vie*, 10–18.

49. Hecquet, *La Médecine théologique*, 1st part, xlvii–xlviii.

50. Hecquet, *La Médecine théologique*, 2d part, 115.

51. Hecquet, *De l'indécence aux hommes d'accoucher les femmes, et de l'obligation de celles-ci de nourrir leurs enfants* (Trévoux, 1708). Also see Jocelyne Livi, *Vapeurs de femmes: Essai historique sur quelques fantasmes médicaux et philosophiques* (Paris, 1984), 66–69. In *Histoire des mères du Moyen Age à nos jours* (Paris, 1977), 72–73, Yvonne Knibiehler and Catherine Fouquet view Hecquet's opposition to male accoucheurs as an expression of regard and respect for women.

52. Jacques Gélis, *La Sage-femme ou le médecin. Une Nouvelle Conception de la vie* (Paris, 1988), 102–3

53. Jacques-Albert Hazon, *Notice des hommes les plus célébres de la Faculté de médecine en l'Université de Paris, depuis 1110, jusqu'en 1750* (Paris, 1778), 190.

54. Maire, *Les Convulsionnaires*, 87–88. Also see Eliane Gabert-Boche, "Les Miraculés du cimitière Saint-Médard à Paris (1727–1735)," in *Les Miracles miroirs des corps*, ed. Jacques Gélis and Odile Redon (Paris, 1983), 132.

55. Maire, *Les Convulsionnaires*, 106.

56. Ibid., 54.

57. Gabert-Boche, *Les Miraculés*, 132.

58. Maire, *Les Convulsionnaires*, 246.

59. Jean-Claude Pie, "Anne Charlier, un miracle eucharistique dans le faubourg Saint-Antoine," in *Les Miracles miroirs des corps*, ed. Jacques Gélis and Odile Redon (Paris, 1983), 185–86.

60. Gabert-Boche, *Les Miraculés*, 157. Also see Jan Goldstein, " 'Moral Contagion' and Psychiatry," 181–217.

61. Arthur Wilson, *Diderot* (Oxford, 1971), 54–55.

62. Diderot's solicitude for women and impatience with their social plight is expressed in *Bougainville's Voyage*. I am grateful to Professor Raymond Birn for drawing my attention to this aspect of Enlightenment thought.

63. For more on Diderot's view of the way in which women's nervous disorders were exploited by the church, see L. J. Jordanova, "Natural Facts: A Historical Perspective on Science and Sexuality," in *Nature, Culture, and Gender*, ed. Carol MacCormack and Marilyn Strathern (Cambridge, 1980), 50–51. Also see Suzanne Doublet, "La Médecine dans les oeuvres de Diderot" (Université de Bordeaux, Faculté de Médecine, thèse 144, 1933–34), 58, quoting Diderot's *Jacques le Fataliste:* "There comes a moment in which almost all young girls are tormented by

a vague restlessness; they seek solitude; the silence of cloisters appeals to them. . . . They take for the voice of God the first effort of a temperament that is developing, and it is precisely when nature entreats that they embrace a type of life contrary to the voice of nature. The error does not last; the pressing of nature becomes clearer; it is recognized; and the sequestered being falls into regrets, languor, vapors, madness or despair."

64. For more on late eighteenth-century Jansenist claims to miraculous healings in the provinces, see the files concerning the 1785 case of Louise Guélon in the Bibliothèque Municipale de Troyes, Bibliothèque Carteron, 77-I; 144-XIII; 7-XXI; 23-XVIII; 23-XIX; and *Journal de Troyes*, 27 April 1785: 65–66. For the case of Jeanne Caillot of Gien, see the *Journal encyclopédique* 5 (July, 1771): 275–79.

65. Edmond Jean François Barbier, *Journal historique et anecdotique du règne de Louis XV*, 4 vols. (Paris, 1846–56), 4:339–41.

66. Maire, *Les Convulsionnaires*, 20. Also see "Procès-verbal dressé par M. de La Condamine," *Correspondance littéraire*, ed. Grimm et Diderot (Paris, 1878–), 3:18–37 and "Conversations avec M. de La Barre, et journée du Vendredi-Saint 1760, par M. du Doyer de Gastel," *Correspondance littéraire*, 2:382–94.

67. Maire, *Les Convulsionnaires*, 21 and Barbier, 4:298.

68. Voltaire, "Convulsions," *Dictionnaire philosophique*, 267 and Gabert-Boche, *Les Miraculés*, 157.

69. Maire, *Les Convulsionnaires*, 19.

70. Voltaire, *Oeuvres complètes*, Correspondance, 1763–65 (Paris, 1881), 11: 27. Elie Catherine Fréron, *L'Année littéraire*, passim.

Chapter Two. The Debate over Late Births, 1764–1806

1. Paul Delaunay, *Le Monde médical parisien au dix-huitième siècle* (Paris, 1906), 431–40. For more on Gerbier, see B. Haureau, *Catalogue chronologique des oeuvres imprimées et manuscrites de J. B. Gerbier* (Paris, 1863); and Saulnier de la Pinelais, *Le Barreau du parlement de Bretagne, 1553–1790* (Rennes/Paris, 1896), 258–68. In *La Femme au dix-huitième siècle* (Paris, 1982), 204–5, Edmond and Jules de Goncourt find the increasing number of aristocratic and bourgeois women seeking legal separation from their spouses over the course of the eighteenth century remarkable. These women flocked to the Palais to hear the eloquent pleas of Gerbier and Bonnières, apparently seeking rhetorical models as they prepared for their own day in court. In *La Poupliniére et la musique de chambre au XVIIIe siècle* (Geneva, 1971), Georges Cucuel discusses the La Poupliniére case at some length. The courts ruled that birth of a child born after the death of its father could not alter the provisions of the father's will. The case became a cause célèbre because the facts were not presented clearly, and public interest focused on the personalities of the parties involved. The mother excited widespread sympathy while her opponent, Mlle de Vandy, was ridiculed for her heartlessness and excessive modesty. Females were especially touched by the judgment, as the correspondence of the adolescent girl Geneviève de Malboissière reveals. See *Une Jeune Fille au XVIIIe siècle: Lettres de Geneviève de Malboissière à*

Adélaide Méliand 1761–1766, ed. Albert, Comte de Luppé (Paris, 1925), 76.

2. John McManners, *Death and the Enlightenment. Changing Attitudes to Death among Christians and Unbelievers in Eighteenth-Century France* (Oxford, 1981), 397.

3. For more on the causes célèbres literature, see Jean Sgard, "La littérature des causes célèbres," *Approches des Lumières: Mélanges offerts à Jean Fabre* (Paris, 1974), 459–70. Hans-Jurgen Lusebrink studies the large portion of causes célèbres devoted to sexual crimes in "Les Crimes sexuels dans les causes célèbres," *Dix-huitième siècle* 12 (1980): 153–62, while Tracey Rizzo explores "Sexual Violence in the Enlightenment: The State, the Bourgeoisie, and the Cult of the Victimized Women," *Proceedings of the Western Society for French History* 15 (1988): 122–29. Excerpts from the original cases of particular interest to women can be found in Isabelle Vissière, ed., *Procès de femmes au temps des philosophes, ou la violence masculine au XVIIIe siècle* (Paris, 1985). Sarah Maza discusses the revolutionary potential of judicial memoirs in "Le Tribunal de la nation: Les Mémoires judiciares et l'opinion publique à la fin de l'Ancien Régime," *Annales. Economies, Sociétés, Civilisations* 42, no. 1 (1987): 73–90.

4. Louis Petit de Bachaumont, *Mémoires secrets pour servir à l'histoire de la République des Lettres en France, depuis* 1762 jusquâ nos jours, 27 December 1787.

5. For more on these causes célèbres and Voltaire's involvement in them, see Peter Gay, *Voltaire's Politics* (Princeton, 1959), 273–308 and passim.

6. For some barnyard wisdom, see Pouteau, "Recherches pour et contre la possibilité physique des naissances tardives," *Gazette salutaire*, 6 February 1766 and Darcet, "Lettre concernant des poulets d'une même couvée, éclos à des termes fort éloignés les unes des autres," *Journal de medecine, chirurgie et pharmacie* 25 (1766): 59–60. This journal published lengthy exchanges regarding cases of prolonged pregnancies involving Mme Dulignac, the wife of a surgeon in Pont-Sainte-Maxence, and Mme Soyer, a peasant from Harbonnières en Santerre. See 23 (1765): 128–132:25 (1766): 426; and 27 (1766): 539.

7. The Bibliothèque Municipale of Rennes possesses an especially rich collection of judicial memoirs and factums that demonstrate how lawsuits could be drawn out for generations, becoming increasingly complex. See, for example, Bibliothèque Municipale/Rennes, Collection de mémoires et factums—Bretagne:

1. 627, vol. 2, no. 8: 1777 etat du procès regarding the estate of the comtesse de Villeneuve, who had died in 1698. This factum sought to appeal decisions made in 1679, 1734, 1735, 1742, 1743, 1745, 1750, 1753," etc., etc."

2. 627, vol. 2, no. 10: factum of 1761, following factums of 1712, 1713, 1714, 1716, 1721, 1740 regarding the conduct of Louise-Anne de Gouandour (d. 1731), widow of Vincent Jourdain du Conedor (d. 1689) as tutrice of the estate of her 3 children.

3. 627, vol. 2, no. 13: case pleaded in 1753, seeking the appeal of a sentence of 1744 regarding the terms of the marriage contract of 1690 between Messire Jean d'Acigné and Dame Marie Gabrielle de Lescu. The dispute involved neither the original parties nor their immediate descendants, but the third generation. It arose when the daughter of d'Acigné and de Lescu died childless,

leaving the collateral heirs to quarrel over the respective rights of paternal and maternal heirs.

Also see Bibliothèque Municipale de Nevers, 3N. 582: Mémoire pour Dame Marie-Anne Rapine de Sainte-Marie, Veuve de M. de Theillat, demanderesse: contre le sieur Louis François Rapine de Sainte-Marie, 1780. This case, which pitted a poor sister against her rich brother in a dispute over an inheritance from their uncle, was decided in favor of the sister.

And see Yvonne Bézard, *Une famille bourguignonne au XVIIIe siècle* (Paris, 1930) and Léon Abensour, *La Femme et le féminisme avant la Révolution* (Paris, 1923), 146–47, 162–65, 247. Abensour documents cases of women of all social conditions—aristocrat, bourgeoisie, peasant—involved in extensive litigation. The fact that individuals from the lower, as well as higher and middle, ranks of society took an interest in causes célèbres is demonstrated in Maurice Gresset, ed., *Une Famille nombreuse au XVIIIe siècle. Le Livre de raison d'Antoin-Alexandre Barbier, notaire et vigneron bisontin (1762–1776)* (Toulouse, 1981). Barbier was constantly embroiled in lawsuits, including one with his mother-in-law over his daughter's accession to some vineyards following the death of her mother and one with his children over an estate left by their uncle. The only reading outside books of piety which Barbier did was from the journals of causes célèbres, borrowed from a servant. For more on the laws, customs, and royal ordinances regulating inheritance, see Robert Joseph Pothier, *Traité des successions, Oeuvres, contenant les traités du droit français*, ed. M. Dupin (Paris, 1825), vol. 7, and William Doyle, *The Parlement of Bordeaux and the End of the Old Regime 1771–1790* (New York, 1974), chap. 8. Doyle notes that marriage contracts were more important than wills in establishing property rights. A childless marriage was considered truly disastrous, precipitating a crisis that involved all branches of a family and often led to conflicts between wives and collateral heirs. For more on the matter of inheritance in early modern France, see Jonathan Dewald, *The Formation of a Provincial Nobility: The Magistrates of the Parlement of Rouen, 1499–1610* (Princeton, 1980), Margaret Darrow, *Revolution in the House: Family, Class, and Inheritance in Southern France, 1775–1825* (Princeton, 1989), and James Traer, *Marriage and the Family in Eighteenth-Century France* (Ithaca, 1980).

8. Anatole de Gallier, *La Vie de province au XVIIIe siècle. Les Femmes, les moeurs, les usages* (Paris, 1887) contrasts the reserve of life in the provinces with the license in Paris; nevertheless, or perhaps for this reason, factums and scandals had enormous popular appeal in the countryside.

9. Stéphanie-Félicité du Crest de St. Aubin, Comtesse de Genlis, *Souvenirs de Félicie*, in *Bibliothèque des mémoires relatifs à l'histoire de France pendant le XVIIIe et le XIXe siècle*, ed. Jean Barrière (Paris, 1857), 14:137–39.

10. *Une Jeune Fille au XVIIIe siècle*, 253–54.

11. Alice Laborde, *L'Oeuvre de Mme de Genlis* (Paris, 1966), 88–89, Mlle d'Espinassy, *Essai sur l'éducation des demoiselles* (Paris, 1764), 65–69, and Albert, Comte de Luppé, *Les Jeunes Filles à la fin du XVIIIe siècle* (Paris, 1925), 179–81.

12. Léon Abensour, *La Femme et le féminisme*, 420.

13. Jean Astruc, *Traité des maladies des femmes, où l'on a tâché de joindre à une théorie solide la pratique la plus sûre et la mieux éprouvée* (Paris, 1765), 5:284–85.

14. See, for example, the letter of M. Dolignon to M. Dufau regarding the stir Catherine Berna created when the whole village of Cressi en Laonnois witnessed her giving birth to four frogs. ("Prétendu sortilege," *Affiches de Bordeaux,* 6 January 1774, 5–7). This case resembled the Mary Tofts affair occurring in Surrey, England, in 1726 and ridiculed by Voltaire in *Des singularités de la nature,* in *Oeuvres complètes* 3:759–60, though in the Tofts affair, rabbits rather than frogs were pulled from the womb.

15. On difficulties with lactation attributed to gypsy curses, see the case of Françoise Ailler, the young wife of a sailor, described in letters dated *an V* by Bret and Laudun, doctors of Arles-sur-Rhône, SRM Archives, carton 131, nos. 6, 28.

16. The mother whose fetus was born without a neck attributed the deformity to having been startled during pregnancy by an owl bearing a striking resemblance to the fetus. See the letter from Bilon, a surgeon, in the "Avis divers" of the *Affiches du Dauphiné,* 9 April 1779, 109. Other reports of monsters appeared in the *Journal de Nancy,* 1781, 243–45; the *Affiches de Dijon* 22 (28 May 1776): 86–95; and the *Affiches pour les Trois Evêchés et la Lorraine* 21 (27 May 1779): 166–67.

17. Canet, master apothecary in Alby, letter to Lassone of 2 January 1782, SRM Archives, carton 199. Some powders hawked by charlatans to prevent fetal deformities reportedly provoked convulsions strong enough to cause miscarriages. See the report of the surgeons of Villeneuve St. Georges and environs to Vicq d'Azyr, SRM Archives, carton 199.

18. Jean Meyer, *La Noblesse bretonne au XVIIIe siècle,* 2 vols. (Paris, 1966), 2: 1115–18.

19. François Métra, *Correspondance secrète, politique, et littéraire,* 16 vols. (London, 1787–89). Louis Petit de Bachaumont, *Mémoires secrets pour servir à l'histoire de la République des Lettres en France, depuis 1762 jusqu'à nos jours,* 36 vols. (London, 1777–89). For more on Bachaumont, see Charles Aubertin, *L'Esprit public au XVIIIe siècle. Etude sur les mémoires et les correspondances politiques des contemporains. 1715 à 1789* (Paris, 1873) and Robert Tate, *Petit de Bachaumont: His Circle and the Mémoires Secrets,* in *Studies on Voltaire and the Eighteenth Century,* ed. Theodore Besterman, vol. 65 (Geneva, 1968).

20. Claude Grimmer, *La Femme et le bâtard. Amours illégitimes et secrètes dans l'ancienne France* (Paris, 1983), 255–57.

21. Robert, "Traité des principaux objets de médicine, avec un sommaire de la plûpart des thèses soutenues aux ecoles de Paris, depuis 1752 jusqu'en 1764," *Gazette salutaire,* 23 April 1767. A large literature on the effects of a pregnant woman's imagination on fetal development spanned the eighteenth century and included works by Benjamin Bablot, Isaac Bellet, Jacques-Auguste Blondel, J. B. Demangeon, and Louis-Sebastien Saucerotte listed in the bibliography below. For the Encyclopedists' views on the subject, see the *Encyclopédie* articles on "Grossesse" and "Imagination des femmes enceintes sur le foetus."

22. Voltaire, "Monstres" and "Influence des passions des mères sur leur foe-

tus," *Dictionnaire philosophique,* in *Oeuvres complètes,* 9 vols. in 5 (Paris, 1867–69), 1:550, 447. These articles call into question the assertion of Katharine Park and Lorraine Daston in "Unnatural Conceptions: The Study of Monsters in Sixteenth- and Seventeenth-Century France and England," *Past and Present* 92 (August 1981): 53–54 that by the end of the eighteenth century speculation about monsters no longer served as a point of contact between learned culture and popular culture because men of learning were committed to a view of the regular and monolithic activity of nature.

23. Paul Hoffmann, *La Femme dans la pensée des Lumières* (Paris, 1977), 83.

24. Thomas Hankins, *Science and the Enlightenment* (Cambridge, 1985), 134–35. For more on the history of generation, see: Elizabeth B. Gasking, *Investigations into Generation 1651–1828* (Baltimore, 1967). Maryanne Cline Horowitz, "Aristotle and Woman," *Journal of the History of Biology* 9, no. 2 (1976): 183–213. Johannes Morsink, "Was Aristotle's Biology Sexist?" *Journal of the History of Biology* 12, no. 1 (1979): 83–112. "Hippocrates: *Diseases of Women 1,*" trans. Ann Ellis Hanson, *Signs 1* (winter 1975): 567–84. Joyce Irwin, "Embryology and the Incarnation," *Sixteenth-Century Journal* 9, no. 2 (1978): 93–104. Jacques Gélis, *L'Arbre et le Fruit, la naissance dans l'Occident moderne, XVIe–XIXe siècles* (Paris, 1984).

25. Basic biographical information for the primary participants in the debate can be found in J. Hoefer, ed., *Nouvelle biographie générale,* 46 vols. (Paris, 1853–66); L. G. Michaud, *Biographie universelle ancienne et moderne,* 45 vols. (Paris, 1843–65); J. Balteau, M. Barroux, M. Prevost, eds., *Dictionnaire de biographie française,* 18 vols. (Paris, 1939–); P. Grimal, *Dictionnaire des biographies* (Paris, 1958); N. L. M. Desessarts, *Les Siècles littéraires de la France, ou nouveau dictionnaire historique, critique, et bibliographique,* 7 vols. (Paris, *an* VIII–*an* XI); and *Dictionnaire des sciences médicales. Biographie médicale* (Paris: 1820–24). In addition, for Bouvart, see F. Vicq d'Azyr, ed., *Encyclopédie méthodique. Médecine* (Paris, 1792), 4:155–57 and C. Brainne, ed., *Les Hommes illustres de l'Orléanais* (Orléans, 1852), 1:297–300.

26. Antoine Louis: Pierre Huard, ed., *Biographies médicales et scientifiques: XVIIIe siècle* (Paris, 1972), 33–79, 111–16. Frank Kafker and Serena Kafker, *Encyclopedists as Individuals: A Biographical Dictionary of the Authors of the Encyclopédie,* vol. 257 of *Studies on Voltaire and the Eighteenth Century,* (Oxford, 1988), 231–35. Pierre Sue, *Eloge de Louis,* in Antoine Louis, *Eloges lus dans les séances publiques de l'Académie royale de chirurgie de 1750 à 1792,* ed. E. F. Dubois (Paris, 1859), 416–54. E. Bégin, ed., *Biographie de la Moselle* (Metz, 1830), 2:554–76.

Jean Calas was a Protestant put to death for murdering his son to prevent his conversion to Catholicism. Voltaire worked for three years (1762–65) to clear the memory of Calas of the charge. His success was due in part to medical evidence provided by Antoine Louis that the son was not a murder victim, but had committed suicide. For more on the Calas affair, see Peter Gay, *Voltaire's Politics* (Princeton, 1959), 273–308 and David Bien, *The Calas Affair: Persecution, Toleration, and Heresy in Eighteenth-Century Toulouse* (Princeton, 1960).

For more on the Sirven affair, see chapter 3 herein.

27. Jean Astruc: Huard, *Biographies,* 7–30. Adolphe Lods, "Jean Astruc et

la critique biblique au XVIIIᵉ siècle," *Cahiers de la revue d'histoire et de philosophie religieuses* 11 (1924): 1–86. Pierre-Maurice Masson, *Une Vie de femme au XVIIIᵉ siècle: Mme de Tencin (1682–1740)* (Paris, 1909), 183. J. A. Hazon, *Notice des hommes les plus célèbres de la Faculté de Médecine en l'Université de Paris, depuis 1110, jusqu'en 1750* (Paris, 1778), 252–62. *Le Nécrologe des hommes célèbres de France, par une société de gens de lettres* (Paris, 1767), 1:133–35. A. C. Lorry, "Eloge historique de M. Astruc," in Astruc, *Mémoires pour servir à l'histoire de la Faculté de Médecine de Montpellier* (Paris, 1767), xxxiii–liv. C. P. Goujet, *Mémoire historique et littéraire sur le Collège Royal de France* (Paris, 1758), 3:237–41.

28. Antoine Petit: Kafker, *Encyclopedists*, 306–9. Brainne, *Les Hommes de l'Orléanais*, 2:300–304. C. Cuissard, "Notice sur Antoine Petit d'Orléans (1722–1794)," in *Mémoires de la Société d'agriculture, sciences, belles-lettres, et arts d'Orléans*, sér. 5, no. 1 (1901): 127–64.

29. Eight prominent doctors and surgeons cosigned Bouvart's consultation: Baron (the younger), Verdelhan, Poissonnier, Bellot, Borie, MacMahon, Macquart, and Solier. Louis's memoir was cosigned by four surgeons: Houstet, Morand, Foubert, and Barbaut. Twenty-three doctors and surgeons signed Petit's consultation; among them were Barbeu du Bourg, Bourdelin, Du Fouart, Gervais, Moreau, Raulin, and Sue.

30. A number of Petit's cosigners were, or would become, authors of medical self-help books. Le Begue de Presle had published *Le Conservateur de santé* (Paris, 1763) just before Petit's consultation appeared. Barbeu du Bourg would later write a book entitled *Eléments de médecine, en forme d'aphorismes* (Paris, 1780). Sue was the prolific author of such books as *Dictionnaire portatif de santé* (Paris, 1771) and *Essais historiques, littéraires et critiques sur l'art des accouchements* (Paris, 1779). Raulin wrote many books addressed specifically to the subject of the *maladies des femmes*, including *Traité des affections vaporeuses du sexe* (Paris, 1758), *Traité des fleurs blanches* (Paris, 1766), and *Traité des maladies des femmes en couche* (Paris, 1771).

31. Jean Astruc, *Doutes sur l'inoculation de la petite vérole* (Paris, 1756), 10–11.

32. Antoine Petit, *Premier rapport en faveur de l'inoculation de la petite vérole* (Paris, 1766), viii–x, 16–19, 107–8, 132, 143–45. The fact that Petit appealed to the mothers, rather than fathers, of families was significant. The issue of surviving smallpox and living with its hideous aftereffects was a particularly sensitive one for women, for, as the Goncourts have remarked, "An ugly woman is a being who has no position in nature, nor place in the world." The Goncourts calculate that one-fourth of all women were stricken by smallpox; of these, 200,000 were so severely deformed that they had to take the veil. (Edmond and Jules de Goncourt, *La Femme au dix-huitième siècle* [Paris, 1982], 55.) Henry Tronchin has observed that women in the upper ranks of society were especially eager to see the ravages of smallpox brought to an end because of the "cruel and rigorous etiquette which enjoined a wife to go into confinement with her husband as soon as he felt the first symptoms of the disease" (Henry Tronchin, *Un Médecin du XVIIIᵉ siècle: Théodore Tronchin [1709–1781], d'après des documents inédits* [Paris, 1906], 109–10). A wrenching autobiographical account of the emotions

one woman experienced when she and her daughter came down with smallpox can be found in Mme de Gauthier, *Lettres de Mme de G——, contenant plusieurs anecdotes dans son voyage aux eaux de Barège, et quelques particularités échappées aux autres voyageurs en France* (Brussels, 1787), 150–219.

33. Marie Prudence Plisson: A. Delacoux, *Biographie des sages-femmes célèbres, anciennes, modernes et contemporaines* (Paris, 1833), 139–40. Lucien Merlet, *Bibliothèque chartraine antérieure au XIXe siècle* (Orléans, 1882), 356–58. Fortunée Briquet, *Dictionnaire historique, littéraire et bibliographique des Françaises* (Paris, 1804), 265. L. Prudhomme, *Répertoire universel, historique, biographique des femmes célèbres, mortes ou vivantes*, 4 vols. (Paris, 1826), 4:73–74. Letters written by Plisson from 1751 to 1753 are in the municipal library of Chartres, new acquisitions, ms. 225.

34. Marie Prudence Plisson, *Réflexions critiques sur les écrits qu'a produit la question de la légitimité des naissances tardives: Suivies d'une dissertation sur les hommes marins* (Paris, 1765), iv.

35. Mme Corron (pseudonym of Pierre Abraham Pajon de Moncets), *Dissertation en forme de lettre sur la cause qui détermine à neuf mois l'accouchement* (Paris, 1757), 1–2.

36. Plisson, *Réflexions*, iii.

37. Jacques Barbeu du Bourg: J.B.F. Carrère, ed.: *Bibliothèque littéraire, historique et critique de la médecine ancienne et moderne* (Paris, 1776), 1:312–13. J. Pesche, ed., *Biographie et bibliographie du Maine et du département de la Sarthe* (Le Mans, 1828), 37–38. Félix Vicq d'Azyr, "Eloge de Barbeu de Bourg," in *Oeuvres*, ed. J. L. Moreau de la Sarthe (Paris, 1805), 2:181–96. Paul Delaunay, "Vieux Médecins Mayennais: Barbeu du Bourg," *Bulletin de la commission historique et archéologique de la Mayenne* 19 (1903): 15–89.

38. Dufresne, *Journal des audiences* (Paris, 1678), 1:710, quoted in Michel Bouvart, *Consultation contre la légitimité des naissances prétendues tardives* (Paris, 1764), 11.

39. Bouvart, *Consultation*, 30.

40. Ibid., 12–13.

41. Ibid., 28.

42. Jean Astruc, *Traité des maladies des femmes, où l'on a tâché de joindre à une théorie solide la pratique la plus sûre et la mieux éprouvée* (Paris, 1765), 5:301.

43. Michel Bouvart, *Consultation sur une naissance tardive . . .* (Paris, 1765), 67.

44. Jean Le Bas, *Lettre à M. Bouvart . . . au sujet de sa dernière "Consultation sur une naissance prétendue tardive. . ."* (Amsterdam, 1765), 41.

45. The moral significance that the Romans attributed to left and right is embedded in our language: our word *sinister* is derived from the Latin "on the left side." In *The Midwife and the Witch* (New Haven, 1966), Thomas Forbes traces the long history and broad circulation of these ideas.

46. Evidence that fanciful measures for planning the sex of a fetus remain a part of popular culture in the West can be found in a *Chicago Sun Times* article pubished in the 1980s which noted that in Texas men are advised to wear boots during intercourse if they wish to have sons. Dr. Robert Mendelsohn of Evanston,

Illinois, has observed that "Although most doctors will deny it, there is considerable evidence that many parents seek amniocentesis not to determine fetal abnormalities, but to determine sex. Their intention, of course, is to abort the baby if it is not of the sex they prefer, and there isn't much chance that the aborted baby will be a boy."

47. Antoine Petit, "Lettre à M. Bouvart, pour servir de réponse à la critique qu'il a faite de la consultation précédente," *Recueil de pièces relatives à la question des naissances tardives* (Amsterdam, 1766), 126.

48. Antoine Louis, *Mémoire contre la légitimité des naissances prétendues tardives: Dans lequel on concilie les loix civiles avec celles de l'oeconomie animale* (Paris, 1764), 13.

49. Ibid., 24–25.

50. Ibid., 54–55.

51. Antoine Louis, *Supplément au mémoire contre la légitimité des naissances tardives* (Paris, 1764), 107.

52. On this point, see L. W. B. Brockliss, *French Higher Education in the Seventeenth and Eighteenth Centuries* (Oxford, 1987), 437–38.

53. Antoine Petit, "Consultation en faveur de la légitimité des naissances tardives," *Recueil de pièces relatives à la question des naissances tardives* (Amsterdam, 1766), 47.

54. Voltaire, "Monstres" and "Influence des passions des mères sur leur foetus," *Dictionnaire philosophique, in Oeuvres complètes* 1:550, 447. Suzanne Doublet, "La Médecine dans les oeuvres de Diderot" (Université de Bordeaux, Faculté de Médecine, thèse 144, 1933–34), 78–86.

55. Petit, "Lettre à M. Bouvart," 75–76.

56. Jean Le Bas, *Question importante. Peut-on déterminer un terme préfix pour l'accouchement* (Paris, 1764), 21.

57. *Journal encyclopédique à Bouillon* (November) 1765:37. *Mémoires pour l'histoire des sciences et beaux-arts* 1765:76.

58. Cicero, *Tusculanar* 1.35, quoted in Jean Astruc, *Traité*, 287.

59. Le Bas, *Question importante*, 27–28.

60. Jacques Barbeu du Bourg, *Recherches sur la durée de la grossesse, et le terme de l'accouchement* (Paris, 1765), 22.

61. According to the Boston Women's Health Book Collective, *The New Our Bodies, Ourselves* (New York, 1984), 366, we now know a lot about labor, but we still don't know what triggers it. Possibilities include the secretion of hormones, the pressure of the baby's head on cervical nerve endings, and a woman's emotional state and physical position.

62. Astruc, *Traité*, 5:294–95.

63. Ibid., 5:303.

64. Ibid., 5:304.

65. Bouvart, *Consultation*, 82.

66. Emile Littré, *Dictionnaire de la langue française* (Paris, 1874), 2:1639.

67. Pierre Darmon, *Mythologie de la femme dans l'ancienne France* (Paris, 1983), 29–30. Darmon quotes Jacob Sprenger's *Malleus Maleficarum*: "We learn, through the pen of Jacob Sprenger that '*femina* comes from *fe* and *minus*, because she has and preserves less faith.' Contrary to man, she defies even the laws of

nature with such assurance that the body of a drowned woman rises up against the river's current rather than being carried downstream, as any normal cadaver would be."

68. Petit, "Consultation," 72.

69. Martha Ornstein, *The Role of Scientific Societies in the Seventeenth Century* (Chicago, 1928), 54.

70. For example, the *Journal de Nancy* ("Evénement singulier," 1779: 103–4) reported a childless, fifty-year-old wife of a carpenter of La Marche who consulted a local doctor for abdominal pains and was given a number of remedies to no avail. Seven months later, she visited another doctor, who diagnosed the problem as hydropsy and treated it accordingly. Toward the end of the ninth month, the woman began to feel even more intense pains and appealed to her female neighbors for help. These neighbors told the doctor the woman was pregnant, not hydropsic, and were summarily dismissed. He promised to effect a radical healing with violent remedies. Before the doctor could fulfill his promise, however, the woman gave birth to a large baby boy. "This event," the article declared, "created such a stir in the town of La Marche that a number of men, parading like musicians, gathered to escort the newborn to the baptismal font. At the end of the ceremony the parish curé concluded his remarks by giving thanks to God that the child had escaped the clutches of medicine and doctors. After the ceremony the godfather and godmother, mounted on an oxcart carrying the child, went up and down all the streets of the town under the same escort, as if in triumph."

The woman of La Marche was lucky; other, more tragic, incidents of misdiagnosis occurred commonly. One doctor, Lecomte, practicing in Evreux, reported that he had disregarded the claim of his patient to being five months pregnant and prescribed abortifacients anyway. In this case the abortifacients were effective: both the infant and the mother died the day after they were administered. (Lecomte, "Idée de la médecine du peuple," 19 February 1778, SRM Archives, carton 191). While deaths were the most dramatic effect of the administration of abortifacients, no less disturbing was the fact that women who survived remained invalids for years after taking them. News of tragedies like this no doubt increased women's anxiety over pregnancy and childbirth. For other cases, see *Journal de Nancy* 1779: 103–4, 150–51; the letter of Dr. Moulet of Caussade, Montauban dated 7 September 1787 (SRM Archives, carton 137, no. 10); and the letter of Bonnot, surgeon of Toulon sur Arroux, dated 28 September 1786 (SRM Archives, carton 134).

71. Jean Le Bas, *Nouvelles observations sur les naissances tardives; suivies d'une consultation de célèbres médecins et chirurgiens de Paris* (Paris, 1765), 91–92.

72. Delacoux, *Biographie des sages-femmes célèbres*, 142–43.

73. Le Bas, *Nouvelles observations*, 85.

74. Bouvart, *Consultation*, 57.

75. Ibid., 62.

76. Ibid., 49.

77. Ibid., 64–65.

78. Petit, "Lettre," 193.

79. Petit, "Consultation," 68.
80. Astruc, *Traité*, 5:308.
81. Louis, *Mémoire*, 81.
82. Bouvart, *Consultation*, 34.
83. Petit, "Consultation," 86.
84. "Examen d'un mémoire contre la légitimité des naissances prétendues tardives," *Journal des sçavans* (June) 1766: 231–32.
85. Le Bas, *Nouvelles observations*, 135.
86. Plisson, *Réflexions critiques*, 47.
87. Plisson's approach is interesting in light of Carol Gilligan's theory in *In a Different Voice: Psychological Theory and Women's Development* (Cambridge, Mass., 1982), 23, about the different priorities women and men place on the values of compassion and justice.
88. Plisson, *Réflexions critiques*, 49. In *The Question of Rest for Women during Menstruation* (New York, 1886), 17, Mary Putnam Jacobi would similarly argue that medical hypotheses likely to have important and inconvenient practical consequences for women should be rigorously evaluated.
89. William Thomson, *Black's Medical Dictionary* (New York, 1979), 712.

Chapter Three. Medical Causes Célèbres and the Development of Medical Jurisprudence

1. Maurice Méjan, *Recueil des causes célèbres* (Paris, 1809), 6:93.
2. Daniel Roche, *Les Républicains des lettres. Gens de culture et Lumières au XVIIIe siècle* (Paris, 1988), 316–18.
3. Jean Baptiste Denisart, ed., *Collection de décisions nouvelles et de notions relatives à la jurisprudence actuelle* 9 (1790): 534.
4. Pierre Le Ridant, *Code matrimonial ou Recueil des édits, ordonnances et déclarations sur le mariage. Avec une dictionnaire des décisions les plus importantes sur cette matière* (Paris, 1766), 257–58.
5. Sarah Hanley, "Engendering the State: Family Formation and State Building in Early Modern France," *French Historical Studies* 16, no. 1 (1989): 4–27.
6. Le Ridant, *Code*, 320.
7. Léon Abensour, *La Femme et le féminisme avant la Révolution* (Paris, 1923), 18–32.
8. Guy du Rousseau de la Combe, *Recueil de jurisprudence civile du pays de droit écrit et coutumier*, 3d ed. (Paris, 1753), 282.
9. Denisart, *Collection* 8 (1789): 542. Also see Pierre Muyart de Vouglans, *Les Lois criminelles de France dans leur ordre naturel* (Paris, 1781), 2:282, and *Encyclopédie* 13 (1782): 938.
10. David Houard, *Dictionnaire analytique, historique, étymologique, critique et interprétatif de la coutume de Normandie* (Rouen, 1782), 4:205.
11. Hanley, "Engendering the State," 8–20.
12. Suzanne Necker, *Réflexions sur le divorce* (Lausanne, 1794), 28.
13. Ibid., 78–85.
14. Rousseau was not very clear on the point, sometimes arguing from the

laws of nature, at other times asserting that even if women's subordination were not based on the laws of nature, it was socially necessary.

Mme Necker feared that with divorce, women would lose their place in the chain of being as daughters, mothers, and wives and would become an amphibious species guided only by the principle of self-love. Her views on divorce were in opposition to those of a number of philosophes, including Montesquieu, Diderot, and Voltaire. For more on the philosophes' views on divorce, see Dominique Dessertine, *Divorcer à Lyon sous la révolution et l'empire* (Lyon, 1981), 12–33.

15. Hanley, "Engendering the State," 26.

16. Pierre Darmon, *Le Mythe de la procréation à l'âge baroque* (Paris, 1977), 226–29.

17. Houard, *Dictionnaire* (1780), 1:17.

18. Claude-Joseph Ferrière, *Dictionnaire de droit et de pratique, contenant l'explication des termes de droit, d'ordonnances, de coutumes et de pratique avec les jurisdictions de France*, new ed., (Paris, 1771), 2:253.

19. Denisart, *Collection* 9 (1790): 530.

20. Ibid., 521–22.

21. Hans-Jurgen Lusebrink, "Le Droit de la filiation légitime," *Dix-huitième siècle* 12 (1980): 251–69.

22. Dianne Alstad, "The Ideology of the Family in Eighteenth-Century France" (Ph.D. thesis, Yale, 1971), 260–66.

23. Ibid., 263. Alstad draws her quotes from Crane Brinton, *French Revolutionary Legislation on Illegitimacy 1789–1804* (Cambridge, Mass., 1936), 25, 54. For a summary of women's legal position under the Ancien Régime and changes wrought by the Napoleonic Code, see Adrienne Rogers, "Women and the Law," in Samia Spencer, ed., *French Women and the Age of Enlightenment* (Bloomington, Ind., 1984), 33–48.

24. Yvonne Knibiehler and Catherine Fouquet, *Histoire des mères du Moyen Age à nos jours* (Paris, 1977), 123, 166–67.

25. Denisart, *Collection* 12 (1806): 149. In *La Grossesse. Etude de sa durée et de sa variations* (Paris, 1901), 106, L. Bouchacourt notes that although Austrian law paralleled French law on the question of succession rights in cases of prolonged pregnancies, in Russia the limit was set at 302 days, while in England it extended to 311 days. In the United States, a more liberal law set no limit.

26. Félix Vicq d'Azyr, ed., *Encyclopédie méthodique. Médecine* 1 (Paris, 1821), 10:460.

27. Méjan, *Recueil* 6 (1809): 94.

28. Denisart, *Collection* 12 (1806): 149.

29. Méjan, *Recueil* 6 (1809): 94. Twentieth-century advances in reproductive technologies have made the provisions of the Napoleonic Code even more problematic. Take, for example, the 1984 case of Corinne Parpalaix, aged 23, who sued a sperm bank for the right to the sperm of her husband, Alain. He died of testicular cancer two days after they were married. A court in the Paris suburb, Creteil, ruled that the sperm should be given to her appointed agent, her doctor, even though French law did not recognize heirs born more than three hundred days after the death of their father. Medical reaction to the decision was divided. Professor Alexandre Minkowski "rejoiced" in the decision because it "respected

the person," but Professor Hughes Gounelle called the ruling "extremely dangerous." Justice Minister Robert Badinter proposed holding a conference of doctors, lawyers, and philosophers to discuss the problems posed by artificial insemination before legislators considered new legislation. (*Le Monde aujourd'hui*, 29–30 July 1984, IV; *New York Times*, 2 July 1984, A7; *NYT*, 2 August 1984, A8, B1; *NYT*, 5 August 1984, sect. 4, p. 7; Reuters North European Service, 2 August 1984; UPI, 2 August 1984; *San Francisco Examiner*, 2 August 1984, A19.)

30. Méjan, *Recueil* 6 (1809): 93–121. For more on the impact of the Napoleonic Code on marriage, conception, abortion, and infanticide, see June Burton, "Human Rights Issues Affecting Women in Napoleonic Legal Medicine Textbooks," *History of European Ideas* 8, nos. 4–5 (1987): 427–34. On changes in the rules of inheritance, see Margaret Darrow, *Revolution in the House: Family, Class, and Inheritance in Southern France, 1775–1825* (Princeton, 1989), 4–19.

31. Denisart, *Collection* 4 (1771): 107.

32. *Encyclopédie* 21 (1781): 357.

33. Ferrière, *Dictionnaire* 1 (1771): 718.

34. *Encyclopédie* 21 (1781): 357.

35. "Prétendu Sortilège: Extrait d'une lettre de M. Dolignon, Maître-en-Chirurgie à Cressi en Laonnois, à M. Dufau, Médecin-Pensionnaire du Roi et de la ville de Soissons, Démonstrateur de l'art des accouchements," *Affiches de Bordeaux*, 6 January 1774: 5–7.

36. Professeur du Bois, A. D. Ille-et-Vilaine C 2530, Etats de Bretagne, cited in Olwen Hufton, *The Poor of Eighteenth-Century France 1750–1820* (Oxford, 1974), 331.

37. Jean Lecuir, "La Médicalisation de la société française dans la deuxième moitié du XVIIIᵉ siècle en France: Aux Origines des premiers traités de médecine légale," *Annales de Bretagne* 86, no. 2 (1979): 232–34. Pierre Huard, ed.: *Biographies médicales et scientifiques: XVIIIᵉ siècle* (Paris, 1972), 59–62. Pierre Sue, *Apperçu général, appuyé de quelques faits, sur l'origine et le sujet de la médecine légale* (Paris, an VIII), 35.

38. Elie Galland, *L'Affaire Sirven. Etude historique d'après les documents originaux* (Mazamet, 1910), 17–18.

39. Antoine Court de Gebelin, *Les Toulousaines ou Lettres historiques et apologétiques* (Edinburgh, 1763), 353, quoted in Camille Rabaud, *Sirven. Etude historique sur l'avènement de la tolérance* (Paris, 1891), 26.

40. Lacroix, *Mémoire pour le sieur Pierre-Paul Sirven . . . (Toulouse*, 1770), quoted in Galland, *L'Affaire Sirven*, 44.

41. Rabaud, *Sirven*, 32–33; Galland, *L'Affaire Sirven*, 66–68.

42. Rabaud, *Sirven*, 39; Galland, *L'Affaire Sirven*, 90.

43. Rabaud, *Sirven*, 69–70.

44. Galland, *L'Affaire Sirven*, 106–7.

45. Ibid., 208, 126.

46. Voltaire, "Certain, Certitude," *Dictionnaire philosophique*, quoted in Galland, *L'Affaire Sirven*, 234; letter of 16 August 1766 to Leroy, professeur à la Faculté de Médecine de Montpellier, quoted in Galland, *L'Affaire Sirven*, 378.

47. Antoine Louis, *Consultation de M. Louis . . . du* 3 juin 1769, quoted in Galland, *L'Affaire Sirven*, 109. Also see Rabaud, *Sirven*, 60–61.

48. Galland, *L'Affaire Sirven*, 425–27.

49. Sarah Hanley, "Family and State in Early Modern France: The Marriage Pact," in *Connecting Spheres: Women in the Western World, 1500 to the Present*, ed. Marilyn Boxer and Jean Quaetart, (Oxford, 1987), 56. For more information on the Edict of Henri II and a discussion of the cases involving accusations of concealment of pregnancy and infanticide which arose from it, see Denisart, *Collection*: "Grossesse," 2 (1771): 582–83; "Déclaration de grossesse," 6 (1787): 10–15; and "Grossesse," 9 (1790): 519–21. Also see Nicolas Desessarts, ed., *Causes célèbres* 1 (1775): cause 128; 41 (1778): 3; 80 (1781): 183; 81 (1781): 75; 85 (1782): 183; 140 (1786): 177.

50. Desessarts, *Causes célèbres* 26 (1777): cause 67, pp. 170–72; Denisart, *Collection*, 6 (1787): 11.

51. Desessarts, *Causes célèbres* 26 (1777): cause 67.

52. Stéphanie-Félicité du Crest de Saint Aubin, Comtesse de Genlis, *Souvenirs de Félicie*, in *Bibliothèque des mémoires relatifs à l'histoire de France pendant le XVIIIe et le XIXe siècle*, ed. Jean Barrière (Paris, 1857), 14:208–9.

For legislation against infanticide in Prussia, see Hamilton Beck, "Of Two Minds about the Death Penalty: Hippel's Account of a Case of Infanticide," in *Studies in Eighteenth-Century Culture*, ed. John Yolton and Leslie Brown, (East Lansing, Mich., 1988), 18: 123–40. The *Edikt* of 1765 stipulated a six-year sentence for a woman who gave birth without reporting her pregnancy to a woman who had herself given birth. Execution was reserved for those mothers who failed to provide necessary care, attention, and nourishment. Penalties for infanticide dated back to article 131 of Charles V's penal code of 1532 (Beck, n. 7, p. 136 and n. 13, p. 137). Given the high rate of illegitimacy in Konigsberg (one in seven births), it is not surprising that infanticide was a frequent theme in eighteenth-century literary works, including Goethe's *Faust* and Schiller's poem "Die Kindesmorderin" (nn. 5, 6, pp. 135–36). During the Revolution in France, crimes against morality such as infanticide were prosecuted more severely in Prussia, for it was feared that immorality was a contributing cause of revolution (p. 134).

53. La Tournelle, Procedures, Archives départmentales, Rennes 1Bn2218; 1Bn2222; 1Bn2272; 1Bn2277bis.

54. Yvonne Knibielher and Catherine Fouquet, *Histoire des mères du Moyen Age à nos jours* (Paris, 1977), 123–27.

55. Claude Grimmer, *La Femme et le bâtard. Amours illégitimes et secrètes dans l'ancienne France* (Paris, 1983), 227. These figures are lower than those given for the sixteenth and seventeenth centuries by Natalie Davis in *Fiction in the Archives, Pardon Tales and Their Tellers in Sixteenth-Century France* (Stanford, 1987), 86, 195. Davis cites Alfred Soman's study of two hundred cases of infanticide brought to the Parlement of Paris between 1565 and 1640. Two-thirds of the accused women were condemned to death. She notes that Jonathan Dewald's research reveals that the Parlement of Rouen was harsher in this matter: twenty infanticide appeals were heard in twenty years; eighteen of the appellants were executed.

56. Abensour, *La Femme*, 406, 438.

57. Olwen Hufton, *The Poor of Eighteenth-Century France 1750–1789* (Oxford, 1974), 318–51. Also see Cissie Fairchilds, "Female Sexual Attitudes and

the Rise of Illegitimacy: A Case Study," *Journal of Interdisciplinary History* 8, no. 4 (1978): 627–67.

58. Vieillard de Boismartin, avocat au Prue de Lafaille, letter of 18 September 1785, SRM Archives, carton 182. As Agnès Fine notes in "Savoirs sur le corps et procédés abortifs au XIXe siècle," in *Le Corps humain: Nature, culture, sur-naturel*, 110e Congrès national des sociétés savantes, Montpellier, 1985 (Paris, 1985), 81–84, it was also difficult for physicians to determine whether women had taken abortifacients or merely resorted to home remedies to resolve menstrual irregularities. Thus, although the Napoleonic Code made abortion illegal, only eight cases were prosecuted in 1828.

59. Voltaire, "Supplice," *Dictionnaire philosophique*, quoted in Pierre Sue, *Apperçu général appuyé de quelques faits sur l'origine et le sujet de la médecine légale* (Paris, 1799–1800), 27–28.

60. For more on the Famin case, see Antoine Petit, *Deux consultations médico-légales . . . pour Famin . . . accusée de suppression, exposition et homicide de deux enfants* (Paris, 1767). This case was publicized in the *Journal encyclopédique* 1 (1768): 128 and in the *Mémoires pour l'histoire des sciences et beaux-arts* 4 (1767): 544–47. Also see Desessarts, *Causes célèbres* 41 (1778): cause 109 and 85 (1782): cause 257.

61. Details on the Granger case can be found in Cabinet Carteron 798, no. 8 of the Bibliothèque Municipale de Troyes. The dossier on the Granger affair includes the *procès-verbaux* of the *officiers de santé*, Gueniot and Forestier, dated 22 *ventôse an* VII, as well as the opinion of Baudelocque and Bourdois on these *procès-verbaux*. This document is followed by the consultation given at Troyes by the doctors Bouquot, Servat-Pouscarre, Bergerat, Serqueil, Pigeotte (the younger), and the surgeons Pigeotte, Baudin, and Huot, dated 23 *frimaire an* VIII. Fodéré's *Mémoire pour la fille Granger, accusée d'infanticide*, dated 12 *frimaire an* VIII, can also be found here.

Two other cases in which surgeons were rebuked for sharing the public's prejudices about the circumstances surrounding infant deaths rather than basing their opinions on the physical evidence at hand are recorded in Desessarts, *Causes célèbres*, 80 (1781): cause 232 and 140 (1786): cause 511.

62. Dessessarts, *Causes célèbres*, 60 (1779): cause 158, p. 167.

63. *Encyclopédie*, 21 (1781): 354.

64. Lecuir, "La Médicalisation," 233.

65. Suzanne Doublet, "La Médecine dans les oeuvres de Diderot" (thèse, Bordeaux, 1933–34), 20.

66. L. G. Michaud, *Biographie universelle* (Paris, 1843–65); 32: 597.

67. Lecuir, "La Médicalisation," 232.

68. Ibid., 244.

Chapter Four. Science, Medicine, and the Salons: A Struggle for Cultural Authority

1. Charles Paul, *Science and Immortality: The Eloges of the Paris Academy of Sciences (1699–1791)* (Berkeley, 1980), 88–102.

2. Jean-Baptiste Gouriet, *Les Charlatans célèbres: ou, Tableau historique des*

bateleurs, des jongleurs, des bouffons, des opérateurs, des voltigeurs, des esca-
moteurs, des filous, des escrocs, des devins, des tireurs de cartes, des diseurs de
bonne aventure, et généralement de tous les personnages qui se sont rendus célèbres
dans les rues et sur les places publiques de Paris, depuis une haute antiquité
jusqu'à nos jours (Paris, 1819), 1:1–2, 270.

3. Matthew Ramsey, *Professional and Popular Medicine in France, 1770–1830. The Social World of Medical Practice* (Cambridge, 1988), 131–32.

4. Indeed, the comic figure of the philosophe as charlatan was a familiar one on the eighteenth-century stage, appearing most notably in La Montagne's *La Physicienne*, Palissot's *Le Cercle, ou les originaux*, and Cidalise's *Les Philosophes*. See Ira Wade, *The Philosophe in the French Drama of the Eighteenth Century* (Princeton, 1926), 35–45, 77–81, 96–103. Also see Paul, *Science and Immortality*, 103.

5. Richard N. Schwab, "The Chevalier de Jaucourt, Physician and Encyclopedist," *Journal of the History of Medicine and Allied Sciences* 13 (April 1958): 256–59 and Schwab, "The History of Medicine in Diderot's *Encyclopédie*," *Bulletin of the History of Medicine* 32 (1958): 216–23.

6. "Sciences," *Encyclopédie* (1765), 14:787–89.

7. Herbert Dieckmann, "The Concept of Knowledge in the *Encyclopédie*," in *Essays in Comparative Literature*, ed. H. Dieckmann (St. Louis, 1961), 80.

8. Herbert Dieckmann, "Themes and Structure of the Enlightenment," in *Essays in Comparative Literature*, ed. H. Dieckmann (St. Louis, 1961), 60.

9. Dieckmann, "Concept of Knowledge," 92.

10. Edmond Pilon, *La Vie de famille au dix-huitième siècle. Illustrations d'après des estampes du temps* (Paris, 1923), 14. Robert Darnton, *The Great Cat Massacre and Other Episodes in French Cultural History* (New York, 1984), 139.

11. "Discours prononcés à l'Académie Française le jeudi 22 janvier 1767, à la réception de M. Thomas," *Journal des dames* (February, 1767): 82–83.

12. Mme la Baronne Duplessy, *Répertoire des lectures faites au musée des dames* (Paris, 1788), 4–5.

13. Suzanne Necker, *Mélanges extraits des manuscrits de Mme Necker*, ed. Jacques Necker, 3 vols. (Paris, 1798), 3:30–31, 2:345.

14. Edmond and Jules de Goncourt, *La Femme au dix-huitième siècle* (Paris, 1982), 368. Also see Alain Decaux, *Histoire des Françaises. La Révolte* (Paris, 1972), 2:365, who argues that learned women like Geneviève de Malboissière guaranteed the triumph of the *Encyclopédie*.

15. Louis Petit de Bachaumont, *Mémoires secrets pour servir à l'histoire de la République des Lettres en France, depuis 1762 jusqu'à nos jours* (13 November 1765), 287. Bachaumont's *Mémoires* mingled analyses of theatrical productions with anouncements of new books, anecdotes, and eulogies of savants, artists, and men of letters. According to the notice of the editors in the first issue, it was intended to save readers the trouble of reading all the journals available in their totality and was filled with precious anecdotes that couldn't be found elsewhere. For more on Bachaumont and his journal, see Charles Aubertin, *L'Esprit public au XVIIIe siècle. Etude sur les mémoires et les correspondances politiques des contemporains, 1715 à 1789* (Paris, 1873), 374–98 and Robert Tate, Jr., *Petit de*

Bachaumont: His Circle and the Mémoires Secrets, in *Studies on Voltaire and the Eighteenth Century,* ed. Theodore Besterman, (Geneva, 1968), 65:129–211.

16. Martha Ornstein, *The Role of Scientific Societies in the Seventeenth Century* (Chicago, 1928), 160–63.

17. Roger Hahn, *The Anatomy of a Scientific Institution: The Paris Academy of Sciences, 1666–1803* (Berkeley, 1971), 44–45, 100.

18. Jean le Rond d'Alembert, "Essai sur la société des gens de lettres et des grands," in *Oeuvres philosophiques, historiques ou littéraires de d'Alembert,* ed. J. F. Bastien (Paris, 1805), 3:25–32.

19. Hahn, *Anatomy of a Scientific Institution,* 155–58.

20. Keith Baker, *Condorcet, From Natural Philosophy to Social Mathematics* (Chicago, 1975), 263.

21. Bachaumont, *Mémoires secrets* (25 August 1768 and 31 December 1768), 197–98.

22. Daniel Mornet, "La Vie mondaine, les salons," in *La Vie parisienne au XVIIIᵉ siècle: Leçons faites à l'Ecole des hautes études sociales* (Paris, 1914), 121–44.

23. D'Alembert, "La Société des gens de lettres," 52.

24. "Man of Letters," *Encyclopedia: Selections,* ed. John Lough (Indianapolis, 1965), 284–85.

25. Stéphanie-Félicité du Crest de St. Aubin, Comtesse de Genlis, "Souvenirs de Félicie," in *Bibliothèque des mémoires relatifs à l'histoire de France pendant le XVIIIᵉ et le XIXᵉ siècle,* ed. Jean Barrière (Paris, 1857), 14:106.

26. Goncourt, *La Femme,* 301.

27. Albert, Comte de Luppé, *Les Jeunes Filles à la fin du XVIIIᵉ siècle* (Paris, 1925), 166. Londa Schiebinger, *The Mind Has No Sex? Women in the Origins of Modern Science* (Cambridge, Mass., 153–54, cites Lepenies in attributing Buffon's decline in popularity after the Revolution to his close association with the aristocracy and women: "Revolutionaries judged his style pompous and aristocratic, while natural historians sought increasingly to dissociate themselves from the tainted world of literature. Interestingly, Buffon was attacked for being a *coquet,* language usually reserved for women."

28. Schiebinger, *The Mind,* 247–50 and Marie Thiroux d'Arconville, *Pensées et réflexions morales, sur divers sujets* (Paris, 1766), 158–59.

29. Goncourt, *La Femme,* 290–91.

30. D'Alembert, "La Société des gens de lettres," 101–3.

31. Ibid., 74–76. Hahn, *The Anatomy of a Scientific Institution,* 116–33.

32. Simon Linguet, *Annales politiques, civiles, et littéraires du XVIIIᵉ siècle. Ouvrage périodique* (London, 1777), 3:215–17.

33. Wolfgang Van den Daele, "The Social Construction of Science: Institutionalization and Definition of Positive Science in the Latter Half of the Seventeenth Century," in *The Social Production of Scientific Knowledge. Sociology of the Sciences,* ed. Everett Mendelsohn, Peter Weingart, and Richard Whitley (Dordrecht, Holland, 1977), 1:44–47. Joseph Ben-David, *The Scientist's Role in Society: A Comparative Study* (Englewood Cliffs, N.J., 1971), 80–85.

34. Jean Torlais, "Le Collège Royal," and Yves Laissus, "Le Jardin du Roi,"

in *Enseignement et diffusion des sciences en France au XVIIIe siècle*, ed. René Taton (Paris, 1964), 261–341.

35. Laissus, "Le Jardin du Roi," 287–316.

36. Terry Parssinen, "Professional Deviants and the History of Medicine: Medical Mesmerists in Victorian Britain," in *On the Margins of Science: The Social Construction of Rejected Knowledge,* ed. Roy Wallis, Sociological Review Monograph 27 (Keele, U.K., March 1979), 104–5.

37. Jacques-Albert Hazon, *Notice des hommes les plus célèbres de la Faculté de médecine en l'Université de Paris, depuis 1110, jusqu'en 1750* (Paris, 1778), vii.

38. Paul, *Science and Immortality,* 70–79. James McClellan, *Science Reorganized. Scientific Societies in the Eighteenth Century* (New York, 1985), 240–49

39. Victorine de Chastenay-Lanty, *Mémoires, 1771–1815* (Paris, 1896), 42–43.

40. Gaston, Duc de Lévis, *Souvenirs et portraits,* in *Bibliothèque des mémoires relatifs à l'histoire de France pendant le XVIIIe et le XIXe siècle,* ed. Jean Barrière (Paris, 1857), 14:392–93.

41. De Chastenay-Lanty, *Mémoires,* 42–43.

42. *Une Femme d'affaires au XVIIIe siècle: La Correspondance de Mme de Maraise, collaboratrice d'Oberkampf,* ed. Serge Chassagne (Toulouse, 1981), 28.

43. Riballier and Cosson, *De l'éducation physique et morale des femmes* (Paris, 1779), 18–19. A large number of writers on the education of women focused on health as the basis for women's empowerment. See, for example, Marie Thiroux d'Arconville, *Pensées et réflexions morales, sur divers sujets* (Paris, 1766), 158–59, and Anne d'Aubourg de la Bove, Comtesse de Miremont, *Traité de l'éducation des femmes, et cours complet d'instruction,* 7 vols. (Paris, 1770–89), 2:11.

44. Manon Phlipon Roland, "Avis à ma fille, en âge et dans le cas de devenir mère," *Oeuvres de J. M. Ph. Roland, Femme de l'ex-ministre de l'intérieur,* ed. L. A. Champagneux (Paris, an VIII), 1:309–10, 329.

45. *Une Jeune Fille au XVIIIe siècle: Lettres de Geneviève de Malboissière à Adélaide Méliand 1761–1766,* ed. Albert, Comte de Luppé (Paris, 1925), 294–96.

46. Henriette, Marquise de la Tour du Pin-Gouvernet, *Journal d'une femme de cinquante ans 1778–1815* (Paris, 1907), 137–38.

47. *Correspondance littéraire, philosophique et critique, par Grimm, Diderot, Raynal, Meister, etc.,* ed. Maurice Tourneux (Paris, 1879), 6 (November 1765): 420, 8 (December 1769): 403–5. For more on the *Correspondance littéraire,* see Jules Bertaut, *La Vie littéraire au XVIIIe siècle* (Paris, 1954) and Ulla Kolving and Jeanne Carriat, *Inventaire de la Correspondance littéraire de Grimm et Meister, Studies on Voltaire and the Eighteenth Century* (Oxford, 1984), vols. 225–27.

48. Bachaumont, *Mémoires secrets,* 10 May 1769, 261–62.

49. Anne Vincent-Buffault, *Histoire des larmes, XVIIIe–XIXe siècles* (Paris, 1986), 13–16, 74.

50. Bachaumont, *Mémoires secrets,* 12 August 1768, 87–90.

51. Dominique Latour, *Discours prononcé dans la salle des consultations gra-*

tuites de médecine et de jurisprudence d'Orléans à l'occasion de l'inauguration du buste de M. Petit (Orléans, 1792), 4–5, 8–11, 14–15.

52. Charles Cuissard, "Notice sur Antoine Petit d'Orléans (1722–1794)," *Mémoires de la société d'agriculture, science, belles-lettres, et arts d'Orléans*, 5th ser., 1 (1901): 165–74.

53. Tap, *Eloge d'Antoine Petit* (n.p., an III), 5–6, 13.

54. M. A. J. B. M. Guenet, *Eloge historique de Michel-Philippe Bouvart* (Paris, 1787), 82–83.

55. Ibid., 15–17, 55–56.

56. Poinsinet, *Le Cercle ou la soirée à la mode*, ed. Auguste Vitu (Paris, 1887), xxi–xxxiii.

57. Louis-Sebastien Mercier, *Tableau de Paris* (Neufchatel, 1781), 1:155.

58. Guenet, *Eloge historique*, 65.

59. Marie-Jean-Antoine-Nicolas Caritat, Marquis de Condorcet, "Eloge de M. Bouvart," in A. Condorcet O'Conner and M. F. Arago, eds., *Oeuvres de Condorcet* (Paris, 1847), 3:293, 289–90.

60. Paul, *Science and Immortality*, 2–3.

61. Condorcet, "Eloge de M. Bouvart," 283–85.

62. Necker, *Mélanges*, 2:299.

63. Condorcet, "Eloge de M. Bouvart," 280, 287–88.

64. Condorcet, "Eloge de M. Tronchin," in *Oeuvres* 2:505–6, 509–10.

65. De Genlis, "Souvenirs de Félicie," 85–86.

66. *Dictionnaire des sciences médicales. Biographie médicale* (Paris, 1820–24), 2:477–85, 6:397–98.

67. J. Pesche, "Barbeu du Bourg," *Biographie et bibliographie du Maine et du départment de la Sarthe* (n.p., 1828), 38.

68. Pierre Sue, *Essais historiques, littéraires et critiques, sur l'art des accouchemens* (Paris, 1799), 2:128.

69. *L'Année littéraire* (1785), 5:261–65. For an analysis of women as journalists, readers of journals, and subjects of journal articles and of the turbulent history of the *Journal des dames* in particular, see Nina Gelbart's *Feminine and Opposition Journalism in Old Regime France* (Berkeley, 1987).

70. Marie Prudence Plisson, *Maximes morales d'un philosophe chrétien. Ouvrage qui peut servir de suite à la Collection des moralistes anciens* (Paris, 1783), 2–4.

Chapter Five. The Debate over Mesmerism, 1778–1787

1. "Les Docteurs modernes, comédie-parade, en vaudevilles," *Recueil général et complet de tous les Ecrits publiés pour et contre le magnétisme animal* 6, no. 87 (1784): 4–5.

2. Jean Jacques Paulet, *Mesmer justifié*, new ed. (Constance, 1784), 3–5.

3. Claude Quétel and Pierre Morel, *Les Fous et leurs médecins de la Renaissance au vingtième siècle* (Paris, 1979), 67–141.

4. Franz Anton Mesmer, "Mémoire sur la découverte du magnétisme animal," *Recueil* 1, no. 1, (1779): 74–77.

5. Ibid., 79–82.

6. The report edited by the commissioners of the Société Royale de Médecine was entitled: "Rapport des commissaires de la Société Royale de Médecine nommés par le Roi pour faire l'examen du magnétisme animal, imprimé par ordre du Roi, daté du 16 août 1784, signé de Poissonnier, Caille, Mauduyt, Andry," *Recueil,* 5, no. 56 (1784). J. B. Bonnefoy supplies useful précis of all the reports in his "Analyse raisonnée des rapports des commissaires chargés par le Roi de l'examen du magnétisme animal," *Recueil,* 6, no. 76 (1784).

7. The reports edited by members of the commission selected from the Faculté de Médecine de Paris and the Académie Royale des Sciences included:

"Exposé des expériences qui ont été faites pour l'examen du magnétisme animal lu à l'Académie des Sciences par M. Bailly en son nom et au nom de MM. Franklin, Le Roy, de Borty et Lavoisier, le 4 septembre 1784, imprimé par ordre du Roi," *Recueil* 5, no. 55 (1784).

J. S. Bailly, ed., "Rapport des commissaires chargés par le Roi de l'examen du magnétisme animal, imprimé par ordre du Roi," *Recueil* 5, no. 52 (1784).

J. S. Bailly, ed., "Rapport secret sur le mesmerisme, ou magnétisme animal," 1784, in Alexandre Bertrand, *Du Magnétisme animal en France et des jugements qu'en ont portés les sociétés savantes, avec le texte des divers rapports faits en 1784 par les commissaires de l'Académie des Sciences, de la Faculté et de la Société Royale de Médecine* (Paris, 1826), 511–16.

8. "Extrait des registres de la Faculté de Médecine de Paris, 1 décembre 1784," *Recueil,* 7, no. 103 (1784). The authenticity of this document is open to dispute, but it is valuable for the issues it raises in the debate over mesmerism.

9. Ibid., 3.

10. L. W. B. Brockliss, *French Higher Education in the Seventeenth and Eighteenth Centuries* (Oxford, 1987), 436–43.

11. John McManners, *Death and the Enlightenment: Changing Attitudes to Death among Christians and Unbelievers in Eighteenth-Century France* (Oxford, 1981), 434–35. In chapter 1 of *"Shattered Nerves": Doctors, Patients, and Depression in Victorian England* (Oxford, 1991), Janet Oppenheim notes that these problems continued to haunt British investigators of nervous disorders in the nineteenth century. After the Revolution, with the influence of Philippe Pinel, the approach of the French medical community to mental disorders would change dramatically. In his *Treatise on Insanity* (Sheffield, 1806, 4), Pinel noted that many empirics had been singularly successful in their cures but that they had in no way contributed to the advance of medical science by any valuable writings. Pinel didn't renounce the empirics' methods per se; he was intent, however, on understanding and disseminating the principles on which they were based. The numerous case histories he recounted illustrate the great extent to which he incorporated theatrics in treating patients. Pinel referred to these theatrics as "kind treatments" and "dextrous stratagems"; others might wonder about the problem of mendacity.

12. Bailly, "Rapport secret," 514.

13. Ibid., 512.

14. Jean-Jacques Rousseau, *Politics and the Arts: Letter to M. d'Alembert on*

the Theatre, trans. Allan Bloom (Ithaca, 1968), 35. Rousseau's letter was first published in 1758. The last edition to be corrected by Rousseau himself appeared in 1782.

15. See chapter 6 below.

16. For more on this topic, see Diane Alstad, "The Ideology of the Family in Eighteenth-Century France," (Ph.D. dissertation, Yale University, 1971), 59.

17. Susan Okin, *Women in Western Political Thought* (Princeton, 1979), 147.

18. Michel Augustin Thouret, "Recherches et doutes sur le magnétsime animal," *Recueil*, 6, no. 37 (1784): 59.

19. Jean-Pierre Guicciardi, "Between the Licit and the Illicit: The Sexuality of the King," in *"'Tis Nature's Fault". Unauthorized Sexuality during the Enlightenment*, ed. Robert Maccubin (Cambridge, 1987), 88–97. Sarah Maza pursued this theme in her paper "'The Faith placed in Covenants': Adultery and Politics in Prerevolutionary French Culture," presented to the American Historical Association's annual convention in 1986. Also see Jeffrey Merrick, "Social Politics and Public Order in Late Eighteenth-Century France: The *Mémoires secrets* and the *Correspondance secrète*," *Journal of the History of Sexuality* 1, no. 1 (1990): 68–84.

20. Bailly, "Rapport secret," 516.

21. Charles Devillers, "Le Colosse aux pieds d'argille," *Recueil*, 8, no. 108 (1784): 142.

22. "Magnétisme animal dévoilé par un zélé citoyen françois," *Recueil* 8, no. 107 (1784): 24. For more on the cultural acceptance of the centrality of pain to the birth process, see Mireille Laget, "La Naissance aux siècles classiques. Pratique des accouchements et attitudes collectives en France aux XVIIe et XVIIIe siècles," *Annales E.S.C.* 32, no. 5 (1977): 966–67. In *La Femme dans la pensée des Lumières* (Paris, 1977), 18–20, Paul Hoffmann argues that the program of enlightenment called into question the conventional acceptance of the necessity of suffering as a consequence of sin.

23. Thouret, "Recherches," 165–218.

24. Hecquet is quoted by Yvonne Knibiehler and Catherine Fouquet, *Histoire des mères du Moyen Age à nos jours* (Paris, 1977), 90.

25. Coupel, "Lettre au Directeur des Affiches, concernant les maris qui empêchent leurs femmes d'allaiter leurs enfans," *Affiches du Poitou*, no. 28 (11 July 1782): 109–10.

26. Marie Angélique Anel Le Rebours, *Avis aux mères qui veulent nourrir leurs enfants*, 5th ed. (Paris, An VII), 280. Mme Le Rebours was a fashionable Parisian midwife whose works enjoyed favor among the elite, including Mme Roland and Mme de Bombelles. First published in 1767, Le Rebours's text went through a number of editions. Later editions were preceded by a letter from Tissot commending the work and a favorable report by four doctors, including Barbeu du Bourg, of the Faculty of Medicine of Paris. The faculty unanimously approved the book and it was certified by the dean of the faculty, Le Thieullier. George Sussman, *Selling Mother's Milk: The Wet-Nursing Business in France, 1715–1914* (Urbana, Ill., 1982), 28, 81, 89–90.

27. Mme J. M. P. Roland, "A Ma Fille," in *Oeuvres*, ed. L. A. Champagneux (Paris, An VIII) 2:363. For more on the eighteenth-century exaltation of maternity,

see Elisabeth Badinter, *L'Amour en plus. Histoire de l'amour maternel, XVIIIe–XIXe siècles* (Paris, 1980).

28. On Mme de Genlis' misgivings about maternal nursing, see Albert, Comte de Luppé, *Les Jeunes Filles à la fin du XVIIIe siècle* (Paris, 1925), 29. Provincial doctors concerned with the health risks of maternal nursing included Rocques of Beauvais, "Projet d'Etablissement pour l'Administration des Enfants Trouvés," SRM Archives, carton 132 bis, no. 48 and Gastaldi, letter of 29 July 1791, SRM Archives, carton 134. Reacting against the fashionable tendency of labeling natural something that could in fact be harmful, Rocques remarked, "I will observe, however, that the mania for turning all women into nurses has not been thought through carefully. With the words religion and nature the majority of men are seduced, asking no more than to be spared the trouble of coming to the core of things."

29. Jean A. Perkins, "Love, Marriage and Sex in Eighteenth-Century France," *Studies on Voltaire and the Eighteenth Century* 256 (1988): 283–96.

30. In *Man and the Natural World: Changing Attitudes in England, 1500–1800* (London, 1983), 43, Keith Thomas notes that until the eighteenth century, the upper classes usually considered suckling debasing, to be avoided if possible by putting infants out to nurse, and pregnant women were commonly said to be "breeding." Léon Abensour, *La Femme et le féminisme avant la Révolution* (Paris, 1923), 226, quotes Mercier on the bourgeoisie's continued practice of sending children out to nurse.

31. Maurice Garden, *Lyon et les Lyonnais au XVIIIe siècle* (Paris, 1970), chap. 4 and pp. 139–40. On p. 29 of *Selling Mother's Milk*, Sussman concludes that the "primary effect of the campaign against wet-nursing upon the well-to-do, in addition to a short-lived fashion of maternal nursing around Paris and the court, was probably to encourage parents to choose their babies' wet nurses more carefully and to keep them under closer surveillance."

32. Garden, *Lyons*, 122–25. Knibiehler and Fouquet, *Histoire des mères*, 93. According to Sussman, the major effect of the "campaign against wet-nursing on the children of working families in the capital was a significant development of police regulation and surveillance over their wet-nursing. At the same time other French cities, particularly Lyon, tried to introduce police regulations on the Parisian model, without lasting success" (*Selling Mother's Milk*, 32). The inability of institutions to cope with the onslaught of abandoned infants in need of nurses is outlined in vivid detail by Olwen Hufton in *The Poor of Eighteenth-Century France, 1750–1789* (Oxford, 1974), 335–49.

33. See the review of a medical thesis presented to the Faculty of Paris by M. de la Feutrie, "La Saignée faite à la saphène, peu de tems après l'accouchement, est-elle un préservatif sûr et certain chez les femmes qui ne veulent pas allaiter?" *Gazette salutaire*, 30 April 1767.

34. Details of the SRM's experiments on alternatives to maternal nursing conducted at the foundling hospital can be found in SRM Archives, carton 127. A competition was announced for the best memoir on the benefits and hazards of maternal nursing. See SRM Archives, carton 198.

35. Beaumarchais suggested establishing an Institut de Bienfaisance for working mothers in a letter to the *Journal de Paris* reprinted in the *Affiches de Dauphiné*, 27 August 1784. For a report on the 112 infants and nursing mothers who benefited from the Institut de Bienfaisance of Lyon, see "Etat de la recette et de la dépense de l'Institut de Bienfaisance pour les mères-nourrices," *Journal de Lyon*, 1786: 87–91.

36. Valleton de Boissière, "Lettre à M. Thouret, pour servir de réfutation à l'extrait de la correspondance de la Société Royale de Médecine relativement au magnétisme animal," *Recueil*, 10, no. 119 (1784): 86–87. Charles Deslon, "Observations sur les deux rapports de MM. les Commissaires nommés par Sa Majesté, pour l'examen du magnétisme animal," *Recueil*, 5, no. 64 (1784): 21–22. And "Supplément aux deux rapports de MM. les Commissaires de l'Académie et de la Faculté de Médecine de Paris et de la Société Royale de Médecine," *Recueil*, 5, no. 66 (1784): 11.

37. Valleton de Boissière, "Lettre," 176–78.

38. "Réflexions sur le rapport des commissaires nommés pour examiner les principes et les effets curatifs de la doctrine de M. Deslon, et apologie de la conduite de ce médecin," *Recueil*, 5, no. 75 (1784): 10.

39. For analysis of these themes in popular literature, see Jean Paul Oddos, "Bibliothèque bleue: Etude d'une littérature populaire," in *La Littérature de colportage-exposition* (Reims, 1979). Also see Geneviève Bollème, *Les Almanachs populaires aux 17ᵉ et 18ᵉ siècles* (Paris, 1969) and *La Bibliothèque bleue* (Paris, 1971).

40. "*Journal de Paris*, 17 février 1784," *Recueil*, 2, no. 18 (1784): 24.

41. Mesmer, "Copie de la requête à nosseigneurs de Parlement," *Recueil*, 5, no. 59 (1784): 9. Matthew Ramsey, "Traditional Medicine and Medical Enlightenment: The Regulation of Secret Remedies in the Ancien Régime," *Historical Reflections/Réflexions historiques*, 9 (1982): 215–32. Also see Natalie Davis, "Proverbial Wisdom and Popular Errors," *Society and Culture in Early Modern France* (Standford, 1975), 227–67. And William Coleman, "Health and Hygiene in the Encyclopedia: A Medical Doctrine for the Bourgeoisie," *Journal of the History of Medicine and Allied Sciences*, 29 (1974): 399–421.

42. René Descartes, *Discourse on the Method of Rightly Conducting the Reason and Seeking for Truth in the Sciences*, vol. 31 of *Great Books of the Western World*, ed. Robert Hutchins (Chicago, 1952), 61.

43. Joseph Servan, "Doutes d'un provincial, proposés à MM. les médecins-commissaires, chargés par le roi, de l'examen du magnétisme animal," *Recueil*, 6, no. 80 (1784): 126.

44. In 1767 Servan argued against a philandering husband's effort to have his marriage to a Protestant woman declared invalid because the marriage had not been celebrated by a Catholic priest. In 1770 he sought damages against a sixty-year-old dancing instructor who had seduced his fifteen-year-old pupil. In 1772 he defended an aristocrat who reneged on a promise he had made to repay debts owed an actress, accusing her of *captation* (legacy hunting). Although Servan was victorious in the first two suits, public opinion turned against him on the third.

For more on Servan, see Jean Egret, *Le Parlement de Dauphiné et les affaires publiques dans la deuxième moitié du XVIIIᵉ siècle*, vol. 1, *L'Opposition parlementaire (1756–1775)* (Grenoble, Paris, 1942), 145–68.

45. Adolphe Rochas, *Biographie du Dauphiné contenant l'histoire des hommes nés dans cette province* (Geneva, 1971), 1:404–11.

46. Carolyn Merchant, *The Death of Nature: Women, Ecology, and the Scientific Revolution* (New York, 1980).

47. Nicolas Bergasse, "Lettre d'un médecin de la Faculté de Paris, à un médecin du Collège de Londres, ouvrage dans lequel on prouve contre M. Mesmer, que le magnétisme animal n'existe pas," *Recueil*, 2, no. 8 (1781): 66–67.

48. Thouret, "Extrait de la correspondance de la Société Royale de Médecine relativement au magnétisme animal," *Recueil*, 10 (1785): 45–48.

49. An exchange among a local curé, a doctor, and a surgeon regarding the benefits of animal magnetism addressed to the editors of the *Affiches du Dauphiné* in 1785 illuminates the strained relations that the curé's or surgeon's endorsement of an alternative healing could provoke. See the letters of La Condamine and Grandchamp in Joseph Servan, ed., *Lettres adressées au rédacteur des affiches du Dauphiné, sur une cure opérée par le magnétisme animal* (n.p., 1785), 12–23.

50. Maury, letters of 2 octobre 1784 and 5 octobre 1787, SRM Archives, carton 137, no. 8 and *Journal de Nancy*, 1780: 337–45.

51. For a summary of the Société Royale de Médecine's perception of its research rather than regulatory mission, see Geoffroy, "Compte rendu du deux mémoires envoyés par M. Le Comte, médecin à Evreux," of 28 June 1785, in SRM Archives, carton 191. Also see the review of Destieux's letter written by Coquereau and Halle, 25 June 1780, in SRM Archives, carton 194.

52. On the realities behind the myth of absolutism, see James Collins, *The Fiscal Limits of Absolutism. Direct Taxation in Early Seventeenth-Century France* (Berkeley, 1988); Roger Mettam, *Power and Faction in Louis XIV's France* (Basil Blackwell, 1988); and C. B. A. Behrens, *Society, Government, and the Enlightenment: The Experiences of Eighteenth-Century France and Prussia* (New York, 1985).

53. *Affiches pour les Trois-Evêchés et la Lorraine* 19 (6 May 1784): 149 and *Affiches, annonces, et avis divers du Dauphiné* 26 (25 October 1782): 101.

54. Maury, letter of 1 April 1783, SRM Archives, carton 137, no. 8.

55. Bonamy, Doyen de la Faculté de Nantes, letter of 14 September 1784, SRM Archives, carton 195.

56. Pelet, correspondent from Millau en Rouergue, letter of 24 September 1784, SRM Archives, carton 178.

57. Maury, letter of 23 October 1789, SRM Archives, carton 137, no. 8.

58. Robin de Kiervalle, médecin à Josselin, Bretagne, "Projet pour la destruction du charlatanisme en France," 8 October 1784, SRM Archives, carton 184.

59. Doucet, maître chirurgien à Frolois près Ste. Reine en Bourgogne, "Mémoire sur l'état de la chirurgie des campagnes," SRM Archives, carton 131, no. 18.

60. The practice is deplored in *Le Censeur universel anglois, ou revue générale, critique et impartiale de toutes les productions angloises sur les sciences, la littérature, les beaux-arts, les manufactures, le commerce, etc.*, 1 (3 July 1785): 4.

For examples of the phenomenon, see the advertisement of Dame Veros, who described herself as a chemist and promised to heal "all secret illnesses," in *Annonces de Marseilles* 1771: 11, and that of Sieur Deverre, a self-proclaimed botanist who claimed to have the ability to preserve women from miscarriages and abortions, *Annonces de Marseilles* 1773: 170. Also see the advertisement of a surgeon, Sieur Thomas, specializing in feminine disorders and guaranteeing secrecy, *Affiches de la Bourgogne*, 5 June 1787, 123.

61. Barailon, correspondent from Chambon en Combraille, letter of 5 March 1779, SRM Archives, carton 199.

62. *Ancient Medicine: Selected Papers of Ludwig Edelstein*, ed. Oswei Temkin and C. Lilian Temkin (Baltimore, 1967), 13–18, 62–63.

63. Subdelegate to Intendant, letter of 3 September 1788, Archives Départementales de l'Aube, C1164, no. 2.

64. Cazabonnu, chirurgien, "Observations particulières sur les sages-femmes de Toulouse," 23 September 1786, SRM Archives, carton 87. As a letter from Puisais, curé of Savigny-l'Evécault, to the *Affiches du Poitou* 35 (30 August 1781): 137–38 demonstrates, changing mentality was just as important as educating midwives if midwifery were to be considered an honorable occupation. One of Puisais's parishioners, Marguerite Bacon, had served as the village undertaker, wrapping and preparing bodies for burial. She attended a free course in midwifery in Poitiers and received a certificate attesting to her competence. Upon returning to her village, Bacon announced that she had abandoned her previous occupation and was eager to serve her community as midwife. Puisais observed that "despite the fact that the women of this parish and its environs recognize the trustworthiness and other good qualities of this woman, they have declared publicly that they would never allow her to attend their births. They claim that her previous occupation would harm them and their children and that whoever has wrapped the bodies of the dead would bring misfortune to the living whom she would tend in such circumstance." Despite all Puisais's efforts in public and private to dissuade the women from their resolution, this was one popular prejudice he found impossible to destroy.

65. Giordana Charuty, "Le Mal d'amour," in *Le Corps humain: Nature, culture, surnaturel*, Actes du 110ᵉ Congrès national des sociétés savantes, Montpellier, 1985 (Paris, 1985), 87.

66. Alain Lottin, "Naissances illégitimes et filles mères à Lille au XVIIIᵉ siècle," *Revue d'histoire moderne et contemporaine* 17 (April-June, 1970): 280–81. Knibiehler and Fouquet, *Histoire des mères*, 128. Although the medical community encouraged the training of midwives, it did not believe it proper for women to be instructed in all the workings of the human body. The prejudice against women practicing medicine continued during the Revolution and Empire. The letter of Lassus, Peyrilsier, and Sabatier dated 9 messidor an 6 (Archives de la Bibliothèque de la Faculté de Médecine de Paris, ms. 2277) takes up the case of the widow of a doctor who had received an indemnity for giving free medical care to the poor. The widow petitioned the Minister of the Interior to continue receiving the indemnity because she was continuing her husband's practice. Although two doctors had attested to the woman's competence, Lassus, Peyrilsier,

and Sabatier insisted that she be tested. Because, however, it was considered improper for a woman to be tested, she could not be authorized to practice medicine and was thus not qualified to continue receiving the indemnity.

67. Pujol, médecin à Castres (Languedoc), letter of 24 October 1784, SRM Archives, carton 129.

68. Pujol, SRM Archives, carton 129.

69. Meillardet, médecin de l'hôpital militaire de la ville de Gray, "Réponses aux questions faites aux médecins par la cour," 18 November 1775, SRM Archives, carton 124.

70. The content of the provincial journals varied somewhat depending on the personality of their editor and the interests of the audience, though the avowed aim of them all was to distract and to instruct. While some, like the *Journal de Lyon*, assumed a highly literary character, others, like the *Annonces pour la ville de Marseille*, consisted of little more than a variety of announcements and advertisements. The same book announcements and releases from government agencies, such as the Société Royale de Médecine, appeared in many of the journals, as did particularly piquant news items. Some editors, for example, the editor of the *Journal de la ville de Troyes*, believed their journals should provide a forum for debate of issues of regional concern and printed numerous letters from their neighbors. Others, such as the editor of the *Affiches du Poitou*, emphasized the importance of their journals' role in bringing enlightenment to the countryside. Articles on science and medicine, often written by local doctors or clergy, figured prominently in the provincial journals and reaffirmed the positions of these individuals as community leaders. The journal had a limited circulation, particularly compared to the almanacs. Because they were relatively expensive and generally sold by subscription rather than by individual copy, the journals attracted a privileged, bourgeois readership. A good description of these journals can be found in Claude Bellanger et al., eds., *Histoire générale de la presse française*, vol. 1, *Des Origines à 1814* (Paris, 1969), 323–402. Also see Eugène Hatin, *Histoire de la presse en France* (Paris, 1859) and *Bibliographie historique et critique de la presse périodique française* (Paris, 1866).

71. For a striking example of this juxtaposition, see *Annonces de Marseille*, 181. The practice is criticized in "Extrait d'une lettre adressée à l'auteur de cette gazette," *Gazette salutaire*, 28 April 1768. This juxtaposition is also noted by Gilles Feyel in "Médecins, empiriques et charlatans dans la presse provinciale à la fin du XVIIIe siècle," in *Le Corps et la santé*, Actes du 110e Congrès des sociétés savantes, Montpellier, 1985, (Paris, 1985), 1:81.

72. *Affiches, annonces, et avis divers pour les Trois-Evêchés et la Lorraine*, 37 (9 September 1784).

75. Paulet, "Mesmer," passim.

74. *Journal de Troyes et de la Champagne méridional*, 7 July 1784. Also see *Affiches pour les Trois-Evêchés et la Lorraine* 24 (10 June 1784): 187.

75. *Affiches du Dauphiné* 31 (5 December 1783): 130.

76. *Affiches pour les Trois-Evêchés et la Lorraine* 38 (28 July 1785): 234.

77. Nicolas Dessessarts, ed., *Causes célèbres* 144 (1786): 61–65. Also see the "Arrêt du Conseil du Cap qui défend aux gens de couleur l'exercise du magnétisme animal et renouvelle les défenses des attroupemens illicites," 16 May 1786, in

SRM Archives, carton 176. And Henri Carré, *La Noblesse de France et l'opinion publique au XVIIIe siècle* (Paris, 1920), 148–53. Also David Epstein, "Malouet and the Issue of Slavery in Saint Domingue, 1767–1802," *Proceedings of the Western Society for French History* 15 (1988): 179–80.

78. Joseph Servan, *Discours sur les moeurs, prononcé au parlement de Grenoble en 1769* (Lyon, n.d.), 5.

79. François Furet and Denis Richet, *La Révolution française* (Paris, 1973), 45, quoted in Pierre Guicciardi, "Between the Licit and Illicit," 97. Also see Robert Darnton, "Philosophy under the Cloak," in *Revolution in Print. The Press in France 1775–1800*, ed. Robert Darnton and Daniel Roche (Berkeley, 1989), 27–49.

Chapter Six. Ignorant and Superstitious or Overly Refined? The Convulsive Female in Physicans' Critiques of Culture

1. See Michel Foucault, *Folie et déraison: Histoire de la folie* (Paris, 1961), 660–70, for a list of the medical works on the subject of convulsions. Advertisements for remedies for convulsions as well as any number of other disorders appeared regularly in the *Affiches de Marseille* in the 1770s. The advertisers were often unmarried women and widows.

2. See the review of Robert Whytt's *Observations sur la nature, les causes et le traitement des maladies qu'on nomme communément nerveuses, hypocondriaques ou hystériques* in *Gazette salutaire*, 10 October 1766. Also see Claude Quétel and Pierre Morel, *Les Fous et leurs médecins de la Renaissance au vingtième siècle* (Paris, 1979).

3. L. J. Jordanova, "Natural Facts: A Historical Perspective on Science and Sexuality," in *Nature, Culture, and Gender*, ed. Carol MacCormack and Marilyn Strathern (Cambridge, 1980), 48.

4. Suzanne Doublet, "La Médecine dans les oeuvres de Diderot" (Université de Bordeaux, Faculté de Médecine. thèse 144, 1933–34), 44.

5. See Moublet-gras of Tarascon en Provence, "Mémoire sur la question proposée par la Société Royale de Médecine: 'Exposer quels sont les caractères des maladies nerveuses proprèment dittes, telles que l'hystéricisme et l'hypocondriacisme, et jusqu'à quel point elles différent des maladies analogues, telles que la mélancolie; quelles sont leurs causes principales, et quelle méthode l'on doit employer en général dans leur traitement" (1785), 46, in SRM Archives, carton 197.

6. The competition was announced in the *Histoire . . . avecs les mémoires de médecine et de physique médicale* of the Société Royale de Médecine (Paris, 1782–83), 17. Further details can be found in SRM Archives, carton 198.

7. *Encyclopédie* 16 (1765): 836–37.

8. For more on the repressive panic displayed by doctors when confronted with female sexuality, see Yvonne Knibiehler, "Les Médecins et la 'nature féminine' au temps du Code Civil," *Annales. Economies, Sociétés, Civilisations* 31, no. 4 (1976): 840.

9. Edmond and Jules Goncourt, *La Femme au dix-huitième siècle* (Paris, 1982), 223–24.

10. "Causes physiques et morales des maladies des nerfs," *Gazette salutaire*, 6 October 1768.

11. For more on eighteenth-century art and engraving, see Jean Adhémar, *La Gravure originale au XVIIIᵉ siècle* (Paris, 1963), Baron Roger Portalis and Henri Béraldi, *Les Graveurs du dix-huitième siècle*, 3 vols. (Paris, 1880–82). Thomas Crow, *Painters and Public Life in Eighteenth-Century Paris* (New Haven, 1985), and Paul Lacroix, *XVIIIᵉ siècle. Lettres, sciences, arts. France 1700–1789* (Paris, 1878). On representations of women, see Carol Duncan, "Happy Mothers and Other New Ideas in French Art," *The Art Bulletin* 55 (December 1973): 570–83. On the portrayal of medicine in art, see Léon Binet and Pierre Vallery-Radot, *Médicine et art de la Renaissance à nos jours* (Paris, 1968), and Jean Rousselot, *Medicine in Art: A Cultural History* (New York, 1967). On p. 210, Rousselot describes the charming frontispiece of Joseph Raulin's *De la conversation des enfants* (1768); it depicts a mother caring for her children under the watchful eye of Hippocrates.

12. Anne d'Aubourg de la Bove, Comtesse de Miremont, *Traité de l'éducation des femmes, et cours complet d'instruction* (Paris, 1779–89). Riballier et Cosson, *De l'éducation physique et morale des femmes, avec une notice alphabétique de celles qui se sont distinguées dans les différentes carrières des sciences et des beaux-arts, ou par des talens et des actions mémorables* (Paris, 1779). Marie Thiroux d'Arconville, *Pensées et réflexions morales, sur divers sujets, par l'auteur du traité de l'amitié, et de celui des passions* (Paris, 1766). Alice Laborde, *L'Oeuvre de Mme de Genlis* (Paris, 1966). Mme la Baronne Duplessy, *Répertoire des lectures faites au musée des dames* (Paris, 1788). Louise F. P. Tardieu d'Esclavelles d'Epinay, *Les Conversations d'Emilie* (Leipzig, 1774). Mlle d'Espinassy, *Essai sur l'éducation des démoiselles* (Paris, 1764).

13. Thiroux d'Arconville, *Pensées*, 106–10.

14. *Une Jeune Fille au XVIIIᵉ siècle: Lettres de Geneviève de Malboissière à Adélaide Méliand, 1761–1766*, ed. Albert, Comte de Luppé (Paris, 1925), 35–36, 205–8.

15. *Encyclopédie* 16 (1765): 836–37.

16. Charmeil, "Observations nosologiques," SRM Archives, carton 146.

17. Spielman, SRM Archives, carton 132bis, no. 45; Terrède, letter of 25 October 1777, SRM Archives, carton 137, no. 21; Boillin, "Topographie médicale," 13 October 1777, SRM Archives, carton 195.

18. Dablaing, letter of autumn, 1783, SRM Archives, carton 135, no. 3; Borde, memoir of 1783, SRM Archives, carton 134.

19. Louis Merle, "La Vie et les oeuvres du Dr. Jean-Gabriel Gallot," *Mémoires de la société des antiquaires de l'Ouest*, 4th ser., 5 (Poitiers, 1962): 1–262.

20. Compare the "Suite du Journal de M. Gallot, Médecin à St.-Maurice-le-Girard (mois d'octobre)," appearing in the *Affiches du Poitou* 45 (19 November 1778): 193, with the "Observations nosologiques," which he submitted to the SRM on 6 March 1779. See SRM Archives, carton 189.

21. "Médecine: Suite de la lettre de M. Nicolas," *Affiches du Dauphiné*, 4 November 1774, 123.

22. See "Suite de la lettre sur les fleurs," in *Affiches de Toulouse*, 28 March 1781, for Ingen-Housz's letter. For Dufresnoy's letter, see "Médecine: Des pro-

priétés du Narcisse des près, et du succès qu'on en a obtenus pour la guérison des convulsions," in *Journal de Troyes*, 28 January 1789, 18–19. Dufresnoy's letter to the SRM on the same subject can be found in SRM Archives, carton 188. In this letter of 19 April 1787, Dufresnoy discloses the fact that the cure had only been temporary; his patient suffered a relapse of convulsions.

23. The response of Tessier and Neauroi dated 6 February 1778 to Boucher's inquiry of 12 January 1778 can be found in SRM Archives, carton 134.

24. Chifoliau, médecin à St. Malo, "Observation sur la dilation monstrueuse d'un ovaire," 27 July 1781, SRM Archives, carton 190.

25. "Nouvelles de la Province (Nancy, le 6 février)," *Affiches pour les Trois-Evêchés et la Lorraine*, 10 February 1780, 45.

26. Taranget, médecin à Douay, "Constitutions épidémiques de la ville de Douay et de quelques villages circonvoisins," 1790, SRM Archives, carton 182.

27. Isuard, chirurgien à Embrun, "Observation sur une fièvre putride inflammatoire, compliquée d'affection vapeureuse hypochondriaque détérminée par une passion amoreuse," SRM Archives, carton 193.

28. Bonhomme, médecin à Avignon, "Réflexions sur les maladies de l'année et sur la variété des récoltes," 20 November 1790, SRM Archives, carton 195.

29. Ripert, médecin à Apt, letter of 12 January 1785, SRM Archives, carton 184.

30. Revoltat, médecin à Vienne en Dauphiné, "Topographie médicale," 7 April 1778, SRM Archives, carton 167.

31. "Médecine: Maladies occasionnées par la Révolution," *Notice de l'Almanach sous verre* (1792), 619. Philippe Pinel confirms this rise in nervous disorders as a result of the Revolution in his *Treatise on Insanity* (Sheffield, 1806), 9.

32. "Réflexions médicinales sur le mariage, tirées de l'*Encyclopédie*, article mariage," *Gazette salutaire*, 26 February 1767.

33. Ibid.

34. For the medical diatribes against masturbation, see Jean-Paul Aron and Roger Kempf, *Le Pénis et la démoralisation de l'Occident* (Paris, 1978). On the issue of homosexuality in eighteenth-century culture, see Robert Maccubbin, ed., *"Tis Nature's Fault": Unauthorized Sexuality during the Enlightenment* (Cambridge, 1987). Masturbation was thought to be so deleterious that Marigues, the chief surgeon of the royal infirmary at Versailles, held it responsible for the death of a nineteen-year-old girl. He attributed the inefficacy of his treatments to the fact that the girl had hidden the true nature of her disorder from him. See his memoir, "Sur quelques effets de la masturbation sur l'oeconomie animale," 21 May 1782, SRM Archives, carton 124.

35. Cassan, médecin du roi de Ste. Lucie, "De l'épuisement chez les créoles," in "Traité de l'influence des climats chauds sur les corps animés," 5 February 1790, SRM Archives, carton 179. Cassan acknowledged taking Tissot as his guide on the subjects of masturbation and convulsions.

36. *Une Jeune Fille*, 44.

37. Marie-Claire Grassi, "La Naissance et la mort dans le discours intime," in *Le Corps humain: Nature, culture, surnaturel*, Actes du 110e Congrès national des sociétés savantes, Montpellier, 1985 (Paris, 1985), 112.

38. Giordana Charuty, "Le Mal d'amour," in *Le Corps humain*, 87. Also see

Dominique Le Cunf's analysis of hysteria in Jean-Claude Pie, "Anne Charlier, un miracle eucharistique dans le faubourg Saint-Antoine," in *Les Miracles miroirs des corps*, ed. Jacques Gélis et Odile Redon (Paris, 1983), 189. A clinical psychologist, Le Cunf interprets hysterical symptoms as expressions of unconscious conflicts. A paralysis could be simultaneously a defense against, and a substitute for, reprehensible sexual activity. Hysterical symptoms frequently begin to manifest themselves soon after marriage or the birth of the first child. When the symptoms lose their secondary benefits, they become negligible, and what appears to be a sudden, even miraculous, healing may take place.

39. "Observation sur une démence causée par une frayeur, par M.——, *Gazette salutaire*, 16 February 1769.

40. "Evénement singulier," *Affiches du Dauphiné*, 25 November 1774, 134.

41. Jacques Rossiaud, "Prostitution, jeunesse et société dans les villes du Sud-est au XVᵉ siècle," *Annales. Economies, Sociétés, Civilisations* 31, no. 2 (1976): 289–325.

42. Maret, médecin à Dijon, "Vingtième observation," 1779, SRM Archives, carton 124; Maury, médecin à Sezanne, letter of 3 July 1781, SRM Archives, carton 137, no. 8; Marx, médecin à Hanovre, "Maladie nerveuse assez particulière," SRM Archives, carton 124; Peraud de Laurignai, médecin à Noirmoutier, letter of 30 August 1776, SRM Archives, carton 189.

43. Mercadier, chirurgien de Paris, "Observation sur une abstinence de près de six mois, guérie par le bain d'eau froide," *Gazette salutaire*, 26 September 1765.

44. Ardent, médecin à Gap, letter of 12 August 1776, SRM Archives, carton 140, no. 2.

45. Ibid.

46. Marie-Claude Phan and Jean-Louis Flandrin, "Les Métamorphoses de la beauté féminine," *L'Histoire* 68 (June, 1984): 48–57.

47. Alison Lingo, "Santé et beauté féminines dans la France de la Renaissance," in *Le Corps human: Nature, culture, surnaturel*, Actes du 110ᵉ Congrès national des sociétés savantes, Montpellier, 1985 (Paris, 1985), 191–99. H. G. Ibels, "Le Costume et le Meuble," *La Vie parisienne au XVIIIᵉ siécle: Leçons faites à l'Ecole des hautes etudes sociales* (Paris, 1914), 107.

48. Duvernin, médecin a Clermont-Ferrand, doyen du collège de médecine de Clermont, "Mémoire sur les maladies observées à Clermont-Ferrand et aux environs depuis près de 5 ans," 1777, SRM Archives, carton 170bis, no. 127.

49. Claude Grimmer, *La Femme et le bâtard. Amours illégitimes et secrètes dans l'ancienne France* (Paris, 1983), 219.

50. Tavernier, médecin à Pontcartier, letter of 24 October 1785, SRM Archives, carton 186.

51. Hardouineau, ancien médecin des hôpitaux militaires de Namur, et médecin de l'Hôtel-Dieu d'Orléans, "Observation sur une maladie convulsive," *Gazette salutaire*, 31 July 1767.

52. Mathieu, à Couze près Lasende en Perigord, letter of 22 September 1783, SRM Archives, carton 195; "Observation sur une manie à la suite d'un accouchement," *Gazette salutaire*, 19 May 1768; "Observation sur une mélancolie à la suite d'un accouchement," *Gazette salutaire*, 5 May 1768.

53. M. F. Aublet, médecin des hôpitaux militaires, "Topographie médicale de la ville de St. Jean d'Angély en Saintonge," SRM Archives, carton 177.

54. "Extraits du *Journal de médecine* du mois de mars: Observation sur une manie survenue à une femme le huitième jour de ses couches," par M. Planchon, *Gazette salutaire*, 26 May 1768.

55. La Brossière, médecin, "Topographie médicale de la ville de St. Malo," 12 January 1790, SRM Archives, carton 181.

56. Didelot, chirurgien à Remirement en Lorraine, "Dissertation sur la constitution médicale de l'année 1788 à celle de 1789," SRM Archives, carton 181.

57. Doublet, *La Médecine*, 50.

58. Claudine Herzlich and Janine Pierret, *Illness and Self in Society*, trans. Elborg Forster (Baltimore, 1987), 112.

59. Léon Abensour, *La Femme et le féminisme avant la Révolution* (Paris, 1923), 182, 417.

60. Achard, médecin à Marseille, "Essai sur les maladies des chapeliers," 1781, SRM Archives, carton 139.

61. Ramel, médecin, "Topographie médicale de la Ciolat, Ceireste, Cassis, Aubagne, Luges, Gemenos, Roquevaire et autres lieux," 26 August 1788, SRM Archives, carton 175.

62. Aublet, "Topographie médicale de St. Jean d'Angély," SRM Archives, carton 177.

63. Flangergues, "Observations sur l'influence des travaux relatifs à la fabrication des étoffes de laine sur la santé des ouvriers qui y travaillent dans les manufactures de la ville de Viviers en Vivarais," 10 October 1779, SRM Archives, carton 131, no. 21

64. Desmery, médecin à Amiens, letter of 3 December 1781, SRM Archives, carton 194. For more on Desmery, see Vicq d'Azyr, "Notice sur la vie et les oeuvres . . . Desmery," in *Eloges lus dans les séances publiques de la Société Royale de Médecine* (Paris, 1778–1798), 179–81.

65. "Extrait de *l'English Chronicle*, Preston, Comté du Lancastre," 8 March 1787, SRM Archives, carton 134.

66. Doublet, *La Médecine*, 60.

67. Flangergues, "Observation," SRM Archives, carton 131, no. 21.

68. Alain Lottin, "Naissances illégitimes et filles mères à Lille au XVIIIe siècle," *Revue d'histoire moderne et contemporaine* 17 (April–June 1970): 278–322. Also see Didier Riet, "Les Déclarations de grossesse dans la region de Dinan à la fin de l'Ancien Régime," *Annales de Bretagne et des pays de l'Ouest (Anjou, Maine, Touraine)* 88 (1981): 181–87. And Olwen Hufton, *The Poor of Eighteenth-Century France, 1750–1789* (Oxford, 1974), 318–29. And Cissie Fairchilds, "Female Sexual Attitudes and the Rise of Illegitimacy: A Case Study," *Journal of Interdisciplinary History* 8, no. 4 (1978): 627–67.

69. Sarah Maza, *Servants and Masters in Eighteenth-Century France: The Uses of Loyalty* (Princeton, 1983), 89–91.

70. Abensour, *La Femme*, 209.

71. Arnaud, médecin, "Mémoire sur la topographie médicale du canton du Puy, précédé d'une idée générale des districts du Puy et de Monistrol, département de la haute Loire," SRM Archives, carton 176.

72. Odile Arnold, *Le Corps et l'âme. La Vie des religieuses au XIXᵉ siècle* (Paris, 1984), 319. In "L'Ouvrière," in Jean-Paul Aron, ed., *Misérable et glorieuse. La Femme du XIXᵉ siècle* (Paris, 1980), 67–68, Madeleine Rebérioux remarks on the repressive tenor that the rules of the convent gave to factories in the nineteenth century. In some instances, women were forbidden from speaking at work, meals, and even in their dormitories.

73. Achard, "Essai," SRM Archives, carton 139.

74. Beerenbrock, médecin à Montpellier, letter of 18 May 1780, SRM Archives, carton 140, no. 5.

75. Morgue de Montredum, "Observations sur les naissances, les mariages, et les morts à Montpellier pendant dix années consécutives, de 1772 à 1781," SRM *Histoire* (1780–81): 378–92. For more on the *médecine du travail*, see Arlette Farge, "Work-related Diseases of Artisans in Eighteenth-Century France," in *Medicine and Society in France: Selections from the Annales. Economies, Sociétés, Civilisations* (Baltimore, 1980), 89–103. Farge argues that doctors regarded the health problems connected with labor with a combination of compassion and resignation. While poverty was thought to be necessary, wretchedness was not.

76. Yvonne Knibiehler and Catherine Fouquet, *Histoire des mères du Moyen Age à nos jours* (Paris, 1977), 931.

77. Martin, médecin de l'Hôtel-Dieu, Narbonne, en Languedoc, "Réflexions et observations sur un point relatif à l'éducation physique et au traitement des maladies des enfants," 1783, SRM Archives, carton 193.

78. Eugenii Tarlé, *L'Industrie dans les campagnes en France à la fin de l'Ancien Régime* (Paris, 1910), 22. Abensour, *La Femme*, 183–200, notes that in certain regions patrons appealed to intendants and curés to aid in recruiting women to rural industry. The intendant Imbert de Saint-Paul organized a spinning school in Picardy which curés urged girls to attend. By the second year, the school at Roye had ninety-two students. Certificates and money prizes were distributed to the best students. Solemn award ceremonies were held to attract women from neighboring villages. Still, much remained to be done in instructing female workers, especially in the Lyon silk industry, where masters complained of their workers' ignorance.

79. Tarlé, *L'Industrie*, 19, 22.

80. Ibid., 9. Abensour, *La Femme*, 192–94, notes that large numbers of women were drawn from the countryside to the silk industry in Lyon. His statistics for the beginning of the nineteenth century indicate that 80 percent of the workers in the majority of spinning establishments in the northeast were young girls, women, and children.

81. Tarlé, *L'Industrie*, 37.

82. Alain Decaux, *Histoire des Françaises*, vol. 2. *La Révolte* (Paris, 1972), 427–28.

83. Jacques Ballexserd, "Dissertation sur cette question: Quelles sont les causes principales de la mort d'un aussi grand nombre d'enfants, et quels sont les préservatifs les plus éfficaces et les plus simples pour leur conserver la vie?" *Affiches pour les Trois Evêchés et la Lorraine*, 19 February 1778, 31. Barbeu du Bourg reports that Ballexserd's book was dedicated to Antoine Petit.

84. Knibiehler and Fouquet, *Histoire des mères*, 237.

85. Barthez, "Dix-huitième Consultation," in "Recueil de Consultations," Bibliothèque Municipale de Troyes, ms. 2675.

86. Ayrau, médecin à Mirabeau, "Observations particulières: mélancolie hystérique dégénerée en manie guérie par les douches d'eau froide," SRM Archives, carton 143, no. 1.

87. Meglin, médecin à Guebeviller, petite ville de la Haute Alsace, letter of May 1786, SRM Archives, carton 175.

88. Ripert, médecin à Apt, letter of 12 January 1785, SRM Archives, carton 184.

89. Cornefroy, letter of 13 April 1780, SRM Archives, carton 122, no. 17.

90. Doublet, *La Médecine*, 51.

91. "Jugement de la Faculté de Médecine en l'Université de Paris au sujet des pierres sorties du corps d'une fille du village de S. Geosmes, Diocèse de Langres," ms. 6772, Bibliothèque de l'Arsenal. A similar case pitted a young servant, Catherine Stickrin, against her master. At given intervals Stickrin fell into convulsions and evacuated pins, explaining that robbers had stuffed a pin cushion down her throat to silence her as they robbed the house. Stickrin's master, believing her an accomplice, appealed to the doctors and surgeons of Neufchâteau. While they supported the master, and Stickrin was convicted of fraud and imprisoned in Nancy as a result, their colleagues in Nancy sided with Stickrin. (*Journal de Nancy*, 1779: 159–62; *Journal de Lorraine et Barrois*, 1778: 63–67, 175–81; and Jadelot, "Histoire d'une maladie singulière," in SRM Archives, carton 188).

92. "Extrait d'une lettre de Tain, dans la Bretagne septentrionale, datée du 1 août 1767," *Gazette salutaire*, 1 September 1768. Details and analysis of a number of similar cases occurring in continental Europe, England, and America from the seventeenth through the nineteenth centuries can be found in Joan Jacobs Brumberg's *Fasting Girls. The Emergence of Anorexia Nervosa as a Modern Disease* (Cambridge, Mass., 1988).

93. St. André, médecin, Tarascon, "Mémoire historique de l'abstinence et de l'inappétence d'une fille âgée de 31 ans qui vit en conservant l'embonpoint depuis 14 années," 3 May 1784, SRM Archives, carton 167.

94. Patricia Crawford, "Attitudes to Menstruation in Seventeenth-Century England," *Past and Present* 91 (May 1981): 47–73.

95. Erna Hellerstein, "Women, Social Order, and the City: Rules for French Ladies, 1830–1870" (Ph.D. dissertation, University of California, Berkeley, 1980), 210.

96. Caroline Walker Bynum, "Fasts, Feasts, and Flesh: The Religious Significance of Food to Medieval Women," *Representations* 11 (summer 1985): 1–25. Rudolf Bell, *Holy Anorexia* (Chicago, 1985).

97. In those rare instances when SRM correspondents recommended methods successfully employed by empirics to combat convulsions, they were severely castigated by the SRM. See, for example, the report edited by Fourcroy and Jeannois of Le Monnier's "Observations sur quelques maladies convulsives guéries par un singulier topique en forme d'amulette," 1781, SRM Archives, carton 191. Fourcroy and Jeannois remarked that chemistry and observation were to be preferred to inexplicable remedies that had "fallen into disuse and become the resort

of women in secret." Also see Boillin, médecin à Dole en Franche-Comté, "Topographie médicale," 13 October 1777, SRM Archives, carton 195.

98. "Lettre anonyme aux Messieurs de l'Académie Royale de Médecine," SRM Archives, carton 132bis, no. 64.

99. "Evénement remarquable," *Journal de Troyes et de la Campagne méridionale*, 5 November 1873, 181. Also see the canard entitled "Evénement tragique, arrivé dans le Bourg de Cériziers, Diocèse de Sens, le 25 octobre; confirmé par le procès-verbal des officiers de justice du lieu, et le rapport du sieur Colombier, Maître en Chirurgie," bound with this journal in the Bibliothèque Municipale de Troyes.

100. Cormont, curé de Trémilly, "Lettre adressée à l'auteur de ce journal," *Journal politique* (de Bouillon), 1st fortnight August 1779, 47–50.

101. *Journal politique*, 1st fortnight September 1779, 54–56.

102. "Evénemens intéressans de la ville et du diocèse de Troyes pendant l'année 1779," *Almanach de la ville et du diocèse de Troyes, capital de la Champagne pour l'année bissextile 1780*, 131–35.

103. Ibid.

104. *Mélanges extraits des manuscrits de Mme Necker*, ed. Jacques Necker, 3 vols. (Paris, 1798), 1:355; 3:11, 199–202. Hellerstein, "Women, Social Order, and the City," argues that, in recoil from the modern city, physicians projected their fears about its unnaturalness onto the bodies of women (250). Their diagnoses reinforced the public/private dichotomy, effectively excluding women from activity in the public sphere. For more on how notions of gender influenced the definition and treatment of disorders in the nineteenth century, see Elaine Showalter, *The Female Malady* (New York, 1985).

105. Herzlich and Pierret, *Illness and Self*, 26–28.

106. Sander Gilman, *Difference and Pathology: Stereotypes of Sexuality, Race and Madness* (Ithaca, N.Y., 1985).

Conclusion: The Legacy of the Enlightenment

1. Daniel Roche, *Les Républicains des lettres. Gens de culture et Lumières au XVIIIe siècle* (Paris, 1988), 214–15.

2. Ibid., 327.

3. Carolyn Merchant, *The Death of Nature: Women, Ecology, and the Scientific Revolution* (New York, 1980), 188.

4. Ibid., 164.

5. Londa Schiebinger, *The Mind Has No Sex? Women in the Origins of Modern Science* (Cambridge, Mass., 1989), 228.

6. Thomas Hankins, *Science and the Enlightenment* (Cambridge, 1985), 161.

7. Haydn Mason, *French Writers and their Society* (London, 1982), 194.

8. Diderot, "Encyclopedia," in *Rameau's Nephew and Other Works*, trans. Jacques Barzun and Ralph Bowen (Indianapolis, 1982), 304.

9. Voltaire's influence on the development of science was mixed. He frequently attacked new scientific ideas, including Needham's eels, spontaneous generation, the notion of preestablished harmony, and organic molecules. That he was himself subject to attack for some of his positions can be seen in Bachaumont's *Mémoires*

secrets's review of *De la singularité de la nature* (4 February 1769), 220–21. The review referred to Voltaire as a poet turned philosopher, physician, and metaphysician who, while combatting a number of errors, had introduced others. On 14 July 1769 (301–2), the journal chastised him for being a hypochondriac and *femmelette* in matters of illness and health. For more on Voltaire and science, see Margaret Libby, *The Attitude of Voltaire to Magic and the Sciences* (New York, 1935), Emile Saigey, *Les Sciences au XVIIIᵉ siècle. La Physique de Voltaire* (Paris, 1873), and Colm Kiernan, *The Enlightenment and Science in Eighteenth-Century France*, vol. 59A in *Studies on Voltaire and the Eighteenth Century*, ed. T. Besterman (Oxfordshire, 1973), 49–53. On Voltaire and medicine, see Renée Waldinger, "Voltaire and Medicine," *Studies on Voltaire and the Eighteenth Century*, ed. T. Besterman (Genève, 1967), 58: 1777–1806, and R. Galliani, "Voltaire, Astruc et la maladie vénérienne," *Studies on Voltaire and the Eighteenth Century*, ed. Haydn Mason (Oxford, 1983), 219:19–36.

10. Sander Gilman, *Difference and Pathology: Stereotypes of Sexuality, Race and Madness* (Ithaca, N.Y., 1985), 24.

11. In "Empirics and Charlatans in Early Modern France: The Genesis of the Classification of the 'Other' in Medical Practice," *Journal of Social History* 19 (summer 1986): 588, Alison Lingo traces the etymology of the word *charlatan*. Possible derivations include the Turkish, "who has some one speak, promulgate loudly"; and the Italian, "to chatter." In sixteenth-century France, the word was applied to "those who acted in the open air"—great talkers and storytellers who "captured the hearts, bodies, and money of their audience." Kathleen Wellmann, "Medicine as a Key to Defining Enlightenment Issues: The Case of Julien Offray de la Mettrie," in *Studies in Eighteenth-Century Culture*, ed. John Yolton and Leslie Brown (East Lansing, 1987), 17:81–82, documents how the philosophes used the term *charlatan* against their critics. La Mettrie's satire on the Faculty of Medicine, originally published in 1747 under the title, *La Faculté vengée*, was republished in 1762 under the title, *Les Charlatans démasqués*. In this text, however, the definition of charlatanry differed from that described by Lingo: the charlatanry of doctors lay not in their theatrical impulses, but in their "venality, arrogance, and ignorance."

12. Discrediting a movement by focusing on its appeal to women was a tactic that did not end in the eighteenth century. See, for example, Adrian Desmond's account of the way in which social conservatives sought to discredit Lamarckian ideas in the nineteenth century by arguing that they threatened to undermine the patriarchal family. "Women," he argues, "were acknowledged to have played a crucial role in the Owenite program and to have retained an active presence in the Halls of Science. So it is not surprising that the anonymous *Vestiges* should have been so denigrated by Adam Sedgwick and David Brewster for appealing to women. The serpent was tempting Eve, and through her poisoning the family and respectable society." (Adrian Desmond, "Artisans and Evolution in Britain, 1819–1848," *Osiris*, 2d ser., 3 (1987): 109.)

13. Joan Landes, *Women and the Public Sphere in the Age of the French Revolution* (Ithaca, 1988), 111.

14. John Lesch, *Science and Medicine in France. The Emergence of Experimental Physiology, 1790–1855* (Cambridge, Mass., 1984), 32.

15. Ian Maclean, *The Renaissance Notion of Woman. A Study in the Fortunes of Scholasticism and Medical Science in European Intellectual Life* (Cambridge, 1980), 25, 44, 60, 82–83, 92. In "Royal Bees: The Gender Politics of the Beehive in Early Modern Europe," in *Studies in Eighteenth-Century Culture*, ed. John Yolton and Leslie Brown (East Lansing, 1988), 18:10, Jeffrey Merrick explores the scientific distortions that resulted when classical, medieval, and early modern authors "compared the hive to the microcosmic kingdom of the household and the macrocosmic household of the kingdom." Because women were held to be subordinate by nature to men, it took a very long time for the notion of a queen bee to gain acceptance. "Microscopic discoveries about bees, which necessitated some rethinking of conventional truisms about nature, encountered outright resistance and caused considerable confusion for decades." The fact that the queen bee was also demonstrated to be sexually promiscuous further undermined efforts to prescribe rules of human behavior on the basis of microcosm/macrocosm analogies.

16. For more information on changes in women's position following the Revolution, see Margaret Darrow, "French Noblewomen and the New Domesticity, 1750–1850," *Feminist Studies* 5, no. 1 (1979): 41–65.

17. See, for example, Carol MacCormack and Marilyn Strathern, eds., *Nature, Culture and Gender* (Cambridge, 1980); Marian Lowe and Ruth Hubbard, eds., *Woman's Nature. Rationalizations of Inequality* (New York, 1983); and Ruth Bleier, *Science and Gender: A Critique of Biology and Its Theories on Women* (New York, 1984). On p. viii, Bleier argues that "biological determinist ideas emerge as dominant explanations for economic, social, and political inequality during periods of unrest and struggles for autonomy."

18. On social Darwinism, see Cynthia Russett, *Sexual Science: The Victorian Construction of Womanhood* (Cambridge, Mass., 1989). On sociobiology, see Barry Schwartz, *The Battle for Human Nature, Science, Morality and Modern Life* (New York, 1986).

19. For analysis of the variety of approaches one might take toward the topic of women and science/medicine, see Cécile Dauphin et al., "Culture et pouvoir: Essai d'historiographie," *Annales. Economies, Sociétés, Civilisations* 41, no. 2 (1986): 271–93. Also see Londa Schiebinger, "The History and Philosophy of Women in Science: A Review Essay," *Signs* 12, no. 2 (1987): 305–32 and Elizabeth Fox-Genovese, "Culture and Consciousness in the Intellectual History of European Women," *Signs* 12, no. 3 (1987): 529–47.

20. The challenges of sorting out such matters of truth versus falsehood are explored in Natalie Davis, *The Return of Martin Guerre* (Cambridge, Mass., 1983) and in Robert Finlay, "The Refashioning of Martin Guerre," *American Historical Review* 93, no. 3 (1988): 553–71.

21. See, for example, Roy Porter and Dorothy Porter, *In Sickness and Health: The British Experience 1650–1850* (London, 1988); Elborg Forster, "From the Patient's Point of View: Illness and Health in the Letters of Liselotte von der Pfalz (1652–1722)," *Bulletin of the History of Medicine* 60 (1986): 297–320, and Peter Gay, *The Bourgeois Experience, Victoria to Freud.* Vol. 1, *Education of the Senses* (Oxford, 1984), 149.

22. Matthew Ramsey, *Professional and Popular Medicine in France, 1770–*

1830. The Social World of Medical Practice (Cambridge, 1988), 222, suggests looking more closely at women's diverse roles as medical practitioners. For examples of recent work in this area, see Roy Porter, "Female Quacks in the Consumer Society," *The Clark Newsletter* (spring 1989), 1–4; Colin Jones, *The Charitable Imperative. Hospitals and Nursing in Ancien Régime and Revolutionary France* (London, 1989); and Nina Gelbart, "Mme du Coudray's Manual for Midwives; The Politics of Enlightenment Obstetrics," *Proceedings of the Annual Meeting of the Western Society for French History* (Auburn, Ala., 1989), 16:389–96.

SELECT BIBLIOGRAPHY

Primary Sources

MANUSCRIPTS

Académie Nationale de Médecine (Paris)
  Manuscripts 2–16, 33–35, 74, 82, 119
  Cartons (Société Royale de Médecine) 12, 13, 85–90, 99, 102–5, 108–20, 122–25, 127–40, 142, 143, 145, 146, 148, 152–54, 160, 163, 166, 167, 169, 170, 172–200
Archives Départementales de l'Aube (Troyes)
  1B 287, 1B 353A
  C1165–1168
  M1597–1600
Archives Départementales, Rennes
  1Bn2218; 1Bn2222; 1Bn2272; 1Bn2277bis
Archives Nationales (Paris)
  AB XIX 189; AB XIX 441–42; AD VIII 9B, 10, 26, 30, 33, 41, 42; AD XI 21; AD XVIII C296, C384; AD+940–42
  D VI 56; D XXXVIII 3, dossier 47
  F^{15} 441, 1861, 2811, 3963
  F^{16} 936
  F^{17} 1002, 1005A, 1005B, 1006, 1011, 1144–48, 1194 no. 109, 1245–59, 1309–10, 1318, 1319, 1326, 1344–45, 1356, 1359, 2107
  H^{3} 2554, 2586
  M70, 823–24, 848–54
  $X2^{B}$ 1320–29; $X3^{B}$ 2270
  Y 9510, 9511, 10555, 10637–44
Bibliothèque de l'Arsenal (Paris)
  Manuscripts 871, 969, 2509, 2515, 2519, 2542, 2778, 2815–17, 2820, 2892, 5306, 5806, 6772
  Archives/Bastille 10.269
Bibliothèque des Arts et Traditions Populaires (Paris)
  Manuscripts 49.65//B70; 67.31//B175; 74.115//B255
Bibliothèque de la Faculté de Médecine (Paris)
  Manuscripts 80 (2069), 154 (5033), 178 (5045), 242 (5116), 343–44 (5142–43), 505–7 (2229–31), 517 (5352), 571 (25), 578 (2006), 658 (5273), 717–19 (2275–77), 723 (2278), 767 (5389)
Bibliothèque Municipale de Chartres
  Letters written by Marie Plisson from 1751–53, NA m.s. 225
Bibliothèque Municipale de Troyes
  Cabinet Carteron 823, 2664, 2675

Bibliothèque Nationale (Paris)
  Manuscripts 24252–53; N.A. fr. 16833; N.A. fr. 17371
  Fonds Joly de Fleury 229, fol. 345; 444, fol. 173; 1689–90; 2415–16; 2425; 2530; 2541–43
Bibliothèque Sainte-Geneviève (Paris)
  Manuscripts 1944, 2275, 3114
Newberry Library (Chicago)
  Recueil de discours de différens Convulsionnaires, 1732–33

PERIODICALS

Medical

Gazette d'Epidaure
Gazette salutaire. Composée de tout ce que contiennent d'intéressant pour l'humanité; les livres nouveaux, les journaux et autres écrits publics, concernant la médecine
Journal de médecine, chirurgie, pharmacie, etc.
Journal du magnétisme

Learned

Annales politiques, civiles, et littéraires du XVIIIe siècle
L'Année littéraire
L'Avantcoureur
Le Censeur universel anglois, ou revue générale, critique et impartiale de toutes les productions angloises sur les sciences, la littérature, les beaux-arts, les manufactures, le commerce, etc.
Correspondance littéraire, philosophique et critique, par Grimm, Diderot, Raynal, Meister, etc. Ed. Maurice Tourneux. 16 vols. Paris, 1877–82.
Correspondance secrète, politique, et littéraire. Ed. François Métra. 16 vols. London, 1787–90.
Journal des dames
Journal des mères de famille
Journal des sçavans, avec extraits des meilleurs journaux de France et d'Angleterre
Journal encyclopédique à Bouillon
Journal politique, ou Gazette des gazettes
Mémoires pour l'histoire des sciences et beaux-arts. Commencés d'êtres imprimés l'an 1701 à Trévoux
Mémoires secrets pour servir à l'histoire de la République des Lettres en France, depuis MDCCLXII jusqu'à nos jours. Ed. Louis Petit de Bachaumont. 36 vols. London, 1777–89.
Le Nécrologe des hommes célèbres de France, par une société de gens de lettres.
Notice de l'Almanach sous-verre . . . contenant les découvertes, inventions, ou expériences nouvellement faites dans les sciences, les arts, les métiers, l'industrie

Provincial

Affiches du Beauvaisis
Recueil des annonces, affiches et avis divers pour la ville de Bordeaux

Journal de Champagne, Reims
Affiches, annonces et avis divers du Dauphiné
Annonces et affiches. Dijon
    Affiches, annonces et avis divers de Bourgogne, Bresse, Bugey et Pays de Gex
    Affiches, annonces et avis divers de Dijon ou Journal de la Bourgogne
Journal de Lyon, ou annonces et variétés littéraires, pour servir de suite aux
    petites affiches de Lyon
Affiches du Maine
Annonces, affiches, avis divers et nouvelles maritimes pour la ville de Marseille
Journal de Lorraine et Barrois (Nancy)
    Journal de Nancy
    Journal littéraire de Nancy
Annonces, affiches, nouvelles et avis divers de l'Orléanois, contenant généralement
    ce qui peut intéresser cette province
Affiches du Poitou
Affiches, annonces, etc. de Toulouse, et du Haut-Languedoc
Affiches, annonces, et avis divers pour les Trois-Evêchés et la Lorraine
Almanach de la ville et du diocèse de Troyes, capitale de la Champagne pour
    l'année bissextile
Annonces, affiches et avis divers de la ville de Troyes, capitale de la Champagne,
    contenant tout ce qui peut l'intéresser
    Journal de la ville de Troyes et de la Champagne méridionale
    Journal d'indications et annonces du Département de l'Aube

OTHER PRINTED WORKS

Les Admirables Secrets d'Albert le Grand. Contenant plusieurs traitez sur la con-
    ception des femmes, des vertus des herbes, des pierres prétieuses, et des
    animaux. N.p., 1729, 1752, 1791, 1818.
Astruc, Jean. *Doutes sur l'inoculation de la petite vérole.* Paris, 1756.
————. *Traité des maladies des femmes, où l'on a tâché de joindre à une théorie*
    solide la pratique la plus sûre et la mieux éprouvée. 6 vols. Paris, 1761–65
Bablot, Benjamin. *Dissertation sur le pouvoir de l'imagination des femmes*
    enceintes, dans laquelle on passe successivement en revue tous les grands
    hommes qui, depuis plus de deux mille ans, ont admis l'influence de cette
    faculté sur le foetus, et dans laquelle on répond aux objections de ceux qui
    combattent cette opinion. Paris, 1788.
Bailly, Jean Sylvain, ed. "Exposé des expériences qui ont été faites pour l'examen
    du magnétisme animal. Lu à l'Académie des Sciences par M. Bailly en son
    nom et au nom de MM. Franklin, Le Roy, de Bory et Lavoisier, le 4
    septembre 1784, imprimé par ordre du Roi." *Recueil général et complet de*
    tous les Ecrits publiés pour et contre le magnétisme animal. 14 vols. 5, no.
    55. Paris, 1784–87.
————. "Rapport des commissaires chargés par le Roi de l'examen du magnétisme
    animal, rédigé par J. S. Bailly, imprimé par ordre du Roi." *Recueil,* 5, no.
    52. 1784.
———— "Rapport secret sur le mesmerisme, ou magnétisme animal." 1784. In

Alexandre Bertrand, *Du Magnétisme animal en France et des jugements qu'en ont portés les sociétés savantes, avec le texte des divers rapports faits en 1784 par les commissaires de l'Académie des Sciences, de la Faculté et de la Société Royale de Médecine.* Paris, 1826.

Barbeu du Bourg, Jacques. *Elémens de médecine, en forme d'aphorismes.* Paris, 1780.

——. *Opinion d'un médecin de la Faculté de Paris sur l'inoculation de la petite vérole.* Paris, 1768.

——. *Petit code de la raison humaine: ou, Exposition succincte de ce que la raison dicte à tous les hommes, pour éclairer leur conduite, et assurer leur bonheur.* Paris, 1789.

——. *Recherches sur la durée de la grossesse, et le terme de l'accouchement.* Amsterdam, 1765.

Barbier, Edmond Jean François. *Journal historique et anecdotique du regne de Louis XV.* 4 vols. Paris, 1846–56.

Bellet, Isaac. *Lettres sur le pouvoir de l'imagination des femmes enceintes.* Paris, 1745.

Bergasse, Nicholas. "Considérations sur le magnétisme animal, ou sur la théorie du monde et des êtres organisés, d'après les principes de M. Mesmer." *Recueil,* 7, no. 95. 1784.

——. "Lettre d'un médicin de la Faculté de Paris, à un médecin du Collège de Londres, ouvrage dans lequel on prouve contre M. Mesmer, que le magnétisme animal n'existe pas." *Recueil,* 2, no. 8. 1781.

Besoigne, Jérôme. *Réfutation d'un second écrit contre la Consultation; intitulé: Exposition du sentiment de plusieurs théologiens défenseurs légitimes de l'oeuvre des convulsions et des miracles.* Paris, 1735.

Blondel, Jacques-Auguste. *Dissertation physique sur la force de l'imagination des femmes enceintes sur le foetus.* Translated by A. Lebrun. Leyde, 1737.

Bonnefoy, Jean. "Analyse raisonnée des rapports des commissaires chargés par le roi de l'examen du magnétisme animal." *Recueil,* 6, no. 76. 1784.

——. "Examen du Compte rendu par M. Thouret, sous le titre de Correspondance de la Société royale de médecine relativement au magnétisme animal." N.p., 1785.

Bougeant, Guillaume-Hyacinthe. *La Femme docteur, ou la théologie tombée en quenouille. Comédie.* Liège, 1731.

——. *La Femme docteur vangée, ou le théologien logé à Bicêtre.* Liège, 1732.

Bouvart, Michel. *Consultation contre la légitimité des naissances prétendues tardives.* Paris, 1764

——. *Consultation sur une naissance tardive, pour servir de réponse 1) à deux écrits de M. Le Bas, Chirurgien de Paris; l'un intitulé: "Question importante," l'autre: "Nouvelles observations;" 2) à une consultation de M. Bertin; 3) à une autre de M. Petit, tous les deux de l'Académie Royale des Sciences, et Docteurs-Régents de la Faculté de Médecine de Paris.* Paris, 1765.

——. *Lettres pour servir de réponses à un écrit qui porte pour titre: "Lettre à M. Bouvart," par A. Petit.* Amsterdam, 1769.

Chastenay-Lanty, Victorine de. *Mémoires de Mme de Chastenay, 1771–1815.* Edited by Alphonse Roserot. 2d. ed. Paris, 1896.

Condorcet, Marie-Jean-Antoine-Nicolas Caritat, Marquis de. *Oeuvres de Condorcet.* Edited by A. Condorcet O'Connor and M. F. Arago. 12 vols. Paris, 1847–49.

"Confession d'un médecin, académicien, et commissaire d'un rapport sur le magnétisme animal, avec les remonstrances et avis de son Directeur." *Recueil,* 10, no. 122. 1785.

Consultation sur les convulsions. Paris, 1735.

Corron, Mme (pseudonym of Pajon de Moncets, Pierre Abraham). *Dissertation en forme de lettre sur la cause qui détermine à neuf moi l'accouchement.* Paris, 1757.

d'Alembert, Jean le Rond. "Essai sur la société des gens de lettres et des grands." In *Oeuvres philosophiques, historiques ou littéraires de d'Alembert.* Edited by J. F. Bastien. Vol. 3. Paris, 1805.

d'Artois, Comte. "Lettre à M. Deslon." *Recueil,* 5, no. 65. 1784.

Demangeon, Jean. *Considérations physiologiques sur le pouvoir de l'imagination maternelle durant la grossesse.* Paris, 1807.

Denisart, Jean Baptiste, ed. *Collection de décisions nouvelles et de notions relatives à la jurisprudence actuelle.* 12 vols. Paris, 1771–1806.

d'Epinay, Louise F. P. Tardieu d'Esclavelles. *Les Conversations d'Emilie.* Leipzig, 1774.

Descartes, René. *Discourse on the Method of Rightly Conducting the Reason and Seeking for Truth in the Sciences.* Vol. 31 of *Great Books of the Western World.* Edited by Robert Hutchins. Chicago, 1952.

Desessarts, Nicolas Toussaint Lemoyne, ed. *Causes célèbres, curieuses et intéressantes, de toutes les cours souveraines du royaume avec les jugemens qui les ont décidées.* 165 vols. Paris, 1775–87.

Deslon, Charles. "Lettre à M. Philip, ancien doyen de la Faculté de Médecine de Paris." *Recueil,* 2, no. 12. 1782.

———. "Observations sur le magnétisme animal." *Recueil,* 1, no. 3. 1780.

———. "Observations sur les deux Rapports de MM. les commissaires nommés par sa majesté, pour l'examen du magnétisme animal." *Recueil,* 5, no. 64. 1784.

d'Espinassy, Mlle. *Essai sur l'éducation des demoiselles.* Paris, 1764.

Devillers, Charles. "Le Colosse aux pieds d'argile." *Recueil,* 8, no. 108. 1784.

Diderot, Denis. *Entretien entre d'Alembert et Diderot. Le Rêve de d'Alembert; Suite de l'entretien.* Edited by Jacques Roger. Paris, 1965.

Diderot, Denis, and Jean le Rond d'Alembert, eds. *Encyclopédie, ou Dictionnaire raisonné des sciences, des arts et des métiers, par une société des gens de lettres.* Neufchastel, 1765–81.

Dinouart, Joseph. *Abrégé de l'embryologie sacrée, ou Traité des devoirs des prêtres, des médecins, des chirugiens et des sages-femmes envers les enfans qui sont dans le sein de leurs mères.* Paris, 1775.

"Les Docteurs modernes, comédie-parade, en vaudevilles." *Recueil,* 6, no. 87. 1784.

d'Onglée, Thomas. "Rapport au public de quelques abus auxquels le magnétisme animal a donné lieu." *Recueil,* 10, no. 115. 1785.

Doppet, François. "Traité théorique et pratique du magnétisme animal." *Recueil,* 7, no. 98. 1784.

Duplessy, Mme la Baronne. *Répertoire des lectures faites au musée des dames.* Paris, 1788.

Du Rousseau de la Combe, Guy. *Recueil de jurisprudence civile du païs de droit écrit et coutumier, par order alphabétique.* 3d ed. Paris, 1753.

Eclaircissemens sur les miracles opérez par l'intercession de M. Pâris. Paris, 1733.

Entretiens sur les miracles des derniers temps, ou les Lettres de M. le Chevalier——. N.p., 1732.

"Examen sérieux et impartial du magnétisme animal." *Recueil,* 4, no. 44. 1784.

Exposition du sentiment de plusieurs théologiens défenseurs légitimes de l'oeuvre des convulsions et des miracles au sujet de la consultation des docteurs du 7 janvier 1735. N.p., 1735.

"Extrait des Registres de la Faculté de Médecine de Paris, 1 décembre." *Recueil,* 7, no. 103. 1784.

"Extrait du *Journal de Médecine,* Cahier de mars, v. 63, p. 334." *Recueil,* 5, no. 68. 1785.

"Extrait du *Journal de Médecine,* sept.-oct., v. 54, p. 289." *Recueil,* 1, no. 4. 1780.

Une Femme d'affaires au XVIIIᵉ siècle: La Correspondance de Mme de Maraise, collaboratrice d'Oberkampf. Edited by Serge Chassagne. Toulouse, 1981.

Ferrière, Claude-Joseph. *Dictionnaire de droit et de pratique, contenant l'explication des termes de droit, d'ordonnances, de coutumes et de pratique. Avec les jurisdictions de France.* New ed. 2 vols. Paris. 1771.

Fodéré, François Emmanuel. *Traité de médecine légale et d'hygiène publique, ou de police de santé, adapté aux codes de l'empire français et aux connaissances actuelles.* 6 vols. Paris, 1813.

Fournel, Jean. "Remonstrances des malades aux médecins de la Faculté de Paris." *Recueil,* X: 123.

Gauthier, Mme de. *Lettres contenant plusieurs anecdotes dans son voyage aux eaux de Barège, et quelques particularités échappées aux autres voyageurs en France.* Brussels, 1787.

Genlis, Stéphanie-Félicité du Crest de St. Aubin, Comtesse de. "Souvenirs de Félicie." Vol. 14 of *Bibliothèque des mémoires relatifs à l'histoire de France pendant le XVIIIᵉ et le XIXᵉ siècle.* Edited by Jean Barrière. Paris, 1857.

Gouriet, Jean-Baptiste. *Les Charlatans célèbres: ou, Tableau historique des bateleurs, des jongleurs, des bouffons, des opérateurs, des voltigeurs, des escamoteurs, des filous, des escrocs, des dévins, des tireurs de cartes, des diseurs de bonne aventure, et géneralement de tous les personnages qui se sont rendus célèbres dans les rues et sur les places publiques de Paris, depuis une haute antiquité jusqu'à nos jours.* Vol. 1. Paris, 1819.

Hecquet, Philippe. *De l'indécence aux hommes d'accoucher les femmes, et de l'obligation de celles-ci de nourrir leurs enfants.* Trévoux, 1708.

———. *Divers ouvrages sur la petite vérole.* Paris, 1722.

———. *La Médecine, la chirurgie et la pharmacie des pauvres.* 3 vols. Paris, 1740.

———. *La Médecine théologique, ou La Médecine créée, telle qu'elle fait voir ici, sortie des mains de Dieu, créateur de la nature, etc., et régie par ses loix.* 2 vols. Paris, 1733.

———. *Le Naturalisme des convulsions dans les maladies de l'épidémie convulsionnaire.* Soleure, 1733.

———. *Le Naturalisme des convulsions démontré par la physique, par l'histoire naturelle, et par les événemens de cette oeuvre, et démontrant l'impossibilité du divin qu'on lui attribue dans une lettre sur les secours meurtriers.* 2d part. Soleure. 1733.

———. *Raisons de doute contre l'inoculation de la petite vérole.* Paris, 1724.

———. *Réponse à la "Lettre à un confesseur touchant le devoir des médecins et des chirurgiens, au sujet des miracles et des convulsions."* Paris, 1733.

Hippocrates. *"Diseases of Women, 1."* Translated by Ann Ellis Hanson. *Signs,* 1, no. 2 (1975): 567–84.

Houard, David. *Dictionnaire analytique, historique, étymologique, critique et interprétatif de la Coutume de Normandie.* 4 vols. Rouen, 1780–82.

Une Jeune Fille au XVIIIe siècle: Lettres de Geneviève de Malboissière à Adélaïde Méliand 1761–1766. Edited by Albert, Comte de Luppé. Paris, 1925.

Jussieu, Antoine de. "Rapport de l'un des commissaires chargés par le roi de l'examen du magnétisme animal, Paris, 12 septembre 1784." *Recueil,* 5, no. 62.

La Tour du Pin-Gouvernet, Henriette Lucie (Dillon), Marquise de. *Journal d'une femme de cinquante ans, 1778–1815.* Paris, 1907.

Le Bas, Jean. *Lettre à M. Bouvart, Docteur en Médecine de la Faculté de Paris, au sujet de sa dernière "Consultation sur une naissance prétendue tardive pour servir de réponse. . ."* Amsterdam, 1765.

———. *Nouvelles observations sur les naissances tardives; suivies d'une consultation de célèbres médecins et chirurgiens de Paris.* Paris, 1765.

———. *Question importante. Peut-on déterminer un term préfix pour l'accouchement?* Paris, 1764.

Le Rebours, Marie-Angélique Anel. *Avis aux mères qui veulent nourrir leurs enfants.* Paris, 1775.

Le Ridant, Pierre. *Code matrimonial; ou Recueil des édits, ordonnances et déclarations sur le mariage. Avec un dictionnaire des décisions les plus importantes sur cette matière.* Paris, 1766.

Le Thieullier, Louis Jean. Doyen-Régent de la Faculté de Médecine de Paris. *Lettre à M.L.N.* N.p., 27 December 1735.

Lettre à un confesseur touchant le devoir des médecins et chirurgiens au sujet des miracles et des convulsions. N.p., 23 March 1733.

"Lettre de M. A.—— à M. B.——, sur le livre intitulé: 'Recherches et doutes sur le magnétisme animal de M. Thouret.' " *Recueil,* 4, no. 41. 22 August 1784.

"Lettre du chef du traitment de Versailles; à M. Gentil . . . sur les Rapports de l'Académie des Sciences et de la Société Royale, contre le magnétisme animal." *Recueil,* 5, no. 70. 1784.

Lettre d'un catholique français à un anglais sur les miracles de M. Pâris. N.p., 1733.

"Lettres sur le magnétisme animal; où l'on discute l'ouvrage de M. Thouret." *Recueil*, 5, no. 70. 1784.

Le Vasseur, maître chirurgien juré de S. Côme, and Clerambourg, apotiquaire. *Lettre*. N.p., 1735.

Lévis, Gaston, Duc de. *Souvenirs et portraits. Bibliothèque des mémoires relatifs à l'histoire de France pendant le XVIIIe et le XIXe siècle*. Edited by Jean Barrière. Paris, 1857.

Lignac, de. *De l'homme et de la femme, considérés physiquement dans l'état du mariage*. Lille, 1772.

Louis, Antoine. *Mémoire contre la légitimité des naissances prétendues tardives; dans lequel on concilie les loix civiles avec celles de l'oeconomie animale*. Paris, 1764.

————. *Supplément au mémoire contre la légitimité des naissances prétendues tardives*. Paris, 1764.

"Magnétisme animal dévoilé par un zélé citoyen françois." *Recueil*, 8, no. 107. 1784.

Mahon, Paul. *Médecine légale*. 3 vols. Rouen, 1801.

Médel, Angélique-Séraphine de. "Correspondence de Mme de Médel, 1770–1789." Edited by Henri Carré, *Archives Historiques du Poitou* 47 (1931): 1–165.

Méjan, Maurice, ed. *Recueil des causes célèbres et des arrêts qui les ont décidées*. 18 vols. Paris, 1807–13.

"Mémoire pour servir à l'histoire de la jonglerie, dans lequel on démontre les phénomènes du mesmerisme." *Recueil*, 4, no. 46. 1784.

Mercier, Louis-Sebastien. *Tableau de Paris*. Edited by Gustave Desnoiresterres. Paris, 1853.

Mesmer, Franz Anton. "Copie de la Requête à nosseigneurs de Parlement en la Grande Chambre supplie humblement A. Mesmer." *Recueil*, 5, no. 59. 1784.

————. "Lettre aux Auteurs du *Journal de Paris*." *Journal de Paris*, 19 August 1784.

————. "Lettre aux Auteurs du *Journal de Paris*." *Recueil*, 2, no. 18. 17 February 1784.

————. *Le Magnétisme animal; oeuvres publiées par Robert Amadon*. Paris, 1791.

————. "Mémoire sur la découverte du magnétisme animal." *Recueil*, 1, no. 1. 1779.

————. "Précis historique des faits relatives au magnétisme jusqu'en avril 1781." *Recueil*, 2, no. 9. 1781.

Miremont, Anne d'Aubourg de la Bove, Comtesse de. *Traité de l'éducation des femmes, et cours complet d'instruction*. Paris, 1779–89.

Montesquieu, Charles-Louis de Secondat, Baron de la Brède et de. *Oeuvres complètes de Montesquieu*. Edited by André Masson. 3 vols. Paris, 1955.

Montgeron, Louis-Basile Carré de. *La Vérité des miracles opérés à l'intercession de M. de Pâris et autres appellans, démontrée contre M. l'archevêque de Sens*. Utrecht, 1737–41.

Montjoie, Christophe Félix Louis Ventre de la Touloubre Galart de. "Lettres aux Auteurs du *Journal de Paris*." *Recueil*, 2, no. 18. 13 February 1784, 4 March 1784, 16 February 1784.

Morand, Sauveur-François. *Opuscules de chirurgie*. 2 vols. in 1. Paris, 1768–72.

Mossaron, Marie. *Lettre à Monseigneur l'Archevêque de Paris, au sujet de ce qui est dit dans son Ordonnance du 8 novembre 1735, contre le miracle de sa guérison*. N.p., 1735.

Muyart de Vouglans, Pierre. *Les Lois criminelles de France dans leur ordre naturel*. Paris, 1781.

Necker, Suzanne. *Des Inhumations précipitées*. Paris, 1790.

———. *Hospice de charité*. Paris, 1780.

———. *Mélanges extraits des manuscrits de Mme Necker*. Edited by Jacques Necker. 3 vols. Paris, 1798.

———. *Réflexions sur le divorce*. Lausanne, 1974.

Nigon de Berty, Louis. *Requête du Promoteur Général de l'Archevêque de Paris*. Paris, 1735.

"Observations adressées à MM. les Commissaires . . . par un médecin de province." *Recueil*, 5, no. 73. 1784.

Paulet, Jean Jacques. "L'Antimagnétisme ou Origine, progrès, décadence, renouvellement et réfutation du magnétisme animal." *Recueil*, 4, no. 47. 1784.

———. *Mesmer justifié*. New ed. Constance, 1784.

Petit, Antoine. "Consultation en faveur de la légitimité des naissances tardives." *Recueil de pièces relatives à la question des naissances tardives*. 2 vols. in 1. Amsterdam, 1766.

———. "Lettre à M. Bouvart, pour servir de réponse à la critique qu'il a faite de la consultation précédente." *Recueil*. Amsterdam, 1766.

———. "Observations sur ce que M. Astruc a écrit contre les naissances tardives, dans le chapitre XI du cinquième tome de son 'Traité des maladies des femmes.'" *Recueil*. Amsterdam, 1766.

———. *Premier Rapport en faveur de l'inoculation. Lu dans l'Assemblée de la Faculté de Médecine de Paris, en 1764*. Paris, 1766.

Plisson, Marie Prudence. *Maximes morales d'un philosophe chrétien. Ouvrage qui peut servir de suite à la Collection des moralistes anciens*. Paris, 1783.

———. *Réflexions critiques sur les écrits qu'a produit la question de la légitimité des naissances tardives: suivies d'une dissertation sur les hommes marins*. Paris, 1765.

Poinsinet, Antoine. *Le Cercle, ou La Soirée à la mode; comédie épisodique en un acte et en prose*. Edited by Auguste Vitu. Paris, 1887.

Pothier, Robert Joseph. *Traité des successions*. Vol. 7 of *Oeuvres, contenant les traités du droit français*. Paris, 1825.

Prévost, Claude Joseph. *Principes de jurisprudence sur les visites et rapports judiciares des médecins, chirurgiens, apothicaires, et sages-femmes*. Paris, 1753.

Procès de femmes au temps des philosophes ou la violence masculine au XVIII
siècle. Edited by Isabelle Vissière. Paris, 1985.

Procès-verbaux de plusieurs médecins et chirurgiens, dressés par ordre de Sa
Majesté, au sujet de quelques personnes soi-disantes agitées de convulsions.
Paris, 1732.

"Rapport des commissaires de la Société Royale de Médecine nommés par le Roi
pour faire l'examen du magnétisme animal, imprimé par ordre du Roi, daté
du 16 août 1784, signé de Poissonier, Caille, Mauduyt, Andry." *Recueil,*
5, no. 56.

"Rapport du Rapport de MM. les Commissaires." *Recueil,* 5, no. 67. 1784.

Raulin, Joseph. *Traité des affections vaporeuses du sexe.* Paris, 1758.

———. *Traité des fleurs blanches.* 2 vols. Paris, 1766.

———. *Traité de maladies des femmes en couche.* Paris, 1771.

"Relation de la maladie et de la guérison miraculeuse de Mlle Louise Guélon de
Troyes." *Recueil,* 10, no. 121. 1785.

"Réflexions impartiales sur le magnétisme animal faites après le publication du
'Rapport des Commissaires.' " *Recueil,* 5, no. 71. 1784.

"Réflexions sur le magnétisme animal, d'après lesquelles on cherche à établir le
degré de croyance que peut mériter jusqu'ici le système de M. Mesmer."
Recueil, 4, no.42. 1784.

Réflexions sur l'ordonnance du Roy en date du 27 janvier 1732 qui ordonne que
la porte du petit cimetière de la paroisse de St. Médard sera et demeura
fermée, etc. Sur les procès-verbaux de plusieurs médecins et chirurgiens qui
sont le fondement de cette ordonnance. Et sur les événemens dont l'exercice
de l'ordonnance a été suivie. N.p., 1732.

"Réflexions sur le rapport des commissaires nommés pour examiner les principes
et les effets curatifs de la doctrine de M. Deslon, et apologie de la conduite
de ce médecin." *Recueil,* 5, no. 75. 1784.

Riballier et Cosson. *De l'éducation physique et morale des femmes, avec une*
notice alphabétique de celles qui se sont distinguées dans les différentes
carrières des sciences et des beaux-arts, ou par des talens et des actions
mémorables. Paris, 1779.

Roland, Manon Phlipon. *Oeuvres de J. M. Ph. Roland, femme de l'ex-ministre*
de l'intérieur. Edited by L. A. Champagneux. Vol. 1. Paris, *an* VIII.

Rousseau, Jean-Jacques. *Politics and the Arts: Letter to M. d'Alembert on the*
Theatre. Translated by Allan Bloom. Ithaca, N.Y., 1968.

Saucerotte, Louis-Sebastien. *Examen de plusieurs préjugés abusifs concernant les*
femmes enceintes, celles qui sont accouchées et les enfans en bas âge. Nancy,
1777.

Servan, Joseph. "Doutes d'un provincial, proposés à MM. les médecins-commissaires, chargés par le roi, de l'examen du magnétisme animal." *Recueil,* 6,
no. 80. 1784.

———. *Lettres adressées au rédacteur des affiches du Dauphiné sur une cure*
opérée par le magnétisme animal. N.p., 1785.

———. "Questions du jeune docteur Rhubarbini de Purgandis, adressées à MM.
les docteurs-régens de toutes les facultés de médecine de l'univers, au sujet
de M. Mesmer, et du magnétisme animal." *Recueil,* 7, no. 101, 1784.

Sousselier de la Tour. "L'Ami de la nature, ou matière de traiter les maladies par le prétendu magnétisme animal." *Recueil*, 7, no. 96. 1784.

Sue, Pierre. *Apperçu général, appuyé de quelques faits, sur l'origine et le sujet de la médecine légale. Lu à la cinquième séance publique de la Société de Médecine, du 22 pluviôse an VIII.* Paris, 1799–1800.

———. *Dictionnaire portatif de santé.* Paris, 1779.

———. *Essais historiques, littéraires et critiques, sur l'art des accouchemens.* 2 vols. Paris, 1799.

"Supplément aux deux Rapports de MM. les Commissaires de l'Académie et de la Faculté de Médecine de Paris et de la Société Royale de Médecine." *Recueil*, 5, no. 66. 1784.

Thiroux d'Arconville, Marie Geneviève. *Pensées et réflexions morales, sur divers sujets, par l'auteur du traité de l'amitié, et de celui des passions.* Paris, 1766.

Thouret, Michel. "Extrait de la correspondance de la Société Royale de Médecine relativement au magnétisme animal." *Recueil*, 10. 1785.

———. "Recherches et doutes sur le magnétisme animal." *Recueil*, 4, no. 37. 1784.

Valleton de Boissière. "Lettre à M. Thouret, pour servir de réfutation à l'Extrait de la correspondance de la Société Royale de Médecine relativement au magnétisme animal." *Recueil*, 10, no. 119. 1765.

Varlet, Dominique. *Ouvrages posthumes de Monseigneur l'Evêque de Babylone; où il est principalement traité des miracles contre M. l'Archevêque de Sens.* Cologne, 1743.

Verdier, Jean. *La Jurisprudence de la médecine en France.* 2 vols. Alençon, 1762–63.

Vicq d'Azyr, Félix, ed. *Encyclopédie méthodique, ou par ordre de matières; par une société de gens de lettres, de savants et d'artistes. Médecine.* 13 vols. Paris, 1787–1830.

Vigée Lebrun, Louise Elisabeth. *Souvenirs de Mme Vigée Lebrun.* 3 vols. Paris, 1835–37.

Voltaire, François-Marie Arouet de. *Oeuvres complètes.* Edited by Emile de la Bédouillière and Georges Avenel. 5 vols. Paris, 1867–81.

Secondary Sources

ARTICLES

Allemand-Gay, Marie-Thérèse. "Le Droit de la filiation légitime." *Dix-huitème siècle* 12 (1980): 251–69.

Baker, Keith. "Politics and Public Opinion." In *Press and Politics in Pre-Revolutionary France*, edited by Jack Censer and Jeremy Popkin, 204–46. Berkeley, 1987.

———. "Politique et opinion publique sous l'Ancien Régime." *Annales. Economies, Sociétés, Civilisations* 42, no. 1 (1987): 3–25.

Beck, Hamilton. "Of Two Minds about the Death Penalty: Hippel's Account of a Case of Infanticide." In *Studies in Eighteenth-Century Culture*, edited by John Yolton and Leslie Brown, 18: 123–40. East Lansing, Mich., 1988.

Begue, Pierrette. "Madame de Genlis. Une Éducatrice moderne du XVIIIe siècle." *Le Corps et la santé*. Actes du 110e Congrès national des sociétés savantes, Montpellier, 1985. 1: 119–25. Paris, 1985.

Behlmer, George. "Deadly Motherhood: Infanticide and Medical Opinion in Mid-Victorian England." *Journal of the History of Medicine and Allied Sciences* 34, no. 4 (1979): 403–27.

Blackman, Janet. "Popular Theories of Generation: The Evolution of Aristotle's Works. The Study of an Anachronism." In *Health Care and Popular Medicine in Nineteenth-Century England: Essays in the Social History of Medicine*, edited by John Woodward and David Richards, 56–88. New York, 1977.

Bonney, Richard. "Review Article: Absolutism: What's in a Name?" *French History* 1, no. 1 (1987): 93–117.

Burton, June. "Human Rights Issues Affecting Women in Napoleonic Legal Medicine Textbooks." *History of European Ideas* 8, nos. 4/5 (1987): 427–34.

Bynum, Caroline Walker. "Fasts, Feasts, and Flesh: The Religious Significance of Food to Medieval Women." *Representations* 11 (summer 1985): 1–25.

Cameron, Vivian. "Gender and Power: Images of Women in Late 18th-Century France." *History of European Ideas* 10, no. 3 (1989): 309–32.

Charuty, Giordana. "Le Mal d'amour." *Le Corps humain: Nature, culture, surnaturel*. Actes du 110e Congrès national des sociétés savantes, Montpellier, 1985. 85–87. Paris, 1985.

Coleman, William. "Health and Hygiene in the Encyclopedia: A Medical Doctrine for the Bourgeoisie." *Journal of the History of Medicine and Allied Sciences* 29 (1974): 399–421.

———. "The People's Health: Medical Themes in Eighteenth-Century French Popular Literature." *Bulletin of the History of Medicine* 51 (1977): 55–74.

Crawford, Patricia. "Attitudes to Menstruation in Seventeenth-Century England." *Past and Present* 91 (May 1981): 47–73.

Darrow, Margaret. "French Noblewomen and the New Domesticity, 1750–1850." *Feminist Studies* 5, no. 1 (1979): 41–65.

Dauphin, Cécile, et al. "Culture et pouvoir des femmes: Essai d'historiographie," *Annales. Economies, Sociétés, Civilisations* 41, no. 2 (1986): 271–93.

Davis, Natalie. "Ghosts, Kin, and Progeny: Some Features of Family Life in Early Modern France." *Daedalus* 106, no. 2 (1977): 87–114.

Dieckmann, Herbert. "The Concept of Knowledge in the *Encyclopédie*." In *Essays in Comparative Literature*, edited by H. Dieckmann, 73–107. St. Louis, 1961.

———. "Themes and Structure of the Enlightenment." In *Essays in Comparative Literature*, edited by H. Dieckmann. 41–72. St. Louis, 1961.

Duncan, Carol. "Happy Mothers and Other New Ideas in French Art." *Art Bulletin* 55 (December 1973): 570–83.

Fairchilds, Cissie. "Female Sexual Attitudes and the Rise of Illegitimacy: A Case Study." *Journal of Interdisciplinary History* 8, no. 4 (1978): 627–67.

Farge, Arlette. "Work-Related Diseases of Artisans in Eighteenth-Century France." In *Medicine and Society in France: Selections from the Annales. Economies, Sociétés, Civilisations*, edited by Robert Forster and Orest Ranum, 89–103. Baltimore, 1980.

Favier, René. "Les 'Affiches' et la diffusion de l'innovation en Dauphiné à la fin du XVIIIᵉ siècle (1774–1778)." *Annales du Midi* 97 (April–June 1985): 157–67.

Feyel, Gilles. "Médecins, empiriques et charlatans dans la presse provinciale à la fin du XVIIIᵉ siècle." *Le Corps et la santé*. Actes du 110ᵉ Congrès des sociétés savantes. Montpellier, 1985, 1: 79–100. Paris, 1985.

Fine, Agnès. "Savoirs sur le corps et procédés abortifs au XIXᵉ siècle." *Le Corps humain: Nature, culture, surnaturel*. 110ᵉ Congrès national des sociétés savantes. Montpellier, 1985, 81–84. (Paris, 1985).

Forster, Elborg. "From the Patient's Point of View": Illness and Health in the Letters of Liselotte von der Pfalz (1652–1722)." *Bulletin of the History of Medicine* 60 (1986): 297–320.

Foucault, Michel. "Les Déviations religieuses et le savoir médical." *Hérésies et sociétés dan l'Europe préindustrielle*, 19–29. Conférence, Royaumont, 1962. Paris, 1968.

Fox-Genovese, Elizabeth. "Culture and Consciousness in the Intellectual History of European Women." *Signs* 12, no. 3 (1987): 529–47.

Gabert-Boche, Eliane. "Les Miraculés du cimitière Saint-Médard à Paris (1727–1735)." In *Les Miracles miroirs de corps*, edited by Jacques Gélis et Odile Redon, 127–57. Paris, 1983.

Giesey, Ralph. "Rules of Inheritance and Strategies of Mobility in Prerevolutionary France." *American Historical Review* 82, no. 2 (1977): 271–89.

Goldstein, Jan. "'Moral Contagion': A Professional Ideology of Medicine and Psychiatry in Eighteenth- and Nineteenth-Century France." In *Professions and the French State, 1700–1900*, edited by Gerald Geison, 182–222. Philadelphia, 1984.

———. "The Hysteria Diagnosis and the Politics of Anticlericalism in Late Nineteenth-Century France." *Journal of Modern History* 54 (June 1982): 209–39.

Grassi, Marie-Claire. "La Naissance et la mort dans le discours intime." *Le Corps humain: Nature, culture, surnaturel*, 111–21. Actes du 110ᵉ Congrès national des sociétés savantes, Montpellier, 1985. Paris, 1985.

Guisan, A. "La Médecine judiciare au 18ᵉ siècle, d'après les procédures criminelles vaudoises." *Revue suisse de médecine, ou Schweitzerische Rundschau für Medizin*, no. 10 (February 1913): 421–32 and no. 16 (May 1913): 672–82.

Hanley, Sarah. "Engendering the State: Family Formation and State Building in Early Modern France." *French Historical Studies* 16, no. 1 (1989): 4–27.

———. "Family and State in Early Modern France: The Marriage Pact." In *Connecting Spheres: Women in the Western World, 1500 to the Present*, edited by Marilyn Boxer and Jean Quaetart, 53–63. Oxford, 1987.

Harris, Ruth. "Melodrama, Hysteria, and Feminine Crimes of Passion in the Fin-de-Siècle." *History Workshop* 25 (spring, 1988): 31–63.

Horowitz, Maryanne Cline. "Aristotle and Woman." *Journal of the History of Biology* 9, no. 2 (1976): 183–213.

Kaiser, Thomas. "This Strange Offspring of *Philosophie*: Recent Historiographical Problems in Relating the Enlightenment to the French Revolution." *French Historical Studies* 15, no. 3 (1988): 549–62.

Knibiehler, Yvonne. "Les Médecins et la 'nature féminine' au temps du Code Civil." *Annales. Economies, Sociétés, Civilisations* 31, no. 4 (1976): 824–45.

Lecuir, Jean. "La Médicalisation de la société française dans la deuxième moitié du XVIIIe siècle en France: Aux Origines des premiers traités de médecine légale." *Annales de Bretagne* 86, no. 2 (1979): 231–50.

Lingo, Alison. "Empirics and Charlatans in Early Modern France: The Genesis of the Classification of the 'Other' in Medical Practice." *Journal of Social History* 19 (summer, 1986): 583–604.

———. "Santé et beauté féminines dans la France de la Renaissance." *Le Corps humain: Nature, culture, surnaturel*, 191–99. Actes du 110e Congrès national des sociétés savantes. Montpellier, 1985. Paris, 1985.

Lottin, Alain. "Naissances illégitimes et filles mères à Lille au XVIIIe siècle." *Revue d'histoire moderne et contemporaine* 17 (April–June 1970): 278–322.

Lusebrink, Hans-Jurgen. "Les Crimes sexuels dans les *Causes célèbres*." *Dix-huitième siècle* 12 (1980): 153–62.

McLaren, Angus. "Abortion in France: Women and the Regulation of Family Size, 1800–1914." *French Historical Studies* 10, no. 3 (1978): 461–85.

———. "Some Secular Attitudes toward Sexual Behavior in France: 1760–1860." *French Historical Studies* 8, no. 4 (1974): 604–25.

Maza, Sarah. "Le Tribunal de la nation: Les Mémoires judiciaires et l'opinion publique à la fin de l'Ancien Régime." *Annales. Economies, Sociétés, Civilisations* 42, no. 1 (1987): 73–90.

Merrick, Jeffrey. "Royal Bees: The Gender Politics of the Beehive in Early Modern Europe." In *Studies in Eighteenth-Century Culture*, edited by John Yolton and Leslie Brown, 18: 7–37. East Lansing, Mich., 1988.

———. "Sexual Politics and Public Order in Late Eighteenth-Century France: The *Mémoires secrets* and the *Correspondance secrète*." *Journal of the History of Sexuality* 1, no. 1 (1990): 68–84.

Mitchell, Harvey. "Rationality and Control in French Eighteenth-Century Medical Views of the Peasantry." *Comparative Studies in Society and History* 21, no. 1 (1979): 82–112.

Morel, Marie-France. "Madame Roland, sa fille et les médecins: Prime éducation et médicalisation à l'époque des Lumières." *Annales de Bretagne* 86, no. 2 (1979): 211–19.

Mornet, Daniel. "L'Eveil de la curiosité intellectuelle dans les provinces françaises et ses conséquences (1770–1789)," *Revue de Paris* 4 (1932): 641–64.

———. "La Vie mondaine, Les salons." In *La Vie parisienne au XVIIIe siècle: Leçons faites à l'Ecole des hautes études sociales*, 121–44. Paris, 1914.

Morsink, Johannes. "Was Aristotle's Biology Sexist?" *Journal of the History of Biology* 12, no. 1 (1979): 83–112.

Murphy, Terence. "Medical Culture under the Old Regime." *Historical Reflec-*

tions/Réflexions Historiques 16, nos. 2–3 (1989): 307–50.

Nathans, Benjamin. "Habermas's 'Public Sphere' in the Era of the French Revolution." *French Historical Studies* 16, no. 3 (1990): 620–44.

Palmer, Sophie. "Formation et déformation du corps. Les Méfaits de l'extraordinaire au cours de la grossesse." *Le Corps humain: Nature, culture, surnaturel*, 67–80. Actes du 110ᵉ Congrès national des sociétés savantes, Montpellier, 1985. Paris, 1985.

Park, Katharine, and Lorraine Daston. "Unnatural Conceptions: The Study of Monsters in Sixteenth- and Seventeenth-Century France and England." *Past and Present* 92 (August 1981): 20–54.

Parssinen, Terry. "Professional Deviants and the History of Medicine: Medical Mesmerists in Victorian Britain." In *On the Margins of Science: The Social Construction of Rejected Knowledge*, edited by Ray Wallis, 103–20. Sociological Review Monograph 27. Keele, U.K., 1979.

Peter, Jean-Pierre. "Le Corps du délit." *Nouvelle revue de psychanalyse* 3 (1971): 99–108.

———. "Le Grand Rêve de l'ordre médical en 1770 et aujourd'hui." *Autrement* 4 (1975): 183–92.

———. "Les Mots et les objets de la maladie. Remarques sur les épidémies et la médecine dans la société française de la fin du 18ᵉ siècle." *Revue historique* 246, no. 2 (1971): 13–38.

Phan, Marie-Claude, and Jean-Louis Flandrin. "Les Métamorphoses de la beauté féminine." *L'Histoire* 68 (June 1984): 48–57.

Pie, Jean-Claude. "Anne Charlier, un miracle eucharistique dans le faubourg Saint-Antoine." In *Les Miracles miroirs des corps*, edited by Jacques Gélis and Odile Redon, 161–90. Paris, 1983.

Ramsey, Matthew. "Traditional Medicine and Medical Enlightenment: The Regulation of Secret Remedies in the Ancien Régime." *Historical Reflections/Réflexions Historiques* 9 (1982): 215–32.

Riet, Didier. "Les Déclarations de grossesse dans la region de Dinan à la fin de l'Ancien Régime." *Annales de Bretagne et des pays de l'Ouest* (Anjou, Maine, Touraine) 88 (1981): 181–87.

Rizzo, Tracey. "Sexual Violence in the Enlightenment: The State, the Bourgeoisie, and the Cult of the Victimized Woman." *Proceedings of the Western Society for French History* 15 (1988): 122–29.

Rossiaud, Jacques. Prostitution, jeunesse et société dans les villes du Sud-est au XVᵉ siècle. *Annales. Economies, Sociétés, Civilisations* 31, no. 2 (1976): 289–325.

Schiebinger, Londa. "The History and Philosophy of Women in Science: A Review Essay." *Signs* 12, no. 2 (1987): 305–32.

Scott, Joan. "Survey Articles, Women in History II: The Modern Period." *Past and Present* 101 (November 1983): 141–57.

Sgard, Jean. "La Littérature des causes célèbres." In *Approches des Lumières: Mélanges offerts à Jean Fabre*, 459–70. Paris, 1974.

Tanner, Tony. "Julie and 'La Maison Paternelle': Another Look at Rousseau's *La Nouvelle Héloise*." *Daedalus* 105, no. 1 (1976): 23–45.

Thackray, Arnold. "History of Science in the 1980s." In *The New History: The*

1980s and Beyond, edited by Theodore Rabb and Robert Rotberg, 299–314. Princeton, 1982.

Van den Daele, Wolfgang. "The Social Construction of Science: Institutionalization and Definition of Positive Science in the Latter Half of the Seventeenth Century." In *The Social Production of Scientific Knowledge. Sociology of the Sciences*, edited by Everett Mendelsohn, Peter Weingart, and Richard Whitley, 1: 27–54. Dordrecht, Holland, 1977.

Wellman, Kathleen. "Medicine as a Key to Defining Enlightenment Issues: The Case of Julien Offray de la Mettrie." In *Studies in Eighteenth-Century Culture*, edited by John Yolton and Leslie Brown, 17: 75–89. East Lansing, Mich., 1987.

BOOKS

Abbiateci, André, et al. *Crimes et criminalité en France sous l'Ancien Régime, 17ᵉ et 18ᵉ siècles*. Paris, 1971.

Abensour, Léon. *La Femme et le féminisme avant la Révolution*. Paris, 1923.

Adhémar, Jean. *La Gravure originale au XVIIIᵉ siècle*. Paris, 1963.

Alstad, Diane. "The Ideology of the Family in Eighteenth-Century France." Ph.D. dissertation, Yale University, 1971.

Ariès, Philippe. *Centuries of Childhood: A Social History of Family Life*. Translated by Robert Baldick. New York, 1962.

Ariès, Philippe, and Georges Duby, eds. *Histoire de la vie privée*. Vol. 3. *De la Renaissance aux Lumières*. Paris, 1986.

Arnold, Odile. *Le Corps et l'âme. La Vie des religieuses au XIXᵉ siècle*. Paris, 1984.

Aron, Jean-Paul, *Misérable et glorieuse. La Femme du XIXᵉ siècle*. Paris, 1980.

Aron, Jean-Paul, *Le Pénis et la démoralisation de l'Occident*. Paris, 1978.

Badinter, Elisabeth. *L'Amour en plus. Histoire de l'amour maternel, XVIIIᵉ–XIXᵉ siècles*. Paris, 1980.

Baker, Keith. *Condorcet. From Natural Philosophy to Social Mathematics*. Chicago, 1975.

Barrows, Susanna. *Distorting Mirrors: Visions of the Crowd in Late Nineteenth-Century France*. New Haven, 1981.

Behrens, C. B. A. *Society, Government, and the Enlightenment. The Experiences of Eighteenth-Century France and Prussia*. New York, 1985.

Bell, Rudolf. *Holy Anorexia*. Chicago, 1985.

Bellanger, Claude, et al. *Histoire générale de la presse française*. Vol. 1. *Des Origines à 1814*. Paris, 1969.

Ben-David, Joseph. *The Scientist's Role in Society: A Comparative Study*. Englewood Cliffs, N.J., 1971.

Bezard, Yvonne, *Une Famille bourguignonne au XVIIIᵉ siècle*. Paris, 1930.

Bien, David. *The Calas Affair: Persecution, Toleration, and Heresy in Eighteenth-Century Toulouse*. Princeton, 1960.

Binet, Léon, and Pierre Vallery-Radot. *Médecine et art de la Renaissance à nos jours*. Paris, 1968.

Bleier, Ruth. *Science and Gender: A Critique of Biology and Its Theories on Women.* New York, 1984.

Blumenfeld-Kosinski, Renate. *Not of Woman Born. Representations of Caesarean Birth in Medieval and Renaissance Culture.* Ithaca, 1990.

Bollème, Geneviève, et al., eds. *Livre et société dans la France du XVIIIe siècle,* Paris, 1965.

Brinton, Crane. *French Revolutionary Legislation on Illegitimacy, 1789–1804.* Cambridge, Mass., 1936.

Brockliss, L. W. B. *French Higher Education in the Seventeenth and Eighteenth Centuries.* Oxford, 1987.

Brumberg, Joan Jacobs. *Fasting Girls. The Emergence of Anorexia Nervosa as a Modern Disease.* Cambridge, Mass., 1988.

Bynum, Caroline Walker. *Holy Feast and Holy Fast: The Religious Significance of Food to Medieval Women.* Berkeley, 1987.

Carré, Henri. *La Noblesse de France et l'opinion publique au XVIIIe siècle.* Paris, 1920.

Censer, Jack, and Jeremy Popkin, eds. *Press and Politics in Pre-Revolutionary France.* Berkeley, 1987.

Crow, Thomas. *Painters and Public Life in Eighteenth-Century Paris.* New Haven, 1985.

Darmon, Pierre. *La Longe Traque de la variole: Les Pionniers de la médecine préventive.* Paris, 1986.

————. *Le Mythe de la procréation à l'âge baroque.* Paris, 1977.

————. *Mythologie de la femme dans l'ancienne France.* Paris, 1983.

————. *Le Tribunal de l'impuissance. Virilité et défaillances conjugales dans l'ancienne France.* Paris, 1979.

Darnton, Robert. *The Great Cat Massacre and Other Episodes in French Cultural History.* New York, 1984.

————. *Mesmerism and the End of the Enlightenment in France.* New York, 1968.

Darnton, Robert, and Daniel Roche, eds. *Revolution in Print: The Press in France 1775–1800.* Berkeley, 1989.

Darrow, Margaret. *Revolution in the House: Family, Class, and Inheritance in Southern France, 1775–1825.* Princeton, 1989.

Davis, Natalie. *Fiction in the Archives. Pardon Tales and their Tellers in Sixteenth-Century France.* Stanford, 1987.

————. *The Return of Martin Guerre.* Cambridge, Mass., 1983.

————. *Society and Culture in Early Modern France.* Stanford, 1975.

Decaux, Alain. *Histoire des Françaises.* Vol. 2. *La Révolte.* Paris, 1972.

Delaunay, Paul. *Le Monde médical parisien au dix-huitième siècle.* Paris, 1906.

Delumeau, Jean. *La Peur en Occident, XIVe–XVIIIe siècle: Une Cité assiégée.* Paris, 1978.

Dewald, Jonathan. *The Formation of a Provincial Nobility: The Magistrates of the Parlement of Rouen, 1499–1610.* Princeton, 1980.

Donzelot, Jacques. *The Policing of Families.* New York, 1979.

Doublet, Suzanne. "La Médecine dans les oeuvres de Diderot." Université de

Bordeaux, Faculté de Médecine, thèse 144, 1933–34.

Doyle, William. *The Parlement of Bordeaux and the End of the Old Regime 1771–1790*. New York, 1974.

Duhet, Paule-Marie. *Les Femmes et la Révolution, 1789–1794*. Paris, 1971.

Ehrard, Jean. *L'Idée de nature en France à l'aube des Lumières*. Paris, 1970.

Farge, Arlette. *La Vie fragile: Violence, pouvoirs et solidarités à Paris au XVIII siècle*. Paris, 1986.

———. *Vivre dans la rue à Paris au XVIIIe siècle*. Paris, 1979.

Flandrin, Jean. *L'Eglise et le contrôle des naissances*. Paris, 1970.

Foucault, Michel. *The Birth of the Clinic: An Archaeology of Medical Perception*. Translated by A. M. Sheridan Smith. New York, 1973.

———. *Histoire de la sexualité: La Volonté de savoir*. Paris, 1976.

———. *Madness and Civilization: A History of Insanity in the Age of Reason*. Translated by Richard Howard. New York, 1965.

Freidson, Eliot. *Professional Powers: A Study of the Institutionalization of Formal Knowledge*. Chicago, 1986.

Gallagher, Catherine, and Thomas Laqueur, eds. *The Making of the Modern Body: Sexuality and Society in the Nineteenth Century*. Berkeley, 1987.

Galland, Elie. *L'Affaire Sirven*. Paris, 1911.

Gallier, Anatole de. *La Vie de province au XVIIIe siècle. Les Femmes, les moeurs, les usages*. Paris, 1887.

Garden, Maurice. *Lyon et les Lyonnais au XVIIIe siècle*. Paris, 1970.

Gasking, Elizabeth B. *Investigations into Generation, 1651–1828*. Baltimore, 1967.

Gay, Peter. *The Enlightenment: An Interpretation*. Vol. II. *The Science of Freedom*. New York, 1977.

———. *Voltaire's Politics*. Princeton, 1959.

Gelbert, Nina. *Feminine and Opposition Journalism in Old Regime France*. Berkeley, 1987.

Gélis, Jacques. *L'Arbre et le Fruit, la naissance dans l'Occident moderne, XVIe–XIXe siècle*. Paris, 1984.

———. *La Sage-femme ou le médecin. Une Nouvelle conception de la vie*. Paris, 1988.

Gillispie, Charles. *Science and Polity in France at the End of the Old Regime*. Princeton, 1980.

Gilman, Sander. *Difference and Pathology: Stereotypes of Sexuality, Race and Madness*. Ithaca, 1985.

———. *Disease and Representation. Images of Illness from Madness to AIDS*. Ithaca, 1988.

Goldstein, Jan. *The French Psychiatric Profession in the Nineteenth Century*. Cambridge, 1987.

Goncourt, Edmond and Jules de. *La Femme au dix-huitième siècle*. Paris, 1982.

Goubert, Jean-Pierre. *Malades et médecins en Bretagne, 1770–1790*. Rennes, 1974.

Goubert, Pierre, and Daniel Roche. *Les Français et l'Ancien Régime*. Vol. 2. *Culture et société*. Paris, 1984.

Grimmer, Claude. *La Femme et le bâtard. Amours illégitimes et secrètes dans l'ancienne France.* Paris, 1983.

Hahn, Roger. *The Anatomy of a Scientific Institution: The Paris Academy of Sciences, 1666–1803.* Berkeley, 1971.

Hankins, Thomas. *Science and the Enlightenment.* Cambridge, 1985.

Hannaway, Caroline. "Medicine, Public Welfare and the State in Eighteenth-Century France: The Société Royale de Médecine of Paris (1776–1793)." Ph.D. dissertation, Johns Hopkins University, 1974.

Harris, Ruth. *Murder and Madness: Medicine, Law and Society in the Fin de Siècle.* Oxford, 1989.

Hatin, Eugène. *Bibliographie historique et critique de la presse périodique française.* Paris, 1866.

———. *Histoire de la presse en France.* Paris, 1859.

Hellerstein, Erna. "Women, Social Order, and the City: Rules for French Ladies, 1830–1870." Ph.D. dissertation, University of California, Berkeley, 1980.

Herzlich, Claudine, and Janine Pierret. *Illness and Self in Society.* Translated by Elborg Forster. Baltimore, 1987.

Hoffman, Paul. *La Femme dans la pensée des Lumières.* Paris, 1977.

Huard, Pierre. *Biographies médicales et scientifiques: XVIIIe siècle.* Paris, 1972.

Hufton, Olwen. *The Poor of Eighteenth-Century France, 1750–1820.* Oxford, 1974.

Imbert, Jean, ed. *Quelques procès criminels des 17e et 18e siècles.* Paris, 1964.

Imbert, Jean, et al. *Le Pouvoir, les juges et les bourreaux.* Paris, 1972.

Jones, Colin. *The Charitable Imperative. Hospitals and Nursing in Ancien Régime and Revolutionary France.* London, 1989.

Jordanova, Ludmilla. *Sexual Visions: Images of Gender in Science and Medicine between the Eighteenth and Twentieth Centuries.* New York, 1989.

Kafker, Serena, and Frank Kafker. *Encyclopedists as Individuals: A Biographical Dictionary of the Authors of the Encyclopédie.* Vol. 257 of *Studies on Voltaire and the Eighteenth Century*, edited by Haydn Mason. Oxford, 1988.

Kaplan, Steven and Cynthia Koepp, eds. *Work in France: Representations, Meanings, Organization, and Practice.* Ithaca, 1986.

Keohane, Nannerl. *Philosophy and the State in France. The Renaissance to the Enlightenment.* Princeton, 1980.

Kiernan, Colm. *The Enlightenment and Science in Eighteenth-Century France*, edited by T. Besterman, Vol. 59A of *Studies on Voltaire and the Eighteenth Century.* Oxfordshire, 1973.

King, Lester. *The Philosophy of Medicine: The Early Eighteenth Century.* Cambridge, Mass., 1978.

Knibiehler, Yvonne, and Catherine Fouquet. *La Femme et les médecins: Analyse historique.* Paris, 1983.

———. *Histoire des mères du Moyen Age à nos jours.* Paris, 1977.

Kreiser, Robert. *Miracles, Convulsions, and Ecclesiastical Politics in Early Eighteenth-Century Paris.* Princeton, 1978.

Laborde, Alice. *L'Oeuvre de Mme de Genlis.* Paris, 1966.

LaCapra, Dominick, and Steven Kaplan, eds. *Modern European Intellectual*

History: Reappraisals and New Perspectives. Ithaca, 1982.

Lacroix, Paul. *XVIIIe siècle. Lettres, sciences, arts. France 1700–1789.* Paris, 1878.

Landes, Joan. *Women and the Public Sphere in the Age of the French Revolution.* Ithaca, 1988.

Laqueur, Thomas. *Making Sex. Body and Gender from the Greeks to Freud.* Cambridge, Mass., 1990.

Lebrun, François. *Les Hommes et la mort en Anjou aux 17e et 18e siècles: Essai de démographie et psychologie historiques.* Paris, 1971.

———. *Médecine, saints et sorciers aux dix-septième et dix-huitième siècles.* Paris, 1983.

———. *La Vie conjugale sous l'Ancien Régime.* Paris, 1975.

Lehoux, Françoise. *Le Cadre de vie des médecins parisiens aux XVIe et XVIIe siècles.* Paris, 1976.

Léonard, Jacques. *Les Médecins de l'Ouest au XIXe siècle.* Paris, 1978.

Lesch, John. *Science and Medicine in France. The Emergence of Experimental Physiology, 1790–1855.* Cambridge, Mass., 1984.

Livi, Jocelyne. *Vapeurs de femmes: Essai historique sur quelques fantasmes médicaux et philosophiques.* Paris, 1984.

Lottin, Alain. *La Désunion du couple sous l'Ancien Régime. L'Exemple du Nord.* Paris, 1975.

Lougee, Carolyn. *Le Paradis des Femmes. Women, Salons, and Social Stratification in Seventeenth-Century France.* Princeton, 1976.

Lough, John. *Writer and Public in France from the Middle Ages to the Present Day.* Oxford, 1978.

Lowe, Marian, and Ruth Hubbard, eds. *Woman's Nature. Rationalizations of Inequality.* New York, 1983.

Luppé, Albert, Comte de. *Les Jeunes Filles à la fin du XVIIIe siècle.* Paris, 1925.

MacCormack, Carol, and Marilyn Strathern, eds. *Nature, Culture and Gender.* Cambridge, 1980.

Maccubbin, Robert, ed. *" 'Tis Nature's Fault": Unauthorized Sexuality during the Enlightenment.* Cambridge, 1987.

Maclean, Ian. *The Renaissance Notion of Woman. A Study in the Fortunes of Scholasticism and Medical Science in European Intellectual Life.* Cambridge, 1980.

McClellan, James. *Science Reorganized. Scientific Societies in the Eighteenth Century.* New York, 1985.

McManners, John. *Death and the Enlightenment. Changing Attitudes to Death among Christians and Unbelievers in Eighteenth-Century France.* Oxford, 1981.

Maire, Catherine-Laurence. *Les Convulsionnaires de Saint-Médard. Miracles, convulsions et prophéties à Paris au XVIIIe siècle.* Paris, 1983.

Marion, Marcel. *Dictionnaire des institutions de la France aux XVIIe et XVIIIe siècles.* Paris, 1923.

Mason, Haydn. *French Writers and Their Society.* London, 1982.

Maza, Sarah. *Servants and Masters in Eighteenth-Century France: The Uses of Loyalty.* Princeton, 1983.

Merchant, Carolyn. *The Death of Nature: Women, Ecology, and the Scientific Revolution.* New York, 1980.

Meyer, Jean. *La Noblesse bretonne au XVIIIe siècle.* 2 vols. Paris, 1966.

Mitterauer, Michel, and Reinhard Sieder. *The European Family: Patriarchy to Partnership from the Middle Ages to the Present.* Translated by Karla Oosterveen and Manfred Hörzinger. Chicago, 1982.

Mornet, Daniel. *Les Sciences de la nature en France, au XVIIIe siècle. Un Chapitre de l'histoire des idées.* Paris, 1911.

Mousnier, Roland. *The Institutions of France under the Absolute Monarchy, 1598–1789.* 2 vols. Chicago, 1979–84.

Muchembled, Robert. *Culture populaire et culture des élites dans la France moderne (XVe–XVIIIe siècles).* Paris, 1978.

———. *L'Invention de l'homme moderne: Sensibilités, moeurs et comportements collectifs sous l'Ancien Régime.* Paris, 1988.

Okin, Susan. *Women in Western Political Thought.* Princeton, 1979.

Oppenheim, Janet. *"Shattered Nerves". Doctors, Patients, and Depression in Victorian England.* Oxford, 1991.

Ornstein, Martha. *The Role of Scientific Societies in the Seventeenth Century.* Chicago, 1928.

Outram, Dorinda. *The Body and the French Revolution: Sex, Class and Political Culture.* New Haven, 1989.

Paul, Charles. *Science and Immortality: The Eloges of the Paris Academy of Sciences, 1699–1791.* Berkeley, 1980.

Pilon, Edmond, *La Vie de famille au dix-huitième siècle. Illustrations d'après des estampes du temps.* Paris, 1923.

Portalis, Roger, Baron, and Henri Béraldi. *Les Graveurs du dix-huitième siècle.* 3 vols. Paris, 1880–82.

Porter, Roy, and Dorothy Porter. *In Sickness and Health: The British Experience, 1650–1850.* London, 1988.

Rabaud, Camille. *Etude historique sur l'avènement de la tolérance.* Paris, 1891.

Ramsey, Matthew, *Professional and Popular Medicine in France, 1770–1830. The Social World of Medical Practice.* Cambridge, 1988.

Roche, Daniel. *Le Siècle des Lumières en province. Académies et académiciens provinciaux.* Paris, 1978.

———. *Les Républicains des lettres. Gens de culture et Lumières au XVIIIe siècle.* Paris, 1988.

Roger, Jacques. *Les Sciences de la vie dans la pensée française du XVIIIe siècle: La Génération des animaux de Descartes à l'Encyclopédie.* Paris, 1963.

Rousseau, G. S., and Roy Porter, eds. *Sexual Underworlds of the Enlightenment.* Chapel Hill, 1988.

Rousselot, Jean. *Medicine in Art: A Cultural History.* New York, 1967.

Russett, Cynthia. *Sexual Science: The Victorian Construction of Womanhood.* Cambridge, Mass., 1989.

Schiebinger, Londa. *The Mind Has No Sex? Women in the Origins of Modern Science.* Cambridge, Mass., 1989.

Sgard, Jean, ed. *La Presse provinciale au XVIIIe siècle.* Grenoble, 1983.

Shorter, Edward. *The Making of the Modern Family.* London, 1977.

Showalter, Elaine. *The Female Malady. Women, Madness, and English Culture, 1830–1880*. New York, 1985.

Smith, Wesley. *The Hippocratic Tradition*. Ithaca, 1979.

Smith-Rosenberg, Carroll. *Disorderly Conduct. Visions of Gender in Victorian America*. New York, 1985.

Sonnet, Martine. *L'Education des filles au temps des Lumières*. Paris, 1987.

Spencer, Samia, ed. *French Women and the Age of Enlightenment*. Bloomington, Ind., 1984.

Sussman, George. *Selling Mother's Milk: The Wet-Nursing Business in France, 1715–1914*. Urbana, 1982.

Tarczylo, Théodore. *Sexe et liberté au siècle des Lumières*. Paris, 1983.

Tarlé, Eugenii. *L'Industrie dans les campagnes en France à la fin de l'Ancien Régime*. Paris, 1910.

Taton, René, ed. *Enseignement et diffusion des sciences en France au XVIIIe siècle*. Paris, 1964.

Temkin, Owsei, and C. Lilian Temkin, eds. *Ancient Medicine: Selected Papers of Ludwig Edelstein. Baltimore*, 1967.

Tilly, Louise, and Joan Scott. *Women, Work, and Family*. New York, 1978.

Traer, James. *Marriage and the Family in Eighteenth-Century France*. Ithaca, 1980.

Vidal, Daniel. *Miracles et convulsions Jansénistes au XVIIIe siècle. Le mal et sa connaissance*. Paris, 1987.

Vincent-Buffault, Anne. *Histoire des larmes, XVIIIe–XIXe siècles*. Paris, 1986.

Wade, Ira. *The Philosophe in the French Drama of the Eighteenth Century*. Princeton, 1926.

INDEX

Abensour, Léon, 145, 179–80n.7
Abortion, 9, 11; charlatan practitioners of,
   118–19; fetal gender and, 184–85n.46;
   French legal prohibition of, 191n.58;
   maternal mortality from, 186n.70
Académie des Belles-Lettres, 91
Académie Française, 90, 91
Académie Nationale de Médecine, 117
"Accouchement" (Houard), 69
Accoucheurs, 30, 171n.51
Adultery, 173–74n.39; mesmerism and,
   11, 110; Napoleonic Code and, 71;
   nursing and, 111, 112
Affiches du Dauphiné, 122, 132, 137
Affiches du Poitou, 111, 131, 202n.70
Affiches de Toulouse, 132
*Affiches pour les Trois Evêchés et la
   Lorraine,* 133, 147
Albert Le Grand, 45
Almanach sous verre, 134
*Almanach de la ville et du diocèse de
   Troyes,* 156–57
Alstad, Diane, 71
Amniocentesis, 184–85n.46
Anatomy, 160
Ancien Régime, 4, 158; hierarchical
   structure of, 16, 17, 87, 129; medical
   jurisprudence and, 8–9; physicians in,
   95, 97; social decay under, 11–12, 103,
   109, 110, 123; women's legal rights in,
   71, 176n.35; women's social position in,
   148, 165, 167, 173–74n.39
Animal magnetism. *See* Mesmerism
Annonces pour la Ville de Marseille,
   202n.70
Anorexia, 152
Ardent (physician), 138–39, 140
Aristocracy, 37, 110; critics of, 93, 97,
   164; women of, 112, 127–28, 148, 149,
   157, 158
Aristotle, 15, 38, 44, 45, 165
Arnold, Odile, 145
Artificial insemination, 188–89n.29
Astruc, Jean, 40, 41; and convulsions, 108;
   on laws of nature, 46, 48; length of
   pregnancy theories, 49, 50–51;
   opposition to possibility of late birth,
   39, 60, 61; religious faith of, 30, 40; and

testimony of women, 51, 52, 59, 60, 166
Augustine, Saint, 19
Aurillac, France, 83
Avicenna, 45

Bachaumont, Louis Petit de, 37, 91,
   96–97, 192–93n.15, 210–11n.9
Bacon, Francis, 161
Bacon, Marguerite, 201n.64
Baer, Carl von, 38
Baker, Keith, 6, 91
Ballexserd, Jacques, 147
Barbeu du Bourg, Jacques, 43, 102; and
   Convulsionary movement, 33; in late-
   birth debate, 41, 45–46, 49–50, 51, 63
Bartholin, Thomas, 57, 69
Baudelocque (physician), 84, 85, 96
Bell, Rudolf, 152
Ben-David, Joseph, 93
Benech, Antoine, 81
Berard, Catherine, 73
Berna, Catherine, 76, 166, 181n.14
Bernardin de Saint-Pierre, Jacques-Henri,
   91
Bible, 162; as basis for medicine, 29, 30;
   Genesis, 111
Bignon, Jean Paul, 90
Boerhaave, Hermann, 88, 144
Bossuet, Jacques-Bénigne (bishop of
   Meaux), 51–52
Bourdois (physician), 84, 85
Bourgeoisie, 1, 112; emulation of
   aristocracy, 127–28, 148, 149, 157, 158
Bourgogne, Parlement of, 83
Bouvart, Michel, 108; as exemplary
   physician, 96, 97, 98, 99–101, 102; in
   inoculation controversy, 41, 100; and
   laws of nature, 44–45, 46, 61, 105, 162;
   on limit of length of pregnancy, 45, 49,
   100; and medical jurisprudence, 74, 85;
   opposition to possibility of late births,
   39, 43, 61, 69, 70, 106, 183n.29;
   rejection of late-birth case histories, 53,
   54, 55, 56–59; rejection of women's
   testimony on pregnancy, 51, 56, 57, 66;
   on reproductive process, 49, 50
Breastfeeding. *See* Nursing
Bremgarten, Switzerland, 82

Index

Brittany, France, 36, 116
Brockliss, L. W. B., 107
Buffon, Georges-Louis Leclerc de, Comte, 40, 48, 94, 128, 193n.27
Bynum, Caroline Walker, 152

Cabanis, Pierre-Jean-Georges, 165
Calas, Jean, 182n.26
Calas affair, 36, 39–40, 77, 79
Charlatans and empirics, 181n.17, 211n.11; as abortionists, 118–19; attempts at regulation of, 10, 16; Convulsionaries equated with, 25; medical community's attempts to discredit, 4–5, 114, 118, 126, 160, 163; mesmerists as, 114, 117, 118, 120, 121; philosophes equated with, 88, 92, 125, 164; similarity of doctors and surgeons to, 74–75, 98, 99, 101; treatment of nervous disorders by, 107, 126, 132, 152–53, 196n.11; women as, 6, 119; women as clientele of, 6, 37, 132, 149, 152
Charlier, Anne, 32
Charuty, Giordana, 136
Chastenay-Lanty, Victorine de, 95
Childbirth: as cause of convulsions, 135–36, 140–41, 156; mesmerists and, 111
Children: abandonment of, 83; convulsions in, 146; illegitimate, 59, 60–61, 71–72, 73, 82; inheritance rights of, 70, 72–73; males preferred to females, 45, 184–85n.46; of Protestants, 79, 81
Christianity, 30, 176n.35; and Hippocratic oath, 119; Jansenist reformers and, 17; and nature of women, 29, 38, 145, 173–74n.39; sacraments of, 18, 82
Cicero, Marcus Tullius, 48
Collège Royal, 94
Comédie Française, 99
Condillac, Étienne Bonnot de, 91, 162
Condorcet, Marie-Jean-Antoine-Nicolas Caritat, Marquis de, 91, 99–101, 103, 115, 139, 162
Contraception, 11
Convulsionaries, 32–33; convulsions of, 18, 22, 24, 25, 26, 28, 126, 150; and Catholic church reform, 9, 17–20; critics of, 13–14, 19–20, 25, 31, 32, 126, 129; dismissed as charlatans, 25, 33; medical experts' judgment on, 8, 9, 12, 13, 20–29, 31, 38, 106, 108, 162, 163, 164; miraculous healings, 12, 17,

20, 22–24, 33, 88; naturalization of convulsions of, 22, 26, 30; women as, 19–20, 28, 31–32, 33, 88, 125, 130, 164; women as commentators on, 15–16, 42
Convulsions, 5, 14, 31, 125–26; as act of reason, 42; charlatans' cures of, 132, 152–53; of Convulsionaries, 18, 22, 24, 25, 26, 28, 126, 150; dismissed as voluntary, 22, 25, 26; emotional stress and, 133, 134; Enlightenment model of, 127, 129–30, 135, 136, 138, 141, 143, 147, 148, 157, 158; as epidemic, 27, 110, 127; marriage and childbirth as causes of, 135–36, 138–39, 140–41, 148, 156, 158; marriage as cure for, 28, 135, 138, 141, 158; in men, 27, 127, 129, 133, 158; mesmerists and, 108, 110, 113–14, 126; naturalization of, 22, 26, 30; occupational causes of, 141, 143–44, 146; physicians' diagnoses of, 22, 24–28, 108, 126, 130–33, 134, 136–37, 142, 148, 150, 156, 157–58; physicians' treatment of, 28–29, 127, 129–30, 131–33, 134, 135, 137–41, 146, 149; provincial doctors' model of, 129–30, 157–58; religious superstition and, 28, 149–50, 152; Revolution and, 134; Royal Society essay competition on, 127, 130; seen as deception by women, 29, 130, 150; sexuality believed to cause, 27, 28, 29, 126, 127, 135, 136, 137, 138–39; as theater, 33; women believed naturally inclined to, 108, 127, 128, 133
Cormont (curé), 154, 155
Correspondance littéraire, philosophique et critique, 96–97
Correspondance secrète, politique, et littéraire, 37, 92
Corron, Mme (Pierre Abraham Pajon de Moncets), 42
Cosson (author), 95–96, 128, 129
Coupel (surgeon), 111–12
Court de Gebelin (mesmerist), 121
Crawford, Patricia, 152
Culture: charlatans in, 117, 149; dechristianization of, 4; feminization of, 103, 109, 114; popular, 149, 158; Rousseau's critique of, 108–9; science and, 97–98, 157, 158–59; women's influence on, 14, 88, 98, 123, 149
Curés, 122, 154

d'Alembert, Jean le Rond, 99, 115; and

Index

Index